ROUTLEDGE HANDBOOK OF WELL-BEING

The *Routledge Handbook of Well-Being* explores diverse conceptualisations of well-being, providing an overview of key issues and drawing attention to current debates and critiques. Taken as a whole, this important work offers new clarification of the widely used notion of well-being, focusing particularly on experiential perspectives.

Bringing together leading authors from around the world, *Routledge Handbook of Well-Being* reflects on:

- What it is that is experienced by humans that can be called well-being.
- What we know about how to understand it.
- How well-being is manifested in human endeavours through a wide range of disciplines, including the arts.

This comprehensive reference work will provide an authoritative overview for students, practitioners, researchers and policy makers working in or concerned with well-being, health, illness and the relation between all three across a range of disciplines, from sociology, healthcare and economics to philosophy and the creative arts.

Kathleen T. Galvin is Professor of Nursing Practice, School of Health Sciences at the University of Brighton, UK.

ROUTLEDGE HANDBOOK OF WELL-BEING

Edited by Kathleen T. Galvin

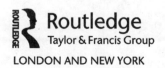

LONDON AND NEW YORK

First published 2018
by Routledge
2 Park Square, Milton Park, Abingdon, Oxon OX14 4RN

and by Routledge
605 Third Avenue, New York, NY 10017

First issued in paperback 2021

Routledge is an imprint of the Taylor & Francis Group, an informa business

Publisher's Note
The publisher has gone to great lengths to ensure the quality of this reprint but points out that some imperfections in the original copies may be apparent.

British Library Cataloguing-in-Publication Data
A catalogue record for this book is available from the British Library

Library of Congress Cataloging-in-Publication Data
A catalogue record for this book has been requested

ISBN 13: 978-0-367-70964-8 (pbk)
ISBN 13: 978-1-138-85010-1 (hbk)

Typeset in Bembo
by Apex CoVantage, LLC

CONTENTS

List of figures   *viii*
Contributor bios   *ix*

Introduction   1

PART 1
The human experience of well-being: what is well-being? Philosophical and theoretical foundations   **15**

1 Residence, identity and well-being   17
  Paul Gilbert

2 A sense of well-being: the anthropology of a first-person phenomenology   23
  Nigel Rapport

3 Cities, well-being, world – a Heideggerian analysis   34
  Robert Mugerauer

4 Dwelling in the world with others as mortal beings: "well-being" in post-disaster Japanese society   51
  Hirobumi Takenouchi

5 Well-being and being-well: a Merleau-Pontian perspective on psychosomatic health   58
  Jennifer Bullington

6 Feminist perspectives on well-being   68
  Charlotte Knowles

Contents

7   Philosophical taxonomies of well-being   76
    Samuel Clark

8   Dwelling-mobility: an existential theory of well-being   84
    Les Todres and Kathleen T. Galvin

9   Capabilities, well-being and universalism   91
    Gideon Calder

PART 2
How are understandings of well-being developing? Disciplinary and
professional perspectives   101

10 Well-being and phenomenology: lifeworld, natural attitude, homeworld
    and place   103
    David Seamon

11 Heritage and well-being: therapeutic places, past and present   112
    Timothy Darvill, Vanessa Heaslip, and Kerry Barrass

12 Disability and ambiguities: technological support in a disaster context 124
    Minae Inahara

13 The existential situation of the patient: well-being and absence   133
    Stephen Burwood

14 Ecological health and caring   141
    Helena Dahlberg and Albertine Ranheim

15 A Jungian contribution to the notion of well-being   154
    Chris Milton

16 A new stance on quality of life   163
    Lennart Nordenfelt

17 "What can't be cured must be endured": living with Parkinson's disease   173
    Virginia Eatough

18 The distribution, determinants and root causes of inequalities in well-being 182
    Eleonora P. Uphoff and Kate E. Pickett

19 Agencies of well-being   194
    Stephen Wallace

20 Embodied routes to well-being: horses and young people   201
    Ann Hemingway

21 Well-being and quality of life in a maternal health context   214
    Julie Jomeen and Colin R. Martin

22 Well-being and self-interest: personal identity, Parfit, and conflicting attitudes
    to time in liberal theory and social policy   222
    Steven R. Smith

23 Values-based practice: at home with our values   230
    K.W.M. (Bill) Fulford and Kathleen T. Galvin

PART 3
How is well-being manifest in human life? The aesthetic nature of well-being   **241**

24 Creativity and aesthetic thinking: toward an aesthetics of well-being   243
    Dorthe Jørgensen

25 Collaborative drawings: blue-prints of conversation dynamics   250
    Deborah Padfield

26 Embodied connectivity through the visual and tactual arts   269
    Catherine Lamont-Robinson

27 Poetry and/as wellness   279
    Monica Prendergast and Carl Leggo

28 Thirteen ways of looking at a clinic   292
    Jennifer Schulz

29 Eudaimonic well-being and education   317
    Denis Francesconi

30 Eighteen kinds of well-being although there may be many more: a conceptual
    framework illustrated with practical direction for caring   324
    Kathleen T. Galvin and Les Todres

Index   *339*

FIGURES

18.1   Gapminder illustrates the gap in teen fertility rates by country GDP per capita   184
18.2   Regions in England with their best and worst scoring child well-being areas   184
18.3   Rainbow diagram by Dahlgren and Whitehead (1991)   186
18.4   The social ladder on the US ship on inequality   189
20.1   Emerging ideas from the literature review   207
20.2   Emotional changes described by the pilot study participants   208
20.3   Ann Hemingway with Arn, their variation of embodiment of the dwelling mobility
       theory of wellbeing   210
23.1   Example triplets of words in feedback from the 'three words' exercise   232
23.2   Three practically challenging features of values   232
23.3   A diagram of values-based practice   233
23.4   Brief definitions of the elements of values-based practice   234
23.5   The Guiding Principles as a framework of shared values   237
25.1   Deborah Padfield with Nell Keddie from the series *perceptions of pain 2001–2006*   256
25.2   Photograph by participant A (clinician) from NPG workshop   259
25.3   Photogram from collaborative drawings on acetate by NPG workshop participants
       W and W5   261
25.4   Photogram from collaborative drawings on acetate by NPG workshop participants
       X and Y   262
25.5   Photogram from collaborative drawings on acetate by NPG workshop participants
       W3 and W4   263
25.6   Photogram from collaborative drawings on acetate by NPG workshop participants
       G and V   265
25.7   Deborah Padfield with Linda Williams from the series *face2face*, 2008–2013   266
26.1   Sweat, Blood and Tears   271
26.2   Meditation   276
30.1   'Dwelling-mobility' lattice   325

CONTRIBUTOR BIOS

Kerry Barrass is a Postgraduate Research Assistant in the Department of Archaeology, Anthropology and Forensic Science, Bournemouth University, UK.

Jennifer Bullington is a Professor at Ersta Sköndal Bräcke, Sweden. She is also a licensed physiotherapist.

Stephen Burwood is a Senior Lecturer in Philosophy at the University of Hull, UK. He considers himself a generalist, though his research interests tend to focus on Wittgenstein, particularly with respect to *On Certainty* and naturalism, philosophy of mind and embodied subjectivity, and the philosophy of education. Happily, these areas occasionally overlap. Recently his interest in embodiment has led to a research project in trans-humanism, immortality and the afterlife.

Gideon Calder is Senior Lecturer in Social Sciences and Social Policy at Swansea University, UK, and works mainly in applied political and ethical theory.

Sam Clark works at the Department of Politics, Philosophy and Religion at Lancaster University, UK.

Helena Dahlberg is a Senior Lecturer at the University of Gothenburg, Sweden. She is a philosopher who currently works with qualitative methods in health care science.

Karin Dahlberg is Professor in Health Sciences, now partly retired. She has been professor of Linnaeus University in Sweden where she developed and directed a doctoral program of health sciences as well as a centre for Lifeworld Research.

Timothy Darvill is Professor of Archaeology in the Department of Archaeology, Anthropology and Forensic Science, Bournemouth University, UK.

Dr Virginia Eatough is a Reader at Birkbeck University of London, UK, in the Department of Psychological Sciences.

Denis Francesconi is Adjunct Professor at University of Verona, Italy, where he teaches group dynamics. Since 2014 he is also Visiting Professor at Humboldt University Berlin, Germany, where he teaches general education.

K.W.M. (Bill) Fulford is a Fellow of St Catherine's College and member of the Philosophy Faculty, University of Oxford, UK; Emeritus Professor of Philosophy and Mental Health, University of Warwick, UK; Founder Editor and Chair of the Advisory Board, Philosophy, Psychiatry, & Psychology; and Director of The Collaborating Centre for Values-based Practice, St Catherine's College, Oxford, UK (valuesbasedpractice.org).

Paul Gilbert is Emeritus Professor of Philosophy at the University of Hull, UK.

Vanessa Heaslip is a Principal Academic in the Department of Nursing and Clinical Science in the Faculty of Health and Social Science, Bournemouth University, UK. She is a Registered Nurse and an experienced Nurse Researcher and Nurse Educator.

Ann Hemingway is Professor of Public Health & Wellbeing, Faculty of Health and Social Sciences, Bournemouth University, UK. Through her involvement in public health research, her interests have focused on the promotion of sustainable well-being through resident involvement in planning and providing services; and capacity building particularly in deprived areas. A principle aim of this work is to actively involve residents in well-being improvement and evaluation work.

Minae Inahara (稲原 美苗) is an Associate Professor in the Faculty of Human Development, Kobe University, Japan.

Julie Jomeen is Professor of Midwifery, and Dean of the Faculty of Health Sciences at the University of Hull, UK.

Dorthe Jørgensen is Professor of Philosophy and the History of Ideas, School of Culture and Society, Aarhus University, Denmark.

Charlotte Knowles is an Associate Research Fellow at Birkbeck. She received her BA in Philosophy and English Literature and her MA in Philosophy from the University of Sussex, UK, before completing her PhD in London in 2016.

Dr Catherine Lamont-Robinson is the curator and creative director of the University of Bristol's Out of Our Heads medical arts website.

Carl Leggo is a poet and Professor of Language and Literacy Education at the University of British Columbia, Canada.

Colin R. Martin is Professor of Mental Health at Buckinghamshire New University, Middlesex, UK. He is a Registered Nurse, Chartered Health Psychologist and a Chartered Scientist.

Chris Milton is a Jungian Analyst and Clinical Psychologist in private practice in Auckland, New Zealand. He is also a Training Analyst of Australian and New Zealand Society of Jungian Analysts (ANZSJA) of which he is currently President.

Robert Mugerauer is a Professor and Dean Emeritus in the College of Architecture and Urban Design at the University of Washington, USA.

Lennart Nordenfelt is Professor of Philosophy of Medicine and Health Care at Linköping University, Sweden.

Deborah Padfield is Teaching Fellow, University College London Culture and Slade School of Fine Art, UCL, London, UK, and is a visual artist specialising in lens-based media and inter-disciplinary practice and research within Fine Art and Medicine.

Kate E. Pickett is Professor of Epidemiology in the Department of Health Sciences at the University of York, UK, and the University's Champion for Research on Justice and Equality.

Monica Prendergast is Associate Professor of Drama/Theatre Education at the University of Victoria, BC, Canada.

Albertine Ranheim has been a Primary Health Care Nurse since 2000. Currently, she is a Lecturer at Karolinska Institutet, Stockholm, Sweden, mainly within the specialist Nursing programmes.

Nigel Rapport is Professor of Anthropological and Philosophical Studies and Head of School of Philosophical, Anthropological and Film Studies, University of St Andrews, UK.

Jennifer Schulz, PhD, is a psychotherapist located in South East Seattle, Washington, US, and a Professor in the English and Interdisciplinary Liberal Studies programs at Seattle University, USA. She teaches a wide variety of courses on creative writing, literature, clinical psychology and interdisciplinary research methods. She also works as a licensed mental health counsellor in private practice. Dr Schulz has written on incorporating creative writing practices in qualitative research methodology.

Steven R. Smith is Professor of Political Philosophy and Social Policy at the University of South Wales, UK. His main research and publications focus on issues concerning social justice, citizenship, and wellbeing, with particular interest in the philosophy of disability, equality and diversity issues, ideologies of the welfare state, and matters concerning the application of abstract principles to the specifics of social policy and professional practice.

David Seamon is an environment-behaviour researcher and Professor of Architecture at Kansas State University in Manhattan, Kansas, USA.

Hirobumi Takenouchi is Professor of Philosophy and Ethics in the Faculty of Agriculture, Shizuoka University, Japan.

Les Todres is Emeritus Professor of Health Philosophy at Bournemouth University, UK. He is author of *Embodied Enquiry: Phenomenological Touchstones for Research, Psychotherapy and Sprituality*, and co-author, with Kathleen Galvin, of *Caring and Well-being: A Lifeworld Approach*.

Eleonora P. Uphoff is a Research Fellow at the University of York working for the Better Start Bradford Innovation Hub at the Institute for Health Research in Bradford, UK.

Stephen Wallace (PhD, MSc, Dip Ed Psych, Dip Ed, BA) retired from full time academic work in 2013 as an Associate Professor. Over a working life of four decades, he had worked (mainly in Australia) as an academic psychologist, researcher, teacher, counsellor and health policy advocate in child abuse, addictions and criminology. (In latter years his developed expertise in clinical sciences led to posts in clinical governance in the NHS and post-graduate medical education in the UK.)

INTRODUCTION

The aim of this *Handbook of Well-Being* is to offer new insights and to revisit perspectives that can move thinking radically beyond the ways in which we have thus far conceptualised well-being, particularly in the disciplines concerned with health and social care. This includes reframing how well-being is in relation to the notion of health and providing accessible philosophical grounding alongside analysis of the state of our knowledge within key disciplinary domains, including engagement with creative approaches to understanding well-being. It is my hope that this text shows and offers emerging new notions of well-being as a multidimensional resource in human life with engagement through for example, the arts, our values, our varied professional and disciplinary perspectives and other means. Well-being has a long history of philosophical exploration, including in the moral and political realm and there are many theories of well-being that span desire-fulfilment, hedonism and eudaimonism to name just a few. The purpose here is not to systematically revisit the range of continuities and discontinuities of ideas about and theories of well-being – other texts have successfully achieved that. Rather, the aim here is to point to some current developments in thinking from a range of applied disciplines that may have the potential to shift and refresh directions in the field.

Therefore the contributing authors seek to address former conceptualisations of well-being, drawing attention to issues and timely critiques with a view to offering new clarification of the notion of well-being, taking a distinctive focus that begins with: *what is it that is experienced by humans that can be called well-being?* Leading authors from an array of disciplines, from across the world, collectively reflect on well-being as multidimensional, attending to a) philosophical clarification, b) the state of our knowledge about well-being, c) emerging and future approaches to understanding well-being and d) well-being as manifest in human endeavours.

The work is timely; well-being as an idea has often been obscured by narratives that have overemphasised the absence of well-being, illness, unhappiness or suffering, and oftentimes the relationship of well-being to its absence has been a troubled one, sometimes separated as if the experience is always an 'either–or'. In the experiential realm well-being is already always in relation to the absence of well-being and each of us knows what the human experience of the presence of well-being is, and we know when it is absent; in other words, well-being is a real experience, concretely lived, that we all have the capacity to know something of. To put it another way, does the ill person, the wealthy person, the impoverished person, the high achiever or the hermit experience well-being? What kind of well-being do they experience? In reflecting on these questions it becomes apparent that there are some complexities about well-being experience that are not sufficiently addressed by equating deficits in aspects of one's life or equating resources such as people and money in one's life to well-being. Well-being is both an individual and a shared notion, and it is neither wholly subjective nor objectively 'out there'. Well-being is not easy to nail down, and it is intertwined with *how things are for you in the world*.

Well-being is also a resource in human life, so what exactly is it that contributes to or constitutes the experience of well-being? What makes well-being possible before we abstractly categorise it into for example, social well-being, mental well-being, physical well-being, spiritual well-being, economic well-being, emotional well-being and so on? In what follows, well-being is shown as not only multidimensional but also transcends disciplinary limits, so that the constraints of conceiving well-being as the absence of illness or the pursuit of 'happiness' through ever increasing consumption become fully apparent. As such, collectively authors point to the deep complexities of well-being, and offer new ways of seeing and understanding well-being to mediate narrowly enframed ideas. This includes, but is not limited to, cultural, ecological, gendered, historical and embodied perspectives, with well-being examined in relation to for example, sense of place and dwelling, sense of connection, sometimes (but not always) being with others, sense of self, identity and body and embraces a range of problems within some key professional and disciplinary contexts.

The chapters in this handbook demonstrate a range of disciplinary concerns both philosophical and applied, examples of current research, and demonstrations and reflections that point to the links between well-being and fields that are far beyond health and social care but which are nonetheless highly relevant. The implicit 'red thread' that runs through the interdisciplinary context offers concerns metaphorically how well-being is allied to a kind of pre- reflective experience of a sense of being deeply at home, in non-literal and literal ways. Examples are provided of all kinds of 'coming home', or not being at home in the deepest sense, of impediments and obstructions, of being on the margins and of finding a way to home, through to, metaphorically speaking, adventures, pathways and possibilities for well-being. Such a text necessarily demands a shift from measurement-oriented instrumental emphases to the timely importance of a multidimensional approach in exploring well-being, with a focus that includes its *meaning* alongside evidence-based exploration of what threatens or makes possible human well-being. This is a shift to well-being as a resource. And if well-being is a resource in human life, what role does well-being have in reclaiming a sense of wholeness in our experiences? Many of the chapters point to a 'reclaiming of wholes', in an applied way in response to a current context of many fragmentations be they physical, historical, social, cultural, technological, economic and ecological. What follows is an overview of each chapter, pointing to the distinctive contribution of each author.

The collection is organised as three parts:

- Part 1: *Human experience of well-being*

  What is well-being? Philosophical and theoretical foundations

- Part 2: *How are understandings of well-being developing?*

  Disciplinary and professional perspectives

- Part 3: *How is well-being manifest in human life?*

  The aesthetic nature of well-being

Part 1: Human experience of well-being: What is well-being? Philosophical and theoretical foundations

Part 1 begins with well-being as a particular way of being in the world, and through an array of disciplines aims to point to the deepest roots of well-being.

It opens with Paul Gilbert's chapter concerning residence, identity and well-being: Gilbert tackles head on the notion that well-being exists in the presence of agreeable feelings and the absence of disagreeable ones. For example, feeling at home in the place where one lives is taken to conduce to well-being and feelings of homesickness to detract from it. He examines some aspects of the relation between feelings and well-being with special reference to feelings about home and the place of home in people's lives arguing that certain pre-reflective relations to home are more important than many reflective feelings about it in conducing to well-being, so that subjective assessments of well-being based on reflective feelings may be deceptive. He points to the complexities of well-functioning as one aspect of well-being that concerns the tone and modes of activity with effortless immersion in the world.

Nigel Rapport begins by posing the question: What does it mean to talk of 'well-being' as against 'health'? As an anthropologist he explores well-being from the comparative standpoint of an individual human body against the world and asks if there is a *human* story of well-being that can be shared or a *cultural* or *social*, *geographical* or *historical* one? In his chapter, as anthropologist questions are raised and considered, hoping to balance the intrinsic bodily state – a sense of well-being – against what might be said to provide contexts for that state: the individual is a member of humankind, also of a society and community (perhaps), also of a local or regional part of the world (perhaps), also of a particular historical period (perhaps).

Robert Mugerauer offers a Heideggerian analysis of cities, well-being and home pointing to how in our anthropocentric era we interpret the phenomena of cities, well-being and home in terms of the value they have for humans, and how we instrumentally or functionally calculate this value in terms of the services that ecosystems or social institutions provide us. Cities are the sites in which the majority of people now attempt to make themselves at home. Cities also are increasingly appreciated as the scene in which we will either manage to attain sustainability or collapse with disastrous results, therefore not only pointing beyond individuals to assemblages of groups and even beyond familiar community to strangers; then further still to the environment that surrounds and pervades them all, that is, beyond the anthropocentric to the eco-centric or even cosmo-centric, wherein, Mugerauer argues, lies the sustainability of local social-natural systems. Rather than embrace a well-rehearsed perspective, that is, to equate well-being with health or economic and material prosperity and to see cities and home as the sites in which we can optimise the net utility, Mugerauer takes a different and radical approach. Drawing on philosophical ideas from Martin Heidegger, he shows us how well-being is deep, highly complex, vast and multidimensional, providing an alternative that has had substantial influence in developing a post-humanistic position that has potential to bear fruit in ecological, urban, psychological and other fields. He offers an interpretation that approximates Heidegger's meaning: 'Well-being would be the Well-being of World – its fruitful unfolding (rather than dissipation or decay)'. Within this framework he argues that we can understand *the forces that enable* social well-being, ecological well-being-sustainability, and individual health, since all individual well-being (of humans and other-than-humans) would be a sub-set of the whole, where, as in complexity theory, all the dimensions are mutually co-constitutive. This is a question of the extent to which, as we say, 'All is right with the world.'

Examining the themes of disaster, disintegration and reconstruction linked to well-being, Hirobumi Takenouchi points to the relation between well-being and dwelling in the land as mortal, offering a reflection on the idea of 'reconstruction' from the disastrous earthquake of March 11, 2011 that assailed Japan. He begins with a critical examination of the dominant ideas of 'reconstruction' and appropriates the idea of 'reconstruction of human being', through reflection on the concrete problems brought to light by the disastrous earthquake. This opens up the problem of how to understand 'social welfare' as well as human 'well-being'. Takenouchi grapples with this problem, paying attention to the significance of the land, and here 'dwelling' comes into view so that the deepest roots of well-being are revealed.

Jennifer Bullington, drawing on Maurice Merleau-Ponty, deals with the body as *lived body*, offering ideas that illuminate notions of health and well-being as multidimensional. She argues that as a shift occurs in our understanding of health and well-being from that of evaluating measurements of material processes in the body towards more holistic conceptualisations, we need theoretical frameworks which enable us to articulate these complex new understandings. She provides such a framework in order to conceptualise health as a *mind-body-world* phenomenon. The dualism between mind and body is circumvented by use of Merleau-Ponty's concept of 'the lived body'. In a similar way, the dichotomy between the experiencing human being (as a mind-body presence to the world) and the experienced world is overcome through his visionary description of the relations between man and world in terms of 'the flesh'. Bullington uses the case of psychosomatic ill health to show how insights on the lived body and the ontological characterisation of 'the flesh' provide a fruitful grounding of health and well-being as a multidimensional phenomenon.

Charlotte Knowles offers a feminist perspective of well-being pointing to one of the key feminist insights, that to live well cannot be a totally individual project. Rather, it must be both an individual and a social pursuit. Yet many feminist accounts appear to struggle to balance the individual and the social aspects of well-being, often emphasising one at the expense of the other. Knowles critically evaluates three feminist approaches to well-being, before developing a new framework that balances individual and social considerations in order to more successfully promote well-being from a feminist perspective. First, she examines an approach from virtue theory, taking note of ethics as a paradigm case in a feminist context. She then turns to an approach with a greater focus on the individual: objective list theories. These suggest that in order to ensure a person's well-being, certain conditions must be met. This approach directs us more clearly to what a person needs in order to flourish and guards against the unintuitive results of some internalist and psychological accounts of human flourishing. However, there is a worry that many conceptions of the good life are not neutral, but inherently masculine. Moreover, she critiques concerns that objective list theories are too prescriptive and too general, failing to offer a pluralistic account of well-being. Accordingly, objective list theories may obfuscate what it will be for *a particular woman* to live well. To counter this worry, she considers a third approach: the account from desire satisfaction. This holds that you are better off to the extent that your desires are satisfied. Such an approach turns the focus to the particular individual and recognises the importance of choice in well-being. However, it takes for granted the idea that people always know what's in their best interests, ignoring the fact that the choices we make are often determined by the (social) situation in which we find ourselves. 'In the context of patriarchy, women's desires are often adapted to their oppressive situation and as a result they may not always express preferences or make choices that promote their own well-being'. Having evaluated these theories and identified their strengths and weaknesses, the final section of Knowles's chapter offers a new approach to well-being that utilises the framework of Heidegger's *Being and Time* in order to incorporate the insights of existing feminist approaches to well-being whilst avoiding their drawbacks and arguing that this new approach is better able to promote flourishing in gendered contexts, as it balances the individual and social aspects of well-being.

Helena Dahlberg and Albertine Ranheim continue a theme allied to the ethics of care in their exploration of ecological perspectives of caring: They point to how, even within the frame of a health and care perspective, everything can be seen as linked together as ecosystem, that for example, decisions within health contexts are all part of a larger continuum. They argue that throughout life, we are part of structures, systems and processes that are substantial to our health, impact how we feel and how we manage to shape our lives. Their chapter addresses the question of how we can deepen our understanding of caring and its focus on health based on the knowledge of our lived contexts, arguing for an expanded comprehensiveness with the aim of illuminating possible ecological perspectives to answer current questions about health and caring. Specifically they introduce what nursing's focus on health in relation to nature, vegetation, the life of animals, nutrition and environment might be and analyse how we understand professional relationship, i.e. between nurses and patients within the context of such an ecological relationship. Drawing on the notion of 'ecosophy', as described by Arne Naess in 1976, they point to ecology as lived wisdom and the need to understand life processes and the development of ecological systems, as well as relations between different organisms and their environment arguing that phenomenology is one approach that is up to the task of engaging with the web of life, offering a philosophy that connects with an ecological ontology. Dahlberg and Ranheim therefore provide a deepened understanding of what an ecological caring could mean drawing on Merleau-Ponty's philosophy and in particular his understanding of corporeal being and flesh. Through this exposition they show us how there is a deep connection, and at the same time an irreducible difference, between the person and her or his body, between human being and nature, and between humans.

Sam Clark provides a philosophical analysis with delineation of a range of taxonomies for well-being. He argues for an expansion in imagination about what well-being could be, pursuing this in two stages. First he sets out and rejects Derek Parfit's influential triad of *Hedonist*, *Desire-Fulfilment*, and *Objective List Theories* of well-being, suggesting instead that there is a need to make multiple, cross-cutting distinctions between theories, with consideration of their interactions. He puts his suggestion into practice by distinguishing between *Empirical* and *Normative*, *Descriptive* and *Revisionary*, *Reflexive* and *Non-Reflexive*, and *Compositional* and *Additive Theories*, and breaks up the incoherent subjective/objective distinction. Out of this second stage he then focuses on questions of political perfectionism.

Continuing a theme of troubling subjective and objective distinctions in notions about well-being, a new *existential* theory of well-being is offered by Les Todres and Kathleen T. Galvin. In this chapter they aim to show how phenomenological-philosophical considerations can open up a productive way of thinking about well-being and which strikes at the question: What is it about the essence of well-being that makes all kinds of well-being possible? Consistent with a phenomenological approach, well-being is both a way of being in the world as well as a felt experience. Drawing on Heidegger's notion of 'Gegnet' (abiding expanse) they characterise well-being as *Dwelling-Mobility*, indicating the adventure of being called into expansive possibilities as well as 'being at home with what has been given'. Eighteen phenomenologically informed intertwined dimensions of well-being are offered.

In the final chapter of Part 1, Gideon Calder explores the insights on well-being emerging in what has come to be called the Capabilities Approach to social justice – with a particular focus on the work of Martha Nussbaum. Calder's overall aim is to offer a balanced assessment of Nussbaum's rich and fertile 'take' on the capabilities approach. He explains that capabilities are opportunities to function: to be or to do fundamentally important things. A capabilities-based approach to well-being sits in a distinct place in relation to two alternative ways of measuring how well we are doing in life. On the one hand, subjective: 'my well-being depends on how well my preferences are satisfied, and so can be assessed on the basis of my feelings and experiences' – my mental state. On the other, objective: 'certain things are good or bad for me, independently (at least in part) of whether I desire them or whether they give rise to pleasurable experiences'. Discussing capabilities, Calder points to how we find ourselves in a complex debate about functionings, and about whether or not some ways we might be, or things we might do, are universal or definitive of the human condition. He indicates that famously,

> Nussbaum's work sits on the "universalist" side of this line, and so she has sought to identify the minimum conditions necessary for truly human functioning – with all the contentiousness that any such project will bring – and on that basis, to develop a specific list of the central human capabilities, from being able to live a life of normal length, to being able to laugh, to play and enjoy recreational activities. Of course, rather than settling the matter, this list – and the very idea that we might devise one – has been the prompt for extensive critique and debate, including among the strongest advocates of a capabilities based approach.

Part 2: How are understandings of well-being developing? Disciplinary and professional perspectives

Part 2 examines some varied disciplinary perspectives on well-being, with inquiries for how we know well-being (or its absence) in a range of situations, contexts and conditions. The social and biomedical sciences have paid increasing attention to well-being, with the goals of this knowledge generation mainly concerned with measurability, value-ladenness, generalisability and the details of constructs that correspond to what we might call well-being. These include but are not limited to satisfaction with life, subjective satisfaction and quality of life approaches that span psychology, economics and health sciences for example. The aim of this section is not to revisit applications of these established and well-rehearsed ideas, but rather to introduce new challenging notions of what may constitute well-being, what can contribute to well-being in funda-mental ways, and what we might learn about well-being when the conditions are not necessarily sufficient or conducive to well-being. On the way some applied research studies are drawn upon in varied contexts that point to new avenues of enquiry. In several chapters in Part 2, examples of things and situations that contribute in a positive resource-oriented way (or in a negative deficit way) to well-being are examined within the context of the latest evidence.

David Seamon opens this second part of the volume inviting us to consider environmental and archi-tectural dimensions of well-being by pointing to the centrality of place and 'homeworld'. His chapter considers the significance of geographical and architectural environments in sustaining or undermining human well-being. Taking a phenomenological perspective, he argues that an integral part of human-being-in-the-world is place – any environmental locus that gathers human experiences, actions and meanings spatially and temporally. Drawing on the phenomenological work of philosophers Edward Casey and Jeff Malpas, he suggests that place is central to human life because, just by being what it is, it gathers worlds spatially and environmentally, marking out centres of human experience, action, meaning and intention that, in turn, contribute to the making of place. He contends that the dynamic reciprocity between place and people-in-place means that the quality of human life is intimately related to the qual-ity of place in which that life unfolds and vice versa. He demonstrates that physical, environmental and spatial qualities play an important role in successful places and illustrate this claim by drawing on recent research and design efforts relating to space syntax, pattern languages, place synergies and universal design covering topics that include the nature of lifeworld and well-being phenomenologically; the nature of place and lived links with human well-being, including the significance of the 'lived body' and 'bodily emplacement'; environmental design as place making and place making as it sustains and undermines human well-being.

Building further on the theme of well-being and place, Tim Darvill, Vanessa Heaslip and Kerry Barrass explore heritage, therapeutic places and well-being links: They begin in places of deep historical signifi-cance such as Stonehenge, UK, and Santiago de Compostela, Spain, that have long been directly associated with healing and the promotion of well-being, a dimension of heritage that continues into the present day. The focus of their chapter contextualises public perceptions and aspirational public policies in relation to heritage and well-being by reviewing the development of interest in therapeutic places, and summarising the achievements of projects that promoted physical and mental well-being through access to heritage landscapes, encounters with museum collections, participation in archaeological fieldwork and journeys around ancient monuments. From their analysis they offer three dimensions that are common to many suc-cessful heritage projects in relation to well-being: the idea of journeying, structured engagements between people and places, and the opportunities offered for human interaction and making sense of empirical experiences.

Minae Inahara examines the ambiguity of technology. She seeks to problematise narratives of disability, disaster and well-being using the context of the Great East Japan Earthquake which struck on March 11, 2011. Following Donna Haraway's 'Cyborg Manifesto' of 1991, Inahara argues that we need to question the normative narratives that inform the development of techno-science for the able-bodied. She explores a case of a home care ALS (amyotrophic lateral sclerosis) patient who required ventilation when the power supply was cut off after the East Japan Earthquake with rapid destruction of exceptional scale, and which involved damage to the Fukushima Daiichi nuclear power plants. This unprecedented disaster, with the loss of more than 15,000 lives, has caused great disorientation in Japan, with its effects still continuing to this day, creating additional difficulties and challenges to daily life for all human beings, perhaps especially those with disabilities or chronic illnesses. All of this has raised serious questions about well-being and what it is to support well-being in human life.

Developing the theme of existential disruption and well-being Stephen Burwood focuses on the existential situation of the patient, drawing on the Dutch phenomenological philosopher Van den Berg: He points us to the philosopher's observations and unfolds an existential analysis to help us think about well-being in embodied, social and environmental ways. Drawing on J. H. van den Berg, *The Psychology of the Sickbed*, Burwood calls our attention to a profound truth embodied in the seminal work about the experience of illness and health that reveals illness, apart from its obvious physiological characteristics, to consist in a number of 'conflicts' – with oneself, one's body, one's environment and with others – which could be said to constitute the existential situation of the patient. This chapter shows us that good health, on the other hand, consists largely, though not entirely, in the absence of these conflicts. In good health, one might say, one is at home with oneself, one's body, one's environment and with others. The experience of good health, because it is largely constituted by the familiar and routine, therefore breeds forgetfulness. Without underplaying the suffering illness visits on the sick, the consolation Van den Berg suggests illness may bring is that it is the 'giver of little things'. After all, it is the little things that often form the wellspring of our sense of well-being. Thus, Burwood highlights that amidst the travail and anguish – or at least within the course of recovery and rehabilitation – we can find a positive reminder of important things familiarity made us forget.

Lennart Nordenfelt examines the notion of quality of life and how it pertains to well-being, offering a new stance on the theory of quality of life in health care. He outlines an introduction to the theory of quality of life in health care with some of the reasons for the incorporation of this concept into medicine and emphasises that quality of life is basically a very general concept which has to be specified and clarified when it takes a place in health care decisions. He discusses some interpretations of quality of life, as used in medicine and health care in general, and then focuses upon and argues for a subjectivist interpretation of the notion where quality of life roughly means happiness with one's life. To this he adds a presentation and discussion of some crucial notions of health and concentrates in particular on a holistic analysis of health. The mentioned concepts of quality of life and health are compared and differences are noted. Finally, with an example taken from actual care, he provides some reasons for keeping the general concept of quality of life in mind in crucial clinical situations making the case that in choosing a narrow disease-oriented notion of quality of life there is a risk of forgetting the whole person and his or her problems in life.

Chris Milton invites us to engage with a Jungian contribution to the notion of well-being. He presents a classical Jungian perspective on individuation as an autochthonous psychic process whereby we develop over the course of our entire lifetime through the evolving living relationship between the ego and the Self. He offers: a presentation of the classical Jungian notion of individuation, a short illustrative case vignette and a fairy-tale in which the individuation processes can be discerned. He concludes with a short phenomenological description of the way-of-being that is reflective of individuation and also of well-being. Overall this chapter attempts to contribute to the discipline of well-being by highlighting a psychology of the unconscious, offering individuation and compensation as formulations of autochthonous processes that lead to well-being with an attempt to provide a nuanced and less individualistic articulation of the experience of well-being.

Virginia Eatough provides phenomenological idiographic analysis of the lifeworld of the person with Parkinson's disease as the demands of Parkinson's disease are lived with for many years and there is a need for knowledge which grasps what this living is like. Many people with long-term conditions such as Parkinson's believe that those involved in their care do not understand well enough the impacts and effects on their daily lives. A detailed understanding of what *matters* to people in situations such as living with Parkinson's requires broadening our ideas of what constitutes evidence to include detailed research-based descriptions of people's lifeworld experiences alongside more conventional measures of users'/patients' views about health care services. Eatough's chapter argues for the value of idiographic enquiry for informing the practice of health care professionals by presenting a phenomenological lifeworld analysis of an

83-year-old woman with Parkinson's disease to demonstrate this value. The focus of idiographic enquiry is the individual but this is always the individual in context, individuality not individualism. The classic dictum that 'Every person is in certain respects a) like all other persons, b) like some other persons and c) like no other person' points to different but equally valid forms of knowledge and this chapter demonstrates the value of knowledge at this third level.

At the same time, a phenomenological focus on the individual opens up a 'way of seeing' which reaches beyond individual specifics. It is a form of empirical enquiry that aims to describe the world as it is lived and experienced with care, rigour and completeness. Eatough's chapter successfully illuminates how the personal idiosyncrasies of Parkinson's disease are lived out and embedded in universal existential features which constitute everyone's lifeworld. These aspects of the lifeworld include embodiment, spatiality, relationality through which the lifeworld of the person with Parkinson's is seen to be both enhanced and diminished. For example, how the body in Parkinson's is conspicuous and no longer capable of skilled flow of action but how strategies can be put into place to regain some ease of movement. Similarly, relationality makes the case for a caring practice based on 'equivalence' to mitigate against a loss of belonging. Finally, this dual focus offers more than simply understanding; it yields knowledge which can strengthen and enrich health care practices as well as contribute to the evidence base that health care professionals draw on in order to make predictions about, and to initiate change in, the lives of *individuals* they care for.

Stephen Wallace draws our attention to and brings out the curiosities of the scholarly treatment of and policy discourse of well-being. For example while it has been generally accepted that oriental cultural practices such as Buddhism, Transcendental Meditation and Yoga have been significant and enduring purveyors of well-being over a long time-scale, he points to how in recent times Aristotle's contribution to the 'good life', are again becoming increasingly influential. He introduces what he terms 'the modernist program of amelioration', resting upon the solid foundations of science and rationality, that has perhaps under-delivered its promissory manifestos, as other cultural programmes of well-being which have emerged over the last century, (such as health psychology, self-help literature, personal development programmes).

He argues that recent political interest in well-being has taken hold of some public imaginaries, and considerable public funding now is invested in all kinds of disparate investigations and measures of well-being. Whereas Eastern philosophies have always asserted the primacy of the individual in well-being-enhancement, nowadays agencies as modest as local governments, and august as the UN and WHO now are attempting to locate themselves centrally within this discourse. Without attempting to explain this emergent interest in well-being, Wallace simply wants to register that well-being has become a topic of considerable scholarly interest and public investment, particularly over the last three decades, and as such deserves some fresh attention in this light. He addresses the question: what are the agencies of well-being? This chapter specifically resonates in a number of ways. It asks how well-being-enhancement may be 'effected' in any describable ways. It asks also about the kinds of agents of well-being-enhancement which may be involved; and it asks how does well-being itself produce effects which might be described and measured in future times.

Eleonora Uphoff and Kate Pickett, taking a population-based approach, discuss the far-reaching impacts of inequalities in well-being. They explain the complex role of social inequality as a determinant of well-being pointing to life expectancies from birth and rates of infant mortality in developing countries: with persistent threats of natural disasters, infectious diseases, poor sanitation, conflict, lack of access to health care and food shortages, combined with an increasing burden of chronic diseases. In parts of the world less affected by many of these threats to well-being, where chronic diseases are the main cause of death for adults, average life expectancy has risen to around 80 years of age. However, large differences in mortality, morbidity and well-being exist both between and within these countries. Among rich countries, the percentage of children reporting poor life satisfaction varies from about 4% to 15%, with obvious implications for the well-being of these children. In countries where children report lower life satisfaction on average, the gap in life satisfaction reported by the poorest compared to those better off is much greater; in other words the social gradient in well-being is steeper. Whereas health behaviours (for example diet, physical activity, sexual activity, smoking, drinking, etc.) are recognised determinants of well-being, they do not explain most of the inequalities in health and well-being. The root causes of inequalities in well-being are more important and perhaps more intractable. Most Western societies measure their success and progress in terms of economic growth, rather than well-being. The dominance of neoliberal so-called 'free market' economic policy and politics has led to sharp increases in income inequality over time. Top incomes in particular have risen dramatically, while lower and middle incomes have stagnated. For the majority of people, the social ladder has become steeper and the rungs are further apart. As social mobility is constrained by inequality, climbing that ladder becomes more and more difficult. In unequal societies, people are less likely to trust each other and to maintain supportive relationships, meaning that the crucial protective role of social relationships as a determinant of health and well-being is compromised. The natural environment, upon which we depend for our well-being, is damaged as people are less likely to be committed to the common good and work collectively towards sustainability. In addition, the daily stress of status anxiety and competition the constant social pressure of seeing ourselves through other people's lives creates chronic biological stress which is associated with a range of health behaviours and morbidities, and which is transferred to future generations through the impact of maternal stress in pregnancy and epigenetic processes. They conclude their chapter with a discussion of the policies and policy directions needed to improve population well-being.

Julie Jomeen and Colin Martin explore well-being and quality of life in a maternal health context with particular reference to psychological aspects of maternal health and what this means for how well-being is conceptualised within maternal care. They point out that in a perinatal context, well-being is a well-used idiom but as in other allied disciplines it is used interchangeably with other terms such as quality of life and general health. Furthermore, quality of life is increasingly shown to play a significant role in the psychological well-being of pregnant and postnatal women and it is argued that the concept of well-being is of particular import in the perinatal period as pregnancy, labour and the postnatal period are recognised as times of physiological and psychological transition. For instance, physiological aspects, such as changing body shape, nausea and fatigue, are perhaps obvious, but are coupled with intense emotional involvement which may not be as transparent, and that the perinatal period requires acknowledgment as a pivotal transition phase in women's lives whereby emotions are ever changing during this time. Jomeen and Martin underscore how the personal and social context within which an individual woman lives, including her economic circumstances and support networks, all influence how well-being has been conceptualised, sometimes in constrained ways in the maternal care field. For instance, as a consequence of the multifactorial nature of women's perinatal experience and the associated intensity of adaptation required, there is a tendency to explore associations with negative psychological consequences and sequelae and to conceptualise well-being in relation to maternal *mental health*.

Ann Hemingway explores embodied and intersubjective routes to well-being through connection with 'the animal other' offering example findings from a recent study with young people. Her chapter pursues two areas, *learning to be well*, and the contribution of animals to such learning. She offers a consideration of what is meant by well-being and then proceeds by outlining the evidence about the positive impacts of interaction with animals in general, followed by more specifically how horses can contribute to the experience of well-being. Detailed research developments related to young people and interaction with horses within this growing area of study are shared alongside a consideration of humans as part of nature, one element within our ecology with attention given to ways that promote well-being which tap into human nature and an ability to learn to be well using our bodies and our emotions. The underpinning philosophy focuses on inter-dependence, intersubjectivity and cooperation with each other and with other species.

Steven R. Smith provides an examination of well-being and self-interest, offering a philosophical analysis that shows tensions that are relevant for policy making. He points us to orthodox liberal accounts of well-being enhancement that depend on particular views of self-interest, attitudes to time, and personal identity. For example, classical liberal views of Adam Smith, Henry Sidgwick and John Rawls all variously argue that a person, acting in her own self-interest, should have a more-or-less neutral attitude to time. For example, consequently, she considers her future self as having similar importance as her present self, and acts accordingly. This consideration facilitates her well-being, as it enables this person to plan for her future – sometimes enduring short-term present pain for long-term future happiness – knowing that overall her life is made better as a result.

However, there are problems for this liberal view, concerning incompatibility with our experience of time which Derek Parfit explores in his book *Reasons and Persons*. The classical view does not recognise other biases we have toward the present and near future, over the past and distant future. For example, typically a person is extremely relieved when her past pain is over, and yet she is filled with trepidation concerning her near-future pain. These very different responses to personal pain are understandable, given how we experience our lives *across* time, but are straining the temporal neutrality recommended by classical liberals. Smith points us to how Parfit exploits this difficulty, arguing that if liberals are to be consistently temporally neutral, then they would need to demonstrate that we are as much concerned about our past, present and future pain, with no special weighting given to any time period. Parfit claims that for most people this seems incredulous given the kind of creatures we are. In his chapter, Smith argues that Parfit's view of personal identity, which girders the critique of liberal self-interest, seems also to oppose key aspects of many contemporary understandings of well-being and so, potentially, may cause significant problems for policy-makers. Parfit's reductionist view of personal identity argues that identity is reducible to the psychological characteristics of 'continuity and connectedness' (as he calls it), which, to lesser or greater degrees, can become increasingly fragile over time. Parfit invites us to consider the large differences between who we *are* now as adults, compared with who we *were* as small children, in order to highlight the fragility of personal identity over time. However, this reductionist view of identity considerably complicates any evaluation made of a person's life concerning their well-being, as reductionism makes it much harder, if not impossible, to practically measure how well a life is going *overall* and to implement policies accordingly. However, using concrete examples throughout, the main proposal in Smith's chapter is to resist plumping for either Parfitian or non-Parfitian propositions concerning personal identity, and to instead hold these propositions *in tension* to enhance well-being. The main claim is that the latter strategy better reflects the human condition given it messily straddles both classical liberal and Parfitian accounts of self-interest, identity and well-being enhancement.

Several chapters in this book attest to the role of values in well-being in areas ranging from health, heritage, residence, professional life and within social contexts and relationships. The final chapter in Part 2 considers the question posed by Bill Fulford and Kathleen T. Galvin: What is well-being without values? Their chapter goes on to outline the potential contribution of a values-based practice to well-being – the very word *well-being* is explicitly value-laden – small wonder then that well-being is challenging, for values themselves are challenging. Values are challenging theoretically and while values have been a focus of philosophical enquiry for over two millennia they are also in various respects challenging practically. Values-based practice has been developed thus far mainly in health care and in this context, as the chapter indicates, has proved effective in supporting balanced clinical decision-making where challenging values issues are in play. This is why values-based practice has potential for well-being, to the extent that the challenges of well-being are, or reflect, values challenges and therefore they should be susceptible to similar values-based approaches.

Part 3: How is well-being manifest in human life? The aesthetic nature of well-being

In this final part of the book a focus is taken on the aesthetics of well-being with some exemplars of aesthetic thinking and includes diverse 'showings' of how well-being may manifest in human experience. Engagement with creative practices and arts-based approaches is a particular feature of this section. As such this part of this book concerns the aesthetic nature of well-being, that is, aesthetic sources, qualities and expressions of well-being.

Dorthe Jørgensen opens with an invitation for us to think aesthetically, outlining an aesthetics of well-being. She begins by asking the question: 'How can philosophical aesthetics contribute to the understanding of well-being?' She proceeds by arguing that aesthetics is not the same as the aesthetic, here aesthetics is theory and the aesthetic is the subject of this theory. Furthermore, the aesthetic is a question not only of art and entertainment, but also of experience and thought. Likewise aesthetics is not identical to art theory or philosophy of art; it is also a question of epistemology and philosophy of existence. So what can the aesthetic view of life offer? What does it mean to think aesthetically, and how is that linked to wisdom? Can concepts such as 'beauty', 'sensitivity' and 'meaning' have a positive value despite critical contemporary interpretations of these concepts? What is the importance for the individual as well as for society of the expanded way of thinking appertained to judgement?

By considering such questions, her chapter aims to lay the philosophical foundation for this final part of the book, that is, to suggest an aesthetics of well-being. In order to do so, she draws upon and discusses elements from various past and contemporary philosophical positions, but the aesthetics she outlines will not least be grounded in her own thought, articulated in works such as e.g. *Skønhed* (Beauty, 2006), *Aglaias dans* (Aglaias' Dance, 2008) and *Den skønne tænkning* (Beautiful Thinking, 2014).

Deborah Padfield shares findings of an arts-based project to focus on the characterisation of 'the aesthetic space'. She begins in a health context and goes onto point to the promotion of well-being through aesthetic engagement. Her chapter explores some of the links between well-being and creativity using image to help to illuminate how we can communicate experiences of pain. She shows us how images and image-making processes can promote discussion of significant experience and personal narrative often felt to be 'not medical' or 'not relevant' by both clinicians and patients, and so frequently omitted from medical discussion.

Her chapter focuses on analyses of selected parts of a project at University College Hospital, London, (*face2face*) set up to explore the value of images to the communication and understanding of chronic pain. The project aimed to bring discussion of the subjective, invisible and multidimensional character of the lived experience of chronic pain into the shared space of the consulting room, using photographic images to elicit pertinent narrative, navigate different perspectives and democratise dialogue. With an emphasis on facial pain and portraiture it did this through a number of routes: delivering art workshops for clinicians and patients to attend to together in association with the National Portrait Gallery (NPG) London, using images from their collection and quick drawing exercises to stimulate dialogue, co-creating photographs with facial pain patients which reflected their unique experience of pain and developing a pilot prototype of 'PAIN CARDS' as an innovative new communication tool for use in NHS clinics alongside the creation of an artist's film reflecting points of intersect and disconnect between patient and clinician perspectives and the role of narrative in pain experience. The chapter explores the ways in which aesthetic spaces appeared to facilitate exchange between different perspectives and generate new language specific to those individuals at that moment in time. Selected examples will be used from the workshops to evidence ways in which images were able to catalyse discussion, and ways in which collaborative image-making processes made visible some of the dynamics of dialogue as they became like conversations through drawing. The consulting room is explored as a physical space within which photographic images of pain can have agency and impact positively on the relationship and the quality of communication happening within it. Using images to elicit and explore aspects of experience relevant to pain's intensity and prolongation can help reduce isolation, improve communication and thus promote healing and well-being.

Monica Prendergast and Carl Leggo provide a showing of poetry as one way to contribute to well-being in their offering of poetry writing as both a way to wellness and as wellness. They make the case that poetry has always served humanity as a means to wellness and this is why we so often turn to poems, prayers and song lyrics in times of great joy (weddings, birthdays, births) and also in times of great sorrow and struggle (illness, trauma, death, bereavement). As 'poetic inquirers' who write poetry for multiple purposes – as literature, as social science research, as autobiography and autoethnography – they also write poetry as a way of being in the world that assists them in the ongoing challenge to gain and maintain a sense of wellness in their complicated lives. In particular, they have written and published poems addressing the question of how to live well within the academy. Their chapter offers a contextual framework about the social function of poetry to sustain and support individuals and communities, especially in regard to providing comfort in times of crisis. They offer some examples from their own poetic enquiry practice that have opened up spaces for becoming 'well in the world' through the investigation of such topics as parental death, fear and vulnerability in academic life, and memory as a site for identity formation and representation.

Following on in the theme of arts-based approaches that can contribute to a sense of well-being, Catherine Lamont-Robinson focuses upon current arts practice that engages with multi-sensory ways of knowing. Her chapter investigates in detail how related sensory/cognitive processing may inform individual well-being. By drawing on the rich languages of sensory engagement in the visual and tactual arts across both medical student and patient communities, her chapter proposes an alternative version of well-being where participatory manifestations of embodiment shape thinking and reveal joint insights around what it is to be human. Drawing on examples of work from medical education and arts-based interventions within rehabilitation of patients recovering from stroke she points to how well-being may be manifest within embodied approaches.

Engaging in reflective and literary writing mode, Jennifer Schulz offers 'Thirteen Ways of Looking at a Clinic': Here, she shares a story about the clinical internship year she spent ten years ago in a community medical clinic working as a therapist-in-training with chronically mentally ill and economically impoverished adults. This is a story that resists conclusions and explanation. It is a story without convention: without protagonist, identifiable conflict, rising action, climax or resolution. It is a story, primarily, about seeing and it is a story that attempts to see. Neither chronological, nor teleological, this story is, instead, phenomenological and speculative. In the words of philosopher Hans-Georg Gadamer (1960/1998), this story is a 'coming to an understanding' (p. 469).

Telling a story of the clinic, rather than a 'written report', necessitates a dialogal structure and a 'speculative' form. Thus, as she considered the form and method for the telling, she turned to Wallace Stevens's poem 'Thirteen Ways of Looking at a Blackbird' as a model. The stanzas that preface each section of this story, *present* reality rather than *represent* reality as the blackbird emerges in thirteen ways as an unfixed being, rather than a fixed object of interpretation. Each section of the story offers its own specific perspective (by means of anecdote, case story, memo or footnote) on the clinic while also drawing from and re-seeing the section that precedes it, and anticipating, or setting a context for, the next. The blackbird is neither subject nor object but *both* observer and observed. Indeed, the first time we see the blackbird, it is its 'moving eye' that we see, not the bird itself. Does it see us before we see it? As it carries us between and among the various sections of this story, the blackbird, like the clinic, emerges as observed and observer in constantly shifting forms. Staff, administration, patients, even the physical space of the clinic, all at different times occupies the role of Stevens's blackbird. Schulz's story, like Stevens's poem, is an attempt to present the whole of the being of, in this case, the clinic. However, the whole of being, as Gadamer would argue, should not imply an exhaustive or totalising study, but rather an opportunity to see the clinic in the lived experience of the clinic.

Her hope is that this story will invite further speculation on what is possible for treating the mentally ill in terms of the whole of their beings and in the lived context of the spaces explicitly designated for treatment; indeed, perhaps we can find more creative possibilities as they emerge in stories.

> *Among twenty snowy mountains,*
> *The only moving thing*
> *Was the eye of the blackbird.*

Denis Francesconi invites us into new ideas about 'a good life' in education. His proposal is about a 'eudai-monic model' for well-being education, a model that he has been developing over the last four years. It derives from educational sciences/phenomenological pedagogy and embodied theory. It is different from positive psychology, human flourishing or the hedonistic model because it has a different epistemology. He uses some old concepts from history of education (*eudaimonia, paideia, cura sui*) and integrates them with modern ideas from embodied cognitive sciences.

Finally Kathleen T. Galvin and Les Todres offer eighteen kinds of well-being that may be relevant to practice and which can be unfolded to perhaps many more kinds and directions. Their chapter offers a conceptual framework by which different kinds and levels of well-being can be named, and as such, pro-vides a foundation for a resource-oriented approach in situations of illness and vulnerability (rather than a deficit oriented approach). Building on Chapter 8 that articulated the philosophical foundations of an existential theory of well-being ('Dwelling-Mobility'), they show how the theory can be further developed towards more practice-relevant concerns. They introduce eighteen kinds of well-being that are intertwined and inter-related, and consider how each emphasis can lead to the formulation of resources that have the potential to give rise to well-being as a felt experience. They argue that by focusing on a much wider range of well-being possibilities, care practitioners may find new directions for care that are not just literal but also at an existential level.

It is my hope that collectively these chapters, albeit brief, indicate the vast ground and depth of scholar-ship concerning well-being. The collective aim has been to shed light on new emerging ideas about well-being, its theory and philosophical application, all which point to interdisciplinary potential and resources that are relevant not just to health and social care, but also to human life beyond these confines.

PART 1

The human experience of well-being

What is well-being? Philosophical and theoretical foundations

1

RESIDENCE, IDENTITY AND WELL-BEING

Paul Gilbert

At the age of 55 the American novelist Henry James, who had lived a somewhat peripatetic life from child-hood, settled down in Lamb House at Rye in England. 'He had found his home, he who had wandered so uneasily, and he longed for its engulfing presence, its familiarity, its containing beauty', as Colm Toibin puts it in *The Master*, his biographical novel about James (Toibin p. 132). One of James's own characters, Strether in *The Ambassadors*, has a different and opposite experience at the same age. This American, when offered a beautiful home by the woman who loves him, Maria Gostrey, rejects it, even though 'it built him softly round, it roofed him warmly over' (James p. 374). As he explains, "I'm not . . . in real harmony with what surrounds me. You are' (James p. 371). Henry James, we may say, feels at home in Lamb House, Strether does not feel at home at Maria Gostrey's. Having a home, rather than being homeless, is in all sorts of ways contributory to one's well-being, but feeling at home also seems an important ingredient. What, though, does it consist in and why does it conduce to well-being? An obvious answer is that feeling at home is an agreeable feeling and that well-being consists in a preponderance of agreeable feelings over disagreeable ones. My aim in exploring homely feelings is to show how such a hedonist account is over simple and throws further light upon well-being.

Feeling at home is a multifaceted phenomenon. It is not only in one's own place of residence that one can feel at home but in other people's too, in some towns, villages or stretches of countryside but not in others, with some people and not with others, and, by a longer metaphorical stretch, with the subjects or activities with which one has a greater familiarity – philosophy and cooking in my case – than with others – physics and carpentry, say. These differences concern the scope of the feeling, but, whatever the scope, feeling at home is always indexical, in the sense that I feel it here in this place, with these people or engaged in this occupation now. It is a feeling directed at the part of the world with which I am currently engaged in some activity or other, so that it characterizes the tone of the activity, so to speak, in relation to features of the context in which it is performed. For example, I might feel at home sitting in my own old room but not in your ultra-modern one. Sitting itself feels different in the two environments.

This is not to say that I necessarily have different sensations in the two situations. Indeed, while feeling at home can often involve characteristic sensations, it is unlikely that I feel any such sensations when sitting in my own room. Rather, what distinguishes this situation from the other is the absence of the sensations that I feel there as I shift uneasily in a modernist chair. We can quickly dismiss, then, the thought that what makes feeling at home contributory to well-being is that it always involves agreeable sensations. It is agreeable to feel at home but not necessarily for this reason. Furthermore, just as someone can feel at home without any particular sensations so they may not be conscious of feeling at home and still be properly

17

ascribed the feeling. In Barbara Pym's novel *Some Tame Gazelle* one of Belinda's guests, the Archdeacon, falls asleep after dinner: 'if the Archdeacon had not been asleep, she could have had some conversation with him, but it was nice to know that he felt really at home, and she would not for the world have had him any different' (Pym p. 127). He was not, of course, conscious of feeling so much at home that he could reasonably fall asleep, nor need he have had any associated sensations; presumably the only sensations he had were of drowsiness. What his feeling at home at Belinda's did involve was that he felt no need to combat his drowsiness and make an effort to remain awake, as he would have tried to do in other people's houses.

Often, however, we are reflectively aware of feeling at home somewhere or among certain people. In many cases our relation to the place or people will be purely indexical, while in others it is not just this place or these people but a place or people with certain characteristics towards which the feeling is directed. Here we can speak of the feeling as conceptualized, since it is directed at an object as falling under certain concepts, and that it falls under them gives my reason for the feeling. This is something of which I can be directly aware, not something I have to learn by observing the situations in which I feel at home, as I might do with other people. Thus I might be struck by how similar someone else's room is to my own and feel at home there in consequence of this. This is not to imply that feeling at home somewhere is always feeling as if I were at home, in a place with some salient properties that my own home has. What makes me feel at home may be quite different properties from those of my own home, for, in unfortunate cases, one's own home may not be one in which one does feel at home. That was the experience for Iris Murdoch when she lived in the house in Hartley Road, Oxford, which her husband, John Bayley, had bought for them. 'She had driven her pen there day after day, and all the more determinedly', he writes, 'because the place was, as I well knew, so uncongenial to her' (Bayley p. 222).

What, then, are the sort of qualities in virtue of which one may feel at home at a place when this is conceptualized as apt for this feeling and how might one's apprehension of it convey these qualities? We can adopt here, I suggest, a notion that Allen Carlson employs in discussing the aesthetic appreciation of the environment. Feeling at home is not exactly an aesthetic response to a place since aesthetic judgments are universalizable, to be shared by all who view the same scene, whereas we have no corresponding inclination to suppose that others ought to feel at home in the same places that we do ourselves. Carlson speaks of a place as having 'expressive qualities' (Carlson p. 113), and he illustrates this by contrasting the way in which traditional farmsteads can be appreciated aesthetically with the repellence felt at the new agricultural landscapes of America. The former are expressive of community and ecologically sound cultivation; the latter express a loss of social stability and environmental integrity (Carlson p. 183). Carlson points out, however, that the very farmsteads that contemporary Americans admire were, when relatively new, viewed by Henry James's brother, William James, as 'hideous, a sort of ulcer, without a single element of artificial grace to make up for the loss of Nature's beauty' (quoted Carlson p. 175). My suggestion is, then, that we can regard feeling at home, when this is a conceptualized feeling, as a response to the expressive qualities we detect in the place.

Carlson's contrast between the responses to traditional and new agricultural landscapes could well be used to illustrate the likely difference between the sorts of places in which one would feel at home and those in which one would not. However, while Carlson takes the expressive qualities to which we should respond aesthetically as 'life values', exemplified by community and environmentally sound agriculture, there is no reason to think that what is responded to when one feels at home in a place is objectively valuable. The qualities taken to be expressed in a place where one feels at home are the qualities of a place where one thinks one could, other things being equal, make a good home for oneself. What these qualities are will depend upon one's conception of what one's home should be like. This is where one may begin to have doubts about whether feeling at home in a place which one conceptualizes in a certain way is necessarily a good thing. It may be an agreeable feeling, but is it a good feeling to have if one's conception of home is open to criticism? For to say that the feeling is not universalizable is not to say that it is beyond criticism. In particular, one can criticize people for not allowing themselves to feel at home in a place because of its failure to correspond to their image of home, and one can do this by showing that the image is inadequate and thereby something which is limiting and thus stands in the way of their well-being. We can go on to consider just one possible example of this.

A familiar way of conceptualizing a particular sort of place as having the properties of home, not just a type of house but types of community and countryside as well, is as the sort of place proper to those of a certain identity, national, regional or ethnic. This sort of place makes an English person, say, feel at home because it has properties that are supposed to be characteristically English, for example those of the English country cottage. While the idea that different sorts of places produce different sorts of people goes back to the Greeks, it is given classic expression by the German Romantic philosopher Johann Gottfried von Herder. 'Every region of the earth', he writes, 'has its peculiar species of animals which cannot live else-where . . . why should it not have its own kind of men? . . . The Arab of the desert belongs to it, as much as his noble horse and indefatigable camel' (quoted Ergang pp. 90–91). People will feel at home, Herder implies, only in the land that shapes them as the sort of people they are. Being there will contribute to their well-being because they would be literally out of place elsewhere. While some vestiges of these ideas may linger on in popular thought I hope that we can dismiss them here without argument. What actually happens when people feel at home in a place that they conceptualize in a way associated with their identity is that they respond as they have been trained to respond when they are inducted into the identity. To feel at home in places that conform to the images they were then given is to feel that this is the right place for one, given who one is, and thus to enact the identity with which the images are associated.

Yet it is not just because of the possible limiting effects I have indicated that we can question whether it is good, say, for someone to feel most at home when they move into the country cottage of their dreams. This is because what is important *to* someone, as we may suppose their having these feelings for the reason given is, is not necessarily what is good *for* them, in the sense that it does actually contribute to their well-being. Having the national identity they espouse and living a life which supposedly reflects this identity may figure large in an individual's scale of values. But it is not thereby objectively valuable. If we are to think of well-being in terms of what is good for someone, irrespective of their views of what this is, then we have to assess their propensities to have such feelings as feeling at home in this light.

However, when we turn to more primitive manifestations of feeling at home than the conceptualized ones we have been discussing we may think of them as more uncomplicatedly good to have and we need to ask why this should be. The most primitive case of feeling at home, I suggest, is the experience of being able to move around unthinkingly in a familiar environment and to get on with activities there without difficulties occasioned by the place. This is what we can usually do in our immediate environment – the house we live in, the streets down which we walk and so on, all of which we do without attending to their layout. One aspect of this manifests what Maurice Merleau-Ponty calls our motor intentionality, whose object is 'that highly specific thing towards which we project ourselves, near which we are in anticipation and which we haunt', rather than its being 'an object represented', so that 'motor intentionality . . . is concealed behind the objective world which it helps to build up, (Merleau-Ponty p. 138 fn.2). Motor intentionality is involved in our commerce with the things we encounter in our everyday activities, the things which Martin Heidegger terms 'things ready-to-hand' (Heidegger p. 98), like the pen with which I write these words. When I put the pen down and reach for it again I do not conceptualize it as a pen in a certain place to be grasped, for my hand goes out for it automatically. Similarly, the large-scale things in our environment are not conceptualized in terms of what I must make certain directional movements towards. It is my body which has, so to speak, learnt my route around house and streets. It is, Merleau-Ponty writes, 'the body which "understands" in the cultivation of habit' (Merleau-Ponty p. 144).

The resident of a place will normally have the sort of familiarity with it that enables them to negotiate it in this habitual, unthinking way. They feel at home there without any sensations or thoughts of feeling so in virtue of this capacity. Similarly with familiar people to whom we can relate without reflection, without minding our 'p's and 'q's as the expression has it. We feel at home with them in virtue of being able to talk and act with them in this easy-going way. The activities with which I feel at home are likewise those that I can engage in without the difficulties of unfamiliar activities – the difficulties of having to constantly monitor my own practice to see if I am acting correctly, rather than simply getting on with the task in hand. Indeed, the case of activities with which I feel at home is in many ways a model for other cases of the feeling, since it brings out how being able to act without a certain sort of reflection and self-appraisal is what enables one to feel at home. We can recall here how in the house in Hartley Road Iris Murdoch had to drive her pen 'determinedly' because 'the place was so uncongenial to her'. She could not get on with things easily because the uncongenial aspects of the house intruded upon her activities like writing.

To feel at home in a place, then, normally requires not only the capacity to negotiate it effortlessly but the ability to pursue one's ordinary activities there without any impediments it causes. We all know how this can be hampered by a light that glares, a dark ceiling that looms over one or by a chair that creaks. In order to get on with our activities the environment needs to be unobtrusive. For it to obtrude is as bad as for one's pen to run out of ink, interrupting the flow of one's work. Then the object is, in Heidegger's words, 'met with as something unusable' and 'enters the mode of *obtrusiveness*. . . . It reveals itself as something present-at-hand and no more' (Heidegger p. 103). We cannot feel at home in an environment that is, as we say anthropomorphically, hostile in this way. We have, as Elaine Scarry puts it, a 'habit of taking *object-awareness as the norm and object unawareness as an aberrant and unacceptable occurrence*' (Scarry p. 293). The objects around us are taken to be aware, so to speak, of our needs and to suit themselves for them, rather than to stand in the way of their satisfaction, because they have been made or chosen for this purpose. It is evident that to be able to feel at home with things that are so aware, like our houses and streets, is conducive to our well-being, for then we can get on with our activities in a trouble-free way. This has nothing to do with having agreeable feelings, though our feelings would be disagreeable if we could not get on with those activities because we did not feel at home.

I said that feeling at home in a place where we can unthinkingly get on with our lives is a primitive feeling, but there is a further aspect to this and to the sort of circumstances in which the feeling is evoked. It is not just ease of action that is involved but, in some sense, safety. Noel Carroll criticizes Carlson's account of the appreciation of the environment in terms of the discernment of expressive qualities – an account which we adapted for the having of conceptualized feelings of homeyness. Carroll's criticism is that this excludes 'responses of a less intellective, more visceral sort', which he illustrates by observing that when 'standing barefoot amidst a silent arbor, softly carpeted with layers of decaying leaves, a sense of repose and homeyness may be aroused in us' (Carroll p. 90). It is precisely such preconceptual feelings that we are now considering. In relation to the arbor Carroll supposes that 'such an emotional state might be caused by our tacit recognition of its refuge potential' (Carroll p. 105), not a conscious recognition of it as such, and he takes such a primitive preconceptual response to be instinctually grounded. We do not need to accept Carroll's evolutionary explanation for such responses to recognize the truth in his account. It captures the way in which feeling at home is not just a state we can be in given the right circumstances, but one which can be triggered by them, and when so triggered involve emotional reactions of the kind that Carroll observes. These are feelings of safety, in the sense of our not needing to be on our guard, though what we do not need to be on our guard against are not predators but elements of the environment which are hostile in the way indicated in the previous paragraph.

If one is fortunate one will normally have these feelings in one's own home, where the environment has been shaped to meet one's needs and where one can act according to one's own rules. The feelings will usually extend beyond one's immediate home to its environs in town or country, even though one does not shape them or the rules that living there require one to abide by. One shapes oneself to the place, and rules that may once have chafed soon become second nature as one becomes an established resident. We can sharply distinguish the role of resident that is taken on by living in a place from the sort of identity involving attachment to it whose dangers we pointed to earlier. Being a resident of a place is not an identity since I may have no inclination to think that the fact that I live there has any bearing on who I am. Nor does it need the sorts of conceptualization of the place that are required by identities constructed in terms of it. All that is needed is the preconceptual familiarity we have discussed and the capacity to get on with my life there to a large extent unreflectively. It is easy to see how this is conducive to well-being, so that feeling at home in the way that residents of a place usually do can be regarded as a manifestation of this aspect of life. It may perhaps never come to consciousness, and one may only realize one had the feeling when it is destroyed by changes to the place that make one no longer feel at home in it.

Philosophical accounts of well-being tend to see it in terms of gaining certain ends. This is the case for the hedonist account we started with, where well-being consists in the presence of agreeable feelings and the absence of disagreeable ones. It is very obviously so for an alternative view that sees well-being as the satisfaction of desires. It is also the case for so-called objective list theories that regard well-being as secured by obtaining such objectively valuable things as health and friendship. I think, however, that our investigation of feeling at home as contributory to well-being suggests that there is an aspect to it that is not captured by reference to ends. The conceptualized feelings we talked about may, indeed, fall into the ends-directed category. Someone who buys a country cottage because they think it is the kind of house they will feel at home in has an end in view, and this is a pleasure which they conceptualize in a certain way. But in the case of preconceptual feeling, which is directed immediately at a place and may or may not involve sensations, no specific end is involved. It is good to feel at home there, I argued, just because this allows for what is in certain respects unreflective action – action in pursuit of other ends. This is to be able to get on with one's life without a variety of factors which involve things or people making this more difficult and requiring of one greater attention, circumspection or effort.

I want to suggest, then, that one aspect of well-being concerns not what ends we can achieve by our actions but the manner of these actions themselves. It seems evident that Iris Murdoch's well-being would have been enhanced if she had not had to drive her pen so determinedly on account of the uncongeniality of the house in Hartley Road. By contrast the Archdeacon's well-being was enhanced by his not having to be on his guard against falling asleep at Belinda's. These are modes of activity which fail or succeed in conducing to well-being just because of the way the activity is engaged in – the tone it has, as I expressed it earlier. This is not, I think, because one mode is less efficient and the other more efficient for getting one's ends realized, though to argue this adequately would require more space than I have here. All I shall say is that the checks to one's activity occasioned by a glaring light or by a potentially censorious fellow occupant of a room do not immediately strike one as impediments to efficiency. What strikes one is that the room is wrong, not homely enough with that bright light, or that the person is unsettling. I do not think first about what I am aiming to achieve and become exasperated with my lack of productivity. That may follow, but in many instances (e.g. the Archdeacon's) nothing like this will matter. Rather, it is the activity itself that is marred by factors like these and greatly improved by their absence.

One might be tempted to say that the activity is 'perfected' by being performed in an atmosphere in which one can feel at home, by analogy with Aristotle's account of pleasure as what perfects the activities we undertake because it manifests our functioning well as human beings. Feeling at home in its primitive preconceptual form can be viewed as a pleasure so understood, and we desire it because we want to function well and not for any ulterior reason. Well-being consists, in part, in just this well functioning.

References

Bayley, J. *Iris* (London: Abacus, 1999).

Carlson, A. *Aesthetics and the Environment* (London: Routledge, 2000).

Carroll, N. 'On Being Moved by Nature: Between Religion and Natural History' in Carlson, A. and Berleant, A. (eds) *The Aesthetics of Natural Environments* (Ontario: Broadview, 2004).

Ergang, R.R. *Herder and the Foundations of German Nationalism* (New York: Columbia University Press, 1931).

Heidegger, M. *Being and Time* translated Macquarrie, J. and Robinson, E. (Oxford: Wiley-Blackwell, 1973).

James, H. *The Ambassadors* (New York: Signet, 1960).

Merleau-Ponty, M. *The Phenomenology of Perception* translated Smith, C. (London: Routledge & Kegan Paul, 1962).

Pym, B. *Some Tame Gazelle* (London: Granada, 1981).

Scarry, E. *The Body in Pain* (New York: Oxford University Press, 1985).

Toibin, C. *The Master* (London: Picador, 2005).

2

A SENSE OF WELL-BEING

The anthropology of a first-person phenomenology

Nigel Rapport

What does it mean to talk of 'well-being' as against 'health'? One refers to something more subjective in its designation and evaluation, less accessible to technological intervention and objective measurement. Well-being is existential rather than metrical, and other adjectives that seem to pertain include personal, momentary, sensorial and variable. I might have a sense of well-being over and against the fact that I know myself to be dying. I have a sense of well-being but is it something of which I can be long assured? Will it abide? My sense of well-being might be connected to the fact that I know the world to be a purely material phenomenon without any supernatural warrant, significance or teleology; my neighbour, contrariwise – or myself at another stage of my life – has felt that well-being attaches to the watchful eye of a personal god. I measure my well-being, perhaps, in terms of my sense of satiation; my neighbour in terms of a sense of devotion. No sense of well-being for me can exceed, perhaps, the feeling I derive from viewing the art of Stanley Spencer; for my neighbour, who is blind, well-being comes from the intellectual assurance that his family is financially catered for. . . . What does this diversity, personalism, sensoriality and contingency tell us? Are there generalities here to elucidate? Is there a *human* story of well-being to tell, or a *cultural* or *social* one, a *geographical* or *historical* one?

In this chapter an anthropologist asks himself these questions, hoping to balance the intrinsic bodily state – a sense of well-being – against what might be said to provide contexts for that state: the individual is a member of humankind, also of a society and community (perhaps), also of a local or regional part of the world (perhaps), also of a particular historical epoch (perhaps). The chapter considers well-being from the comparative standpoint of individual human body against the world.

A department of social anthropology: a survey

I conducted a survey among departmental colleagues at the University of St. Andrews: 'What does "well-being" (or its nearest conceptual equivalent) imply for your research subjects?'. The results are diverse. Here is a sample:

Huon Wardle works in Kingston, Jamaica. Here, human life is conceived of as an individual 'adventure', a movement and a development (Wardle 2001). A sense of well-being derives from 'living good' as one 'passes through', which in turn entails being able to give and receive good things from others – from spirits of the dead, and other beings possibly, as well as humans. 'Good things' might include 'sipping a cup' (of rum), and 'running good jokes' with friends and family at the 'yard' (the family household), or hanging out with contacts at the 'corner'. The 'good life' is also progressive, where one increases the esteem in which one is held and can imagine moving further afield; also where 'pressure' and the physical, mental or social impairments it causes are avoided. Pressure may derive from the 'bad mind' (malicious intent) of neighbours but also from the 'downpression' (oppression) of those in control of society's political and economic resources: government, big business, the police. Well-being is a matter of negative relationships as well as positive personal capabilities.

Mette High conducts research in Mongolia, on its extensive steppes, its growing capital city and its burgeoning mining industry (of minerals including gold). The local expression that best captures the concept 'well-being', High suggests, is *saihan amdral*, meaning a 'wonderful life'. *Saihan amdral* occurs when humans and non-humans – animals and spirit-beings – carefully and respectfully balance their interests and actions, allowing good fortune in fertility, prosperity and longevity to flow unhindered both between them and among them. The opposite of well-being occurs when one part of nature denies the existence of another – with the (eventual) result that it comes to deny itself (see High 2013).

Mark Harris's work explores the historical and social identity of Caboclo fisher folk who live on the banks of the River Amazon in Brazil, a 'floodplain peasantry'. Rather than identifying his research subjects in collective, ethnic and class terms, however, he is concerned to focus on their practical engagement with their environment and how they manage and negotiate this – and have done since the times of the Portuguese colonization and settlement (Harris 2000). Life beside the Amazon is literally a matter of flow, of shifting between land and water, between economic and social and religious adaptations. For Harris's research subjects, well-being is closely connected to a sense of being 'at ease' (*ficar a vontade* is the phrase in Portuguese), which means being one's own boss – *vontade* carries a sense of willingness or will. In essence, 'well-being' implies a sense of being able to come and go as one pleases.

Recent research of my own has concerned well-being at work, as an aspect of professional accomplishment: specifically, senses of well-being among porters in a large, hospital in Scotland (Rapport 2009). Here, 'well-being' derives from ways in which porters feel they move through the hospital plant on their daily rounds – ways that they largely control; also from the way in which they might move between work-site and home according to shifts that they determine; also from the way in which they might themselves move between the statuses of 'porter' and 'patient' without obstacle – working in a hospital it is their 'perk' to be routinely sick. Finally, well-being derives from a sense that hospital-portering need not be their lot always: they might move on. Belying the hospital's image as a total institution with a hierarchical management, the porters' well-being, individually and collectively, is a matter of negotiated movement.

Nominally extending this department of social anthropology, as it were, so as to include contributions from anthropologists based elsewhere than St. Andrews, the survey continues to deliver a diversity of results:

John Gray's research subjects are members of a clan of high caste 'Chhetris' living in the hamlet of Kholagaun in the southern Kathmandu Valley, Nepal. Their aim, he explains (2009), is to prosper not just in the narrow sense of material wealth but also in a wider sense that is conveyed in the Nepali word *samŕddhi*: an abundance of those things that characterize the 'good life'. This includes the well-being of children, health and peaceful relations with oneself, other human beings and the deities. At the same time, 'Chhetris' are enjoined to remain detached from these manifold worldly attachments and to resist 'enslavement' by them so as to achieve 'liberation' and see through the veil of illusion that conceals the fundamental unity of the cosmos. The goal of a good life and the route to well-being is to live in detached attachment, in passionless passion.

Anne-Katrine Brun Norbye has explored the summer 'pilgrimages' that take families of Norwegians 'back' from city to country, to revisit old homes and sample 'country produce'. For instance, *Kyrost*, a type of dairy cheese made of sweet, skimmed milk, for centuries provided Norwegian farmers with protein during winter. It is today sold at rural 'Women's Fairs', having been made in the traditional way at *støler* (mountain summer dairy-farms). City visitors buy this cheese, and serve it to friends and family, and so display a 'modern' attitude to 'local', 'authentic' and 'healthy' food, nature and tradition. There remains a generational divide, however, Brun Norbye explains (2010). For many Norwegian young adults and their children the symbolic relevance of the cheese does not mean they actually *like* to eat it. Only older Norwegians once raised on *Kyrost* cheese find that the taste sustains memories of identities and way of life: for this generation, once more eating *Kyrost* cheese for dinner provides a sense of well-being that derives (however briefly) from a return home.

David Shankland's research subjects are Alevis, members of a heterodox Muslim minority in Turkey. The group is hierarchical, both men and women varying in rank according to the status of the lineage into which they are born. The highest rank is *efendi*, people regarded as being descended from Ali and thus from the Prophet Muhammed. Next in status is the rank of *dede*, and typically it is *dedes* who preside over a series of communal rituals that are regarded as essential for the well-being of village communities as a whole. The rituals are known as *cems*; without *dedes* there can be no *cems*, and without the *cems* the teachings of Ali have not been fulfilled. This sense of interconnection extends to the temporal as well, Shankland explains (2004): unless all are at peace within the assembly of villagers, the *cem* cannot take place. Well-being entails village peacefulness, an absence of dispute, and *cems* officiated by *dedes*.

Leo Coleman's research concern is political activism in the North Indian state of Uttarkhand. For many years, residents of the region – mountainous and under-developed – have agitated for the right to govern their own affairs. Political sovereignty is felt to be a prerequisite to well-being in a competitive global environment. Coleman's interlocutors impress upon him that the real problem is a lack of roads, construction of which would not only make their state the kind of traversable space that the rest of 'modern India' represents, but more importantly would almost magically connect this remote area to distant centres of wealth and prosperity. This single-minded focus on roads as route to well-being should be understood as more than a misguided fixation on the goods and Gods of modernity, Coleman insists (2014), a rustic false consciousness. The fervent embrace of these promises is to be understood as an aesthetics through which the world is known and grasped, certain connections to power and authority are made realizable, and a sense of well-being is hence secured.

Allison James's research subjects are British school-age children, and thence 'childhood health' as a globally authentic phenomenon. The issue for James (2004) concerns the ways and extents to which children may be enabled to take charge of their own health and well-being as subjects in their own right. For the very collective category of 'children' seems premised on questionable assumptions of fact and value: 'children' are identified as if objects 'at risk' and in need of others' constant guidance. It is the case, however, James argues, that any human child is capable of furnishing themselves with a sense of their own well-being. The human body is a work in process, and that of the child especially so: the child is capable, as part of its experience, of taking on the unfinished nature of its the body – of coming to terms with the shapes, sizes and proclivities of its embodiment – and finding its own meanings in them, its own ratios and sense of normalcy.

Michael Jackson's canvas is broader again: 'human beings'. Extensive long-term fieldwork in Aboriginal Australia and also among the Kuranko of Sierra Leone lead him to argue for a pan-human way of our being-in-the-world across these seeming cultural and social divides. 'Being' is precarious and unstable, Jackson concludes (2005): each human being possesses a fluid consciousness which oscillates between solitude and sociality, speech and silence, reflection and habit, aimlessness and purposiveness, body and imagination, passion and calm. A human sense of 'well-being' derives from the equilibrium that can be achieved amid this instability, and the equanimity with which one deals with subtle oscillations – such as one's perception of another's glance, gesture or remark.

The commonality of human being, finally, is intrinsic to an anthropological methodology of participant-observation in which the consciousness of the anthropologist is his or her key tool in gaining an understanding of the lives of those others who are the research subjects. In Trevor Marchand's case, for instance, working among stone-masons in Yemen, Nigeria and Mali, apprenticing himself as a member of the building community, transforms him into a practitioner with vested interests in the making of domestic, public and religious places. Much masonic communication is non-propositional in nature, Marchand notes (2010), relying on an intercourse of visual, auditory and somatic forms of information; nevertheless, he is able to achieve empathy with the daily experiences of co-workers through regular reflection upon his own physical strains, emotional states and changing sense of tedium or accomplishment. *His* sense of well-being leads him to know how *they* take pleasure in a 'secure' edifice, in negotiating innovations in tradition, and in embodying the qualities that evince 'mastery'.

Discussion: the character of 'well-being'

'Well-being' appears in the above survey often as a translation of a local term. How precise or adequate can we expect this translation as being? Even if the translation is adequate, the terms commensurate, does a *linguistic* commensuration – the comparable place of concepts in a linguistic matrix – do the work we might wish in attempting to ascertain a commensuration of *sensibilities*? My survey was an attempt to discover the possibly different *senses* of well-being for different people in different places, not the possibly different senses of '*well-being*'; my search was a sensory one not a linguistic one, but how to distinguish the two? Furthermore, what kind of reification or entification has taken place when a conceptual name stands for a sense – whether within *or* between languages? There is translation involved *in any case* when giving a name, and making into a concept, something that is more inchoate in nature: a 'sense', a 'feeling'. What becomes of a *sense* of well-being when it is conceptualized as 'well-being' – what is secured, what invented, what corrupted?

Compounding such uncertainties is the way that very often the anthropologist is describing in the third-person what is essentially a first-person phenomenon. True, Marchand describes his own sense of well-being; it can be argued that Jackson and James, also, propose an understanding of well-being that places them and their research subjects on the same footing – the well-being of human beings and human children as experienced by researcher and research subjects alike. For others above, however, well-being is something that they *qua* researchers assert *on behalf* of their research subjects; 'translation' here concerns not merely the asserting of commensuration between different languages – and between sensory worlds and verbal ones – but also the possible commensuration of the experience of different human individuals. The anthropologist claims, 'This is how my research subjects formulate and experience well-being'; but there can be no certainty here.

Another issue concerns value. It is noteworthy that in their writings on the subject of 'community' anthropologists have found it difficult to make a clear distinction between their *descriptions* of an empirical situation and an implied *prescription* of an empirical situation; so freighted is community as a term of *positive* signification and evaluation – so much a 'hurray-word' – that it has been difficult to write about community without importing a version of the 'good life' as the anthropologist interprets this. In short: anthropologists have found it difficult to write negatively – accurately – of 'community'; however much a negative description might be warranted by facts on the ground (Rapport 1993: 31–39; Amit and Rapport 2002). Does 'well-being' not suffer from a similar difficulty? 'Well-being' appears so fine and positive a thing that its local conceptual equivalent must translate into 'hurray' terms. Can the anthropologist escape the importing of a positive evaluation into a description of what he or she takes to be research subjects' notions of 'well-being'?

Certainly it appears to be the case that well-being in the above anthropological survey is construed as a kind of part-concept: something positive that is paired with an absence and contrast. The positive sense of well-being exists alongside a recognition of how transient this state is. It is also something transactional: well-being is consequent upon a transaction or engagement with a world beyond the self. Edmund Husserl (1962), building on the work of Franz Brentano, famously proposed that 'intentionality' be understood as a transactional concept, always aimed at and focused upon something other: to 'intend' something was necessarily to place the self in relation to what could be wished for and willed. 'Well-being' would seem to be a sister-concept to intentionality, consequent upon what has been intended: if intentionality is a kind of transmission *from* the self, then well-being is a kind of reception *into* the self, the outcome of an intention. Both engage or transact with the world but possessing an opposite directionality.

If well-being connects with something beyond the self, then what that connection entails – and, indeed, what that 'self' entails – are matters of great empirical diversity, as even a brief survey has evinced. For *James* what was key was that a child be allowed to take charge of their own relation to resources that they construe as instrumental in affording a sense of well-being; while for *Harris* being in charge of one's movements through a home environment was key. For *Rapport*, too, movement within the work-place, and between that work-place and domestic and recreational spaces, added up to a sense that one's environment was one's own to determine.

Well-being for *High* was a matter of balance: that the interests and the actions of human beings, and non-human beings alike, should be in equilibrium. Materiality alongside spirituality figured for *Gray*, too, where peace and good health called for a kind of detached attachment to the world; also for *Shankland*, where a village at peace and village rituals officiated by the properly ordained figure were equally necessary. Materiality figured more narrowly in *Coleman's* account where a sense of well-being derived from engaging with the world in modern ways: through a politically independent state and along paved roads. Similarly, for *Brun Norbye* a certain traditional cheese, eaten at home, brought together a sense of past and present: a tasting of memory.

According to *Jackson*, the self sought to achieve a balance between his or her personal desires and the subtle registering of others' responses to him or her, so that there was both solitude and sociality in well-being, outward aims and inward purposes. *Wardle* described a situation of giving and receiving 'good things' (drink, gossip), and of increasing self-esteem while avoiding political and economic stresses. Finally, *Marchand* described first-hand the well-being that derived from mastery of bodily techniques that sat securely within a customary environment of living traditions of practice.

An anthropology of well-being

Given the above methodological and analytical issues – the anthropologist's first-person sense of 'well-being' is difficult to dissociate from any account of the 'well-being' of his or her research subjects – and given the seeming empirical diversity (both sensory and linguistic), how have anthropologists sought to make a general contribution to an understanding of well-being? Three distinct approaches can be identified. The first can be termed a cultural-relativist one which sees difference and method and value as pertaining alike to worlds of cultural construction that are separate from one another and radically distinct (see Mathews and Izquierdo 2009). 'A culture' constructs a world for its members, through its language, its processes of socialization or 'enculturation', its immersing of individual bodies in environing routines of practice. Who its members become, what they become, how they exist in the world, what is 'well' for them, how they think of themselves (if at all) and how they evaluate 'well-being' all derive from what their culture causes them to take as customary and proper. The 'moral', Emile Durkheim concluded, is synonymous with the 'social' at particular times and places. For followers of Durkheim (or of Franz Boas), the diversity of notions of well-being marks the diversity of cultural worlds and the diversity of ways in which human beings are moulded into members. 'Well-being' might include an individual committing suicide, therefore, if this were to accord with what was allocated to that member as a necessary behaviour for the good of the whole (Durkheim 2002).

A powerful modern version of such relativism – beyond the world of academic anthropology – is the 'identity politics' that accompanies policies of multiculturalism. And the relativization of what 'well-being' might mean in a human life bears significant consequences. For instance, in Anne Sigfrid Grønseth's sensitive ethnography of Tamil refugees in northern Norway, the discourse of multiculturalism deployed by the bureaucracy of the apparently liberal Norwegian state leaves 'Tamil' individuals trapped and isolated in a world of 'cultural' difference. Norwegian doctors, labelling their patients as 'Hindu Tamil', focus on their presumed differences as representatives of a cultural category rather than recognizing the individual before them as moral persons equivalent to themselves. The 'culture' is treated rather than the person, Grønseth avers (2001: 509), the result being that her Tamil acquaintances feel they cannot emerge from the group as either individuals or Norwegians. Their 'well-being' remains a hidden quest only.

The second approach favoured by anthropologists to the diversity of ethnographic versions of 'well-being' might be called a social-structuralist one (see Corsin-Jimenez 2007). Here it is perceived as being in the nature of social organization that the functioning whole that is a society, or the congeries of discourses that is a society, contains difference within itself as part of its nature. 'A society' is, at any one time, a complex assemblage of positions and situations and ways of being and knowing, of classes or castes or statuses, of professions and genders and roles, of spheres or domains (domestic, jural, economic, religious). Members of a society will differ according to the spheres and statuses and roles, and so on, to which they are allocated, at birth or through another selective process such as academic examination. However, the sphere (and so on) to which they are allocated will determine their habits, their life-chances, their world-views, their very awarenesses, to a greater or lesser extent. Including what they take, and the wider society takes, to be their 'well-being'. Following Gramsci (and a notion of determining 'hegemonic' ideologies [Gramsci 2000]) or following Bourdieu (and a notion of determining embodied 'habituses' [Bourdieu 1977]) or following Foucault (and a notion of determining discursive ways of seeing, interacting and knowing [Foucault 2006]) might cause anthropologists to differ regarding the extent to which they allow the possibility of human beings freeing themselves from their social-structuration (and whether there *is* an abiding human being that might benefit from being 'free'), but all would concur in their social contextualization of well-being. A sense of 'well-being' derives from what is allocated to and expected from that human being as a result of their being a member of a particular section of a society: 'working class' or 'female' or 'academic' or 'mentally ill' or 'legally individual' or 'religiously orthodox', and so on.

The third approach adopted by anthropologists to the diversity of ethnographic versions of 'well-being' can be called a phenomenological or existential one (Cohen 1994; Jackson 2011; Rapport 1997, 2012). It does not read well-being as a manifestation of something else – a culture, its discourses and traditions; a social structure, its divisions and functionality. According to a phenomenological-anthropological understanding, a diversity of definitions and practices surrounding well-being reflects the diversity, multiplicity, even contrariety that is essentially contained in the sensorium of an individual human life. 'Humanity' describes a certain universal form of embodiment and mortality; humankind is a species with an evolutionary history that gives rise to certain common *capacities*. Those capacities then come to be *substantiated* in particular ways in different individual lives. Humanity presents itself as individuality. The individual substantiation of those universal and intrinsic capacities allows for a wide range of difference, both between individual lives and within individual lives. 'A sense of well-being' describes the way in which an individual human being takes his or her species inheritance and lives it, applies it, substantiates it, at a particular time and place. Between times and between places, an individual might experience different 'senses of well-being'; at the same time and place, different individuals might experience different 'senses of well-being'; at the same time and place, *the same individual* might experience different 'senses of well-being' *at once*, or very nearly 'at once': we human beings have the capacity to be internally diverse, contradictory, inconsistent, conflicted, to derive a sense of well-being, say, from partaking in a religious ritual with other family members *and* from knowing that the entire belief system and set of ritual practices is a shameful anachronism. And what drives these desires and gratifications need not be abstracted from the person, generalized and impersonalized, say as the outcome of social-structural habituations or emotional enculturations. (It is not consequent that humanity and individuality are constructed differently in different cultural worlds or different historical epochs; and it is not true that humanity and individuality derive their natures from positionalities within complex societal structures and discursive assemblages.) To know why and how an individual human being possesses particular senses of well-being is to know them and the life-project they construe for themselves (Rapport 2003).

Moving around as a hospital porter: the well-being of Phil Ward

Phil Ward had a ready grin, and when he smiled he revealed a black front tooth. Combined with his wiry, boyish and compact frame, he reminded me of an 'Artful Dodger', as Dickens might have portrayed him, albeit that Phil Ward must have been in his late thirties. The other porters at Constance Hospital in the Scottish port-city of 'Easterneuk' largely agreed that 'Wardy' was 'a real character'. I did not personally take to him because I was usually annoyed by what appeared to be an inveterate laziness and irresponsibility, and a petulance and belligerence when he did not get his own way. But there was no doubting his popularity. Many other porters – there were some 150 at Constance – seemed to extend towards him a generosity and a solicitude even at the expense of themselves, and this included the portering management. (Constance Hospital is a large, modern teaching-hospital, and the main employer in a post-industrial area of great male unemployment.) Phil Ward was granted the license to act as an artful dodger at the hospital's expense, as it seemed to me, and in the process maintained a routine – movements within the hospital plant and beyond, in the wider Easterneuk urban environment – that successfully fed his sense of well-being. Briefly I rehearse here a longer treatment of 'Wardy' and his place in a portering community (Rapport 2009: 157–182), for a closer examination of what I can understand that well-being to consist in and how Phil Ward achieved it. Some phrases of Virginia Woolf's provide me with an opening. 'The mere process of life is satisfactory', Woolf writes (1983: 177): to have things follow one another in good order – eating then sleeping, walking to work and then walking home, always with things to do next – repeats the same curve of rhythm, and in the process 'spreads the same ripple of wellbeing'. Identity becomes and remains robust, Woolf concludes, when a person's life possesses a certain methodicality and purposiveness. Let me suppose what might be the methodicality of Phil Ward's life.

At first glance, Phil Ward's life appeared anything but orderly or routine – it was barely in control. Other porters enjoyed hearing and imagining what Wardy might be up to now, and they embellished the sagas of his life: there was a thrill in living vicariously the life of the chancer and skiver. There was also a way in which other porters looked out for Wardy because *he* did not: his irresponsibility seemed to extend even to his own life and welfare, as well as that of his 'bairn' – the child of an ex-partner. Drinking, gambling, fornicating, fighting and lying, always short of money and doing his best to avoid income tax office or the Poll Tax, or Child Support, doing his best sometimes to distance the very ones who would show solicitude towards him, Phil Ward seemed content constantly to challenge his consociates into proving that they were his colleagues after all. In abusing his friends Wardy both asserted that the 'abuse' was not serious, and that others' response should be a continuation of solicitude towards him and trust. It was the success of the popularity and strength of Wardy's character that this strategy also seemed usually to work. People liked to be with him, to hear of him and to weave his derring-do into their worlds of gossip. Wardy's inclusion no-matter-what was part of the 'democracy' of the portering community, the way they ('we') engaged with one another in mutual support and in opposition to the impersonal organization, hierarchy and even regimentation of the wider institution of the hospital.

One morning in the porters' lodge – the two cramped rooms in which we gathered between being allocated jobs, and also to gossip, read the newspaper, listen to the radio, make tea and snacks (known by the porters as 'the buckie') – there was talk of new beds and mattresses coming into certain wards, and how the old ones were to be disposed of. Wardy, indeed, was to get one of the latter for the room he was presently occupying in the Nurses' Residences. Not long afterwards I heard a cheery Wardy himself boast how he was now able to come to work 'along the corridor ... didn't even need a jumper!'. I asked him what he meant:

WARDY: I'm living in the Nurses' Residences 'cos I was kicked out of my house. Same old story – normal reason – too many arguments with my wife.

NIGEL: Have you got kids?

WARDY: No, no kids. Well, I do, but I've not seen him for years. I don't see him. Won't see him. He's got a
new daddy now, and a brother, and a sister.
NIGEL: How old?
WARDY: Nine now: 'Little Phil Ward'. But I've not seen him since he was one.
NIGEL: You probably will one day: he'll want to.
WARDY: Aye. Probably see him again in end – when he's 16 and hooked! [He laughs]

It was typical of Wardy that this information was conveyed without emotion, barring the final black
humour. Having fights with one's spouse and being homeless was presented as a normal old story: there
was no shame attached. Wardy would claim normalcy for his life and challenge others to see it differently.

Another porter, Kaj, lived in the Nurses' Residences with his fiancée. Soon there was joking talk in
the buckie about Kaj being kept awake by Wardy: his music blaring through the wall and the noise of him
fornicating. Ian conjured up the picture of Kaj trying to watch television as the picture bounced and there
was an overwhelming squeaking from Wardy having sex on the bed next door. 'Why shouldn't I make a
noise?' was Wardy's straight-faced rejoinder: 'I pay my Council Tax. *I* can hear Kaj watching *Brookside*! [a
soap opera for adolescents]'. The saga of Wardy's marital relations and his sex life was a popular and ongoing one, fuelled both by Wardy's cryptic statements and others' fanciful embellishments. The tattoo on his
right arm, Wardy explained to me, was meant to be a rose with flames rising from it, and then with 'Sharon'
inscribed beneath. (Above the rose and flames, and normally covered by his shirt sleeve, was also 'Sonya'
[presumably the mother of his son].) Soon, Wardy laughingly added, 'there'll be a black panther beneath
the Sharon!' – or not, he reconsidered: she might fight the panther like a wild thing; and 'It's still Sharon
I love'. Not long after, however, Wardy was announcing, in response to a query, that 'Sharon is binned: it's
definitely over between us'.

The uncertainty regarding Wardy's amorous relations, the bachelor status he had reclaimed for himself,
and what might happen next, were a constant source of titillation amid a tedious work-shift:

IAN: You know how that receptionist, Moira, always drapes her leg over yours when she's in here, on the sofa?
Well, she couldn't do that to Wardy 'cos after 30 seconds he'd need to be off to the loo and wanking off!
DAVE: You know what your problem is, Wardy? Too much . . . what's that stuff? Testosterone! [Wardy grins
and moves to make a phone call] There he is now! On the phone to his lover!
IAN: It's that nurse from Ward 16. I can lip-read what Wardy's saying to her 'cos I've seen it so often now:
'You're gonna get it tonight!'.

With his Delphic words and grins, combined with his boasts, Wardy was happy to play The Porter's For-
nicator. Yes, he admitted: he might have had 'a woman' in the Nurses' Residences, keeping Kaj awake with
his 'entertaining'. . . . Yes: he was off work on Sunday, so they would be 'going at it like bunnies' – the last
time they did it, it felt like his 'knob was coming off' . . . . Yes: if Peggy Cox [the portering sub-manager] was
snooping around the buckie earlier, then it was probably to check on the bulge in his trousers. . . . Alongside
this play, however, were moments of truthful admission from Wardy where he claimed a human sympathy:

WARDY: She's not talking to me at all now, Sean! I just made it far worse. . . . You know how you do something as a reaction? Without thinking. Like you do. Then you regret it. So, I said yesterday: 'I'll kill the
both of them!'. Just as a reaction. And I would have done, yesterday. [He leaves the buckie]
SEAN: [explains to others in the buckie] This is about Linda in [Ward] 16. The blond one. You know. Wardy
heard she was at a car-boot sale and had left with a bloke. And he thought the worst. . . .

That Wardy had been accommodated in the Nurses' Residences amid his marital and domiciliary troubles was thanks to the generosity of the portering management. I was struck by how sympathetic the

hospital managers generally were, taking wider social and economic circumstances into account when instrumental considerations alone (of performance at work) would have warranted dismissal. One morning not long after Wardy had acquired his residential sinecure at the hospital, Peggy Cox and her deputy Mark Hodges had come upon him in the buckie looking unshaven and unkempt. Wardy's makeshift style of dress was often an item of note among the porters: he was teased for wearing the same malodorous, wrinkled blue shirt for ages, also for his skin-tight trousers and for his brogues worn with white socks. On this occasion, Mark Hodges announced that being unshaven might look fine for a night out on the town, but not at work. Wardy replied by complaining that the management had not given him the overtime he had requested – and warranted – to pay for his upcoming court case and counsel ('I can't afford insurance on £130 per week!'). Peggy commiserated but asked him nicely, and teasingly, to please, next time, shave on *his* time not the hospital's. 'What am I going to do with you?', she concluded maternally (though not being that much older in terms of years).

Wardy's tone when discussing his plight – financial as well as sentimental – with management as well as fellow porters was in terms of kinds of rights. The factors that had brought him to this plight were 'human' ones, we have heard – 'same old story: normal reason' – and his actions, he wanted us to understand, were 'human' too; he was not differently responsible to the rest of us. Wardy was quite open about his situation, therefore, and openly demanding that he be given the means – by management or anyone else – to improve upon it. If assistance was not forthcoming, Wardy took it as a personal affront: he was not receiving his due; he was surrounded by 'two-faced c★★★s who stab you in the back!'.

I found if difficult to sympathize with Wardy, as I have said, because he seemed to me so blatantly hypocritical, selfish and self-exculpatory. I was always surprised at the license granted Wardy by the other porters as he aggressively lambasted them, and blamed them for his own failings. . . . It was not his fault, Wardy insisted, that numerous hospital wards were desperate for oxygen cylinders that had not been delivered since Monday because it had only been *his* job since Thursday (today was Friday). . . . It was not his fault that his name appeared nowhere in the job-roster book for the past two hours: he had been allocated the job of clearing the rubbish and, knowing he was going on holiday today, Desmond (one of Wardy's friends) had left everything for him to do: rubbish piled up everywhere! . . . Having kept friends waiting 30 minutes when they had generously offered him a ride home, he then asked the chargehand to sign him in for an extra half hour's overtime for the period he had just spent joshing in the locker room. . . .

In part I think the other porters' generosity was a recognition of a genuine innocence on Wardy's part. He did not (always) appear to know he was being cheeky, hypocritical, lazy, self-exonerating. When Wardy returned to the buckie from a job – his first for a while – with the laconic utterance 'Robot!' as he settled himself back to studying the betting pages in *The Sun*, he genuinely seemed to believe that he was being put to work as if an automaton ('Them nurses will be wanting us to give them a rub soon, lying on the beds!'). There was a likeable innocence to Wardy's enjoyments, scams and derring-do. Also, Wardy appeared not able to help himself, needing others to protect him from his own self-destructive (and belligerent) tendencies. When a notice went up in the buckie that a new chargehand (a minor position in portering management) would be taken on and trained and 'all names will get consideration', the name 'Phil Ward' soon appeared on the list – and Wardy seemed genuinely hurt and embarrassed at the general hilarity this caused. When Lee, a current chargehand, even told him he had no chance – 'That's just my opinion, like: you could prove me wrong' – a shocked Wardy retorted: 'Well, why don't you keep your opinions to your f★★★ing self!', before going on to add that the first thing he would do with his new power would be to ban people from going for smoking breaks. . . . Perhaps it was more fun to see what mishap would befall Wardy next, rather than getting (pointlessly) annoyed. The sagas of his life became something of a cherished possession among the porters. He was *their* trickster.

The porters also put up with Wardy, I think, because of a recognition that his troubles could easily be anyone's. There was a kind of integrity to Wardy, an authenticity: there was a recognition that Wardy was who he was, his own person, and could not help being this anymore than anyone else could. This integrity was due respect: amid the institutionalism of the hospital, amid the shaming limitations of broader social and economic aspects of the portering life, Wardy resolutely remained the person he had to be. Indeed, Wardy *demanded* the notice of others, and the porters – if they at all liked him – gave this to him with solicitude and a certain respect.

Moreover, it was the case, as we have seen, that Wardy saw *himself* as normal and average: trying to make do in difficult circumstances but making choices and having priorities that were to be expected, accepted. He insisted on the routineness of his life, and this, too, was something that demanded respect from the other porters. Wardy succeeded in convincing himself – as it seemed to me – and to convince other porters that how he acted was normal, however abnormal the circumstances he was reacting to. It was this claim to normalcy, coupled with the other porters' solicitous responses to the claim, that afforded Wardy the sense of well-being that his life possessed.

Coda: from individual diversity to human universality

In a passage of subtle ethnography, Friedrich Nietzsche in 1889 considered the diversity of ways in which a general concept such as 'peace of soul' – and I take this as a further possible synonym of 'well-being' – might be 'honestly' understood in personal terms:

> 'Peace of soul' can be, for one, the gentle radiation of a rich animality into the moral (or religious) sphere. Or the beginning of weariness, the first shadow of evening, of any kind of evening. Or a sign that the air is humid, that south winds are approaching. Or unconscious gratitude for a good digestion (sometimes called 'love of man'). Or the attainment of calm by a convalescent for whom all things have a new taste and who waits. Or the state which follows a vigorous gratification of our ruling passion, the well-being of a rare satiety. Or the senile weakness of our will, our cravings, our vices. Or laziness, persuaded by vanity to give itself moral airs. Or the appearance of certainty, even a dreadful certainty, after the protracted tension and torture of uncertainty. Or the expression of maturity and mastery in the midst of action, creation, endeavour, volition, a quiet breathing, 'freedom of will' *attained*.
>
> [1979: 44]

I can imagine no better description of the ways in which different individuals might derive a sense of well-being. At the same time I am drawn to the promise held out by John Stuart Mill, from 1859, concerning well-being as a universal human condition:

> As mankind improve, the number of doctrines which are no longer disputed or doubted will be constantly on the increase: and the well-being of mankind may almost be measured by the number and gravity of the truths which have reached the point of being uncontested.
>
> [1963: 168]

The anthropologist meets local individual lives for whom 'a sense of well-being' is a diverse accomplishment of engaging with the world in particular ways at particular moments. But this diversity evinces a commonality, nevertheless. The diversity is the individual substantiation or operationalization of a universal human capacity to 'sense' and to achieve 'well-being'. The very diversity and its individual provenance – the fact that the well-being is a sense of a particular living person and no other – is evidence of a universal humanity. The challenge for a phenomenological and an existential anthropology is to move from Nietzsche's insights to Mill's: from individuality to humanity; from an ethnographic recognition of the diversity of ways in which human beings might experience and conceptualize – substantiate – 'well-being' to a moral-cum-political programme that secures the ontological capacity to substantiate well-being in individual ways as a universal human right. What are the best conditions whereby the universal capacity to possess and exercise a personal sense of well-being may be individually substantiated?

References

Amit, V. and Rapport, N. 2002 *The Trouble with Community: Anthropological Reflections on Movement, Identity and Collectivity*, London: Pluto.

Bourdieu, P. 1977 *Outline of a Theory of Practice*, Cambridge: Cambridge University Press.

Brun Norbye, A.-K. 2010 'Eating Memories: A Taste of Place', in S. Williksen and N. Rapport (eds) *Reveries of Home: Nostalgia, Authenticity and the Performance of Place*, Newcastle: Cambridge Scholars.

Cohen, A. P. 1994 *Self Consciousness: An Alternative Anthropology of Identity*, London: Routledge.

Coleman, L. 2014 'The Imagining Life: Reflections on Imagination in Political Anthropology', in M. Harris and N. Rapport (eds) *Reflections on Imagination*, London: Ashgate.

Corsin-Jimenez, A. (ed) 2007 *Culture and Well-Being: Anthropological Approaches to Freedom and Political Ethics*, London: Pluto.

Durkheim, E. 2002 [1897] *Suicide: A Study in Sociology*, London: Routledge.

Foucault, M. 2006 [1961] *Madness and Civilization*, New York: Random House.

Gramsci, A. 2000 *The Antonio Gramsci Reader* (ed D. Forgacs), London: Lawrence & Wishart.

Gray, J. 2009 'Where truth happens: The Nepali house as Mandala', *Anthropologica* 51(1): 195–208.

Grønseth, A. S. 2001 'In search of community: A quest for well-being among Tamil refugees in northern Norway', *Medical Anthropology Quarterly* 15(4): 493–514.

Harris, M. 2000 *Life on the Amazon: The Anthropology of a Brazilian Peasant Village*, Oxford: Oxford University Press.

High, M. 2013 'Believing in Spirits, Doubting the Cosmos: Religious Reflexivity in the Mongolian Gold Mines', in M. Pelkmans (ed) *Ethnographies of Doubt: Faith and Uncertainty in Contemporary Societies*, London: Tauris.

Husserl, E. 1962 *Ideas: General Introduction to Pure Phenomenology*, London: Collier.

Jackson, M. 2005 *Existential Anthropology*, Oxford: Berghahn.

———. 2011 *Life Within Limits: Well-Being in a World of Want*, Durham, NC: Duke University Press.

James, A. 2004 'The standardized child: Issues of openness, objectivity and agency in promoting childhood health', *Anthropological Journal on European Cultures* 13: 93–110.

Marchand, T. 2010 'Embodied Cognition, Communication and the Making of Place and Identity: Reflections on Fieldwork with Masons', in N. Rapport (ed) *Human Nature as Capacity: Transcending Discourse and Classification*, Oxford: Berghahn.

Mathews, G. and Izquierdo, C. (eds) 2009 *Pursuits of Happiness: Well-Being in Anthropological Perspective*, Oxford: Berghahn.

Mill, J.S. 1963 *The Six Great Humanistic Essays of John Stuart Mill*, New York: Washington Square.

Nietzsche, F. 1979 [1889/1895] *Twilight of the Idols, and The Anti-Christ*, Harmondsworth: Penguin.

Rapport, N. 1993 *Diverse World-Views in an English Village*, Edinburgh: Edinburgh University Press.

———. 1997 *Transcendent Individual: Towards a Liberal and Literary Anthropology*, London: Routledge.

———. 2003 *I am Dynamite: An Alternative Anthropology of Power*, London: Routledge.

———. 2009 *Of Orderlies and Men: Hospital Porters Achieving Wellness at Work*, Durham, NC: Carolina Academic Press.

———. 2012 *Anyone, the Cosmopolitan Subject of Anthropology*, Oxford: Berghahn.

Shankland, D. 2004 'The open society and anthropology: An ethnographic example from Turkey', *Anthropological Journal on European Cultures* 13: 33–50.

Wardle, H. 2001 *An Ethnography of Cosmopolitanism in Kingston, Jamaica*, Ceredigion: Mellen.

Woolf, V. 1983 *The Waves*, London: Granada.

3

CITIES, WELL-BEING, WORLD – A HEIDEGGERIAN ANALYSIS

Robert Mugerauer

Introduction

Thinking about the city and well-being is an enormous task. In our anthropocentric era we interpret the phenomena of cities and well-being in terms of the value they have for humans which we instrumentally or functionally calculate in terms of the services that natural systems or social institutions provide us. Consequently, it is usual to equate well-being with health or economic-material prosperity and to see cities as the locations in which we can optimize the net utility. Heidegger, however, provides an alternative, convincingly explaining how we can't adequately understand (or act upon) any of the constituent dimensions, much less well-being itself, if we start from the taken-for-granted view. Rather, we need to think well-being in terms of World, which he understands as the dynamic gathering together and continuing to come forth of what he calls the fourfold of heavens and earth, immortals and mortals. Well-being would be the Well-being of World – its fruitful unfolding (rather than dissipation or decay).

To frame the project within Martin Heidegger's figure of the gathering of the fourfold might seem to create even more difficulties. But such is not the case because this approach provides both powerful theory and a way to interpret telling case material. The theory would recast well-being as an emergent state arising from the positive, generative dynamic of the gathering itself, which enables the flourishing of each of the mutually co-constitutive dimensions. Finally, those relationships enable individual and social well-being to occur and better explain the multi-dimensional sub-aspects such as basic material and economics for a good life, security, health, good social relations, and freedoms of choice,[1] than can be done if they are seen separately much less if well-being is reduced to one or another of them.[2] Surprisingly then, this no-longer-anthropomorphic approach provides a far more adequate account of human characteristics and needs, of our own journey toward and at least partial dwelling in well-being.

Here the city would be the great artifact which plays a dynamic role in precipitating the simultaneous gathering together of the fourfold that enables us to come into our own.[3] That is, the city would be the historically realized place and means through which we might enact our individual and communal well-being as particular mode of belonging in the world. The phenomena of the city today, here and now, gives us more than enough to consider. Just as operating with an abstract theory without empirical content yields useless generalizations, trying to speak vaguely of "cities" is equally pointless. The task would be to begin the large communal project of undertaking many case studies to investigate the well-being of specific groups if not individuals in particular cities with their often contradictory forces, with their multiple layers from the past which, as Lefebvre observes, do not go away but bear on us today.[4]

The project, then, is to better understand well-being and how it is enriched or impoverished in a particular city. This essay neither tries to prove anything, nor to generalize; rather it explores an approach that respects the singular. I employ the phenomenological process, working out how empirical description and fruitful theory co-constitute one another. This essay provides a case study describing Berlin, through which critical features of well-being emerge; when these are thematized they generate a pattern we recognize as Heidegger's fourfold. At the same time, Heidegger's view that historical-cultural worlds come about as the gathering of the fourfold – mortals, immortals, heavens, and earth – provides the framework for a convincing interpretation of the seemingly disparate urban phenomena.

Remembering that the process of presentation does not normally repeat the process of discovery, I give the three findings here, so as to make the multi-directional unfolding less confusing. First, distinctive features of well-being appear when we examine the way we live with others in community, respond to a spiritual impulse, participate in the rhythms of the heavens, and appreciate the elements and processes of the earth. Second, a more intense well-being can occur when, rather than some of the four dimensions manifesting themselves separately, all four appear as gathered together, resulting in coherent depth and richness of experience. Third, when, in cities, we live within and contribute to the gathering, which in turn feeds back to enrich our existential possibilities, our capacities can be most developed; the gathering provides the site where who you are or can become, what you do or might do, can unfold in multiple dimensions. That is, it is within the dynamic gathering of the fourfold into a concrete, historical world, such as happens in Berlin, that each of us is enabled to come most fully into "one's own" – into the fullest well-being.

Mortals

Walter Ruttmann's great film, *Berlin: Symphony of a City*, powerfully presents the restlessness, the dynamism, of the metropolis. The rhythm of machines, movement, money, people; machines, movement, money, people. Buildings and streets appear as the stable features against which trains, trollies, automobiles, assembly lines, and deliveries show their movement; in which the poor beg, men fight, the bourgeoisie displays its affluence if not decadence, men and women manifest distinct and unequal sexualized behavior, the workers contrast with the powerful and ruling class in differences that hold even across races. The city generates its own atmosphere: machines, money, and people in constant motion.

Berlin has attracted and mixed multiple groups for a long time, groups behaving in heterogeneous ways toward each other across the range of violent hostility, exploitation, indifference, empathy, and cooperation. Its stable base consists of Germans and guestworkers attracted there because of the jobs available in Germany's most industrial city, but then simultaneously subjected to the economic and psychological stresses, often desperate poverty, that characterize capitalized employment (as well as the conflicts that occur when different groups come together in a dense urban setting). Earlier successes in electrical and engineering processes were supplemented by machinery, chemical, metalwork, textile, and food production, as well as by banking, insurance, and legal sectors. Jason Lutes's recent graphic novel, *Berlin: City of Stones*, picks up where Ruttmann's film leaves off. At the turbulent moment of transition to the Weimar Republic a powerful train brings a student and other immigrants to Berlin, "a city in the modern sense" where "communists, socialists, nationalists, democrats, republicans, criminals, beggars [many crippled veterans], thieves, and everything in between, all mixed up together . . . into the flow of it as into a river through warring currents of flesh and smell."[5]

Berlin continued as the principle site of mobility after WWII when a shortage of labor not only drew Germans from all over the country but large numbers of Turks, as well as some Yugoslavians and Italians. As with other industrialized metropolises, housing was always inadequate, with workers typically living in vast blocks of *Mietskasernen* (large tenement blocks, some remaining from the 1860s and 1870, most from between 1880–1900, which often had additional dwelling buildings and light-industry facilities built in the interior spaces), usually in crowded rooms with no interior light and no pluming facilities. Landlords, contractors, and speculators regularly extracted maximum profit and kept workers in harsh conditions.

To oversimplify, the tri-part population making up the bulk of the population (Germans doing adequately well as office workers, civil servants, shopkeepers, or restauranteurs; poor German workers; poor guestworkers) play out core characteristics long associated with cities: the city as the site of meeting and trade, of jobs and the prospect of a better life compared to rural poverty, and thus a magnet of hope. At the same time neither have large numbers of immigrants achieved prosperity nor have different classes and ethnic groups lived in happy intimacy. But for the last 70 years there has been at least a basic getting used to each other and working out ways to stay separate and to interact without unusual levels of violence. In terms of well-being these residents have tried to get what they basically need by leaving each other alone or becoming indifferent to each other, which seems to be realistic and generates a certain hardness as Richard Sennett appreciates about urban life, citing James Baldwin's assessment of interracial relationships in the U.S., "people who can never understand one another, who are permanent strangers, can still live together," though he also believes that "they need not be cut off in mutual indifference" – of which more later.[6]

Complementing the way many diverse groups often stay to themselves, they also regularly develop rich relationships, networks of resources, and small daily satisfactions within their own neighborhoods. With the city as a simple marketplace long gone, replaced by millions engaged in industrial production and consumption, professional and everyday services, with large disparities in enjoyment and suffering in a meshwork of complexly scattered and concentrated factories, housing (from mansions to tenements), offices, stores, and open and overcrowded spaces, Berlin actually is an agglomeration of neighborhoods with distinct characters, all of which constantly are under pressure to "make room" for yet other, new groups. Hence neighborhoods (*Kietz*), with taverns (*Kneipen*) for drinking and sociability, shops operating on a sub-economy with resident-specific goods and locally affordable prices are scenes of "making do." Getting what one needs depends on the city being heterogeneous, not just in population but where goods and services can be accessed.

In fundamentally "anti-establishment" neighborhoods such as Kreuzberg, because of the poverty and relatively low costs of derelict housing, as well as the lack of power to be in control of itself, Turkish guestworkers were joined by members of other "marginal groups": squatters, the unemployed, young men who could avoid the draft during the cold war by living in the isolated city, retirees, and numerous artists and bohemians who had more resources. This clustering does not mean that the more impoverished welcomed the latter groups with open arms but that while managing to get along, they all developed a certain solidarity. Though not at all constituting any coherent social structure they became politically active, advocating at the grass roots level for better housing, open spaces and parks, and an ecological way of building, especially through processes that promoted serious resident participation in the rehabilitation planning as exemplified in IBA (*International Bauausstellung*, International Building/Construction Exposition) of 1984–1987, where the strong local concerns contrasted with the goals of the official Berlin administration. Opposite the official city planners intent on a modernist urban renewal agenda and the Berlin Senate which wanted to develop density by significantly compromising allotment gardens and other open spaces, locally oriented residents supported IBAs' official goal of a "livable city," . . . "careful urban renewal without displacement" as headed by Hardt-Waltherr Hämer.

The local, self-sufficient dimension came to the fore in the way residents coped with the remaining environment of 19th century *Mietskasernen*, often unmaintained for five decades or longer and still regularly without adequate sanitary facilities. (Overall, the housing shortage remained unresolved, even though still larger developments had appeared on the edge of the city).[7] By early 1980s there was substantial resistance, for instance by squatters' daily practices, to the developers and landlords who routinely hired goons to break into and trash occupied apartments in run-down but rent-controlled buildings, ripping out the plumbing so that the owners could legally claim that the unit needed to be renovated, allowing the rent to be raised for the next tenant. In the political arena it was argued and demonstrated that it was socially and economically preferable to renovate dilapidated buildings, allowing the tenants who had already lived there for many years to remain, "retaining their accustomed environment and their social structure."[8]

Activist architects and urban designers, students, artists, immigrants, and counter-culture residents ener-getically worked out details of how attractive buildings could be modulated by alternative, rather than mainline, modes of thinking and used to the end of a healthier environment and increased resident well-being. Professionally sophisticated community members opened up to and engaged with other residents to work out designs and building plans. Finally, in 1983, under pressure, the city authorities and Berlin House of Representatives adopted the Kreuzberg local authority's "Twelve Principles for Urban Renewal," after which thousands of participants conceptually developed the idea and built pilot projects.

> Careful urban renewal is understood as planning in close relationship to the local situation with the aim of harmonizing the overall and individual conditions; decisions relating to the urban space and buildings must, in line with this concept, be linked to the social issues of day-to-day life – provision of affordable housing, preservation and management of jobs, provision of schools and nurseries, and co-ordination of developments in the urban structures.
>
> . . .
>
> [It is possible] to create a basis to [sometimes] enable agreements to be reached between the property owners, tenants, redevelopment corporations, city and local authorities, architects and firms carrying out the work, users and residents' pressure groups.[9]

The increasingly complex political agendas (which include push back against the government's poorly planned and carried out post-war rebuilding and highways cut into the social and physical fabric) as well as the multi-faceted, diverse ecological movements bring to the fore nested dimensions crucial to well-being: adequate material and economic resources, social support, and the ability to make significant choices, which means more than a choice between two places to live, two versions of a product or food to buy, or two places to work or worship – though certainly minimally these. At a deeper level, it includes participation in the deliberative and decision-making processes operative in and on one's life and the possibility of developing multiple dimensions of one's self. Berlin does relatively well as a site to actualize the related underlying values though it still has significant limitations resulting from the structural factors of capital development and vested political power.

When the government was moved from Bonn the many ministries and offices along with the large connected network of foreign embassies and consulates, the support service providers of law firms, copy centers, and information technology consultants came *en masse*, all requiring housing and everything else. At first, when fewer international corporations located in the new Berlin than hoped for, they were coerced, pulled, and pushed by various means in an effort to obtain something like a critical mass that would continue on its own to self-organize economically, socially, and physically. This has happened as skilled professionals have come as residents or consultants in software development, marketing, advertising, and financial consulting. These groups add another dimension of richness to the population, but combined with the development of the new capitol complex and surrounding area including the new main train station have stimulated price increases and opportunities drawing international speculative capital while simultaneously displacing former residents. Within the latter group, the increasing competition, contrasts, and separations involve not only the core of poorer German workers and Turks, Yugoslavians, and Greeks who have been there for a longer time but, since the fall of the wall, the flood of immigrants from Poland, the former Soviet Republics. Not all of these groups appreciated one another as is seen in the initial and still persisting condescension of West Berliners to those coming from East Germany, with its long-internalized "communist" assumptions and expectations of state subsidization. While there is continued displacement in all real estate sectors, this unevenly impacts thousands of diverse residents given the especially notable conversion of modest central property to accommodate highly paid newcomers, including the international clientele wealthy and mobile enough to be able to choose to live in what are touted as the most desirable locations in the latest "hot" city.

In addition to such multiplicity as at least providing the possibility of material prosperity, access to some medical care and social services, there is the equally interesting complexity of the multiple dimensions which each person has and what Berlin – but not every city – offers.

There is a great variety of different places, each with distinctive affordances; further, these places can themselves have multiple uses, especially over the course of a day or week. Correspondingly each person has many aspects at any given time and certainly over the course of a day and lifetime. Multiplying these intersecting personal, spatial, and temporal factors Berlin generates a dizzying set of possibilities.

The variety of places with their offerings matters, but so does the temporal rhythm of availability and uses. Being able to try out or do different things during the course of a day, or a lifetime, depends on the spontaneous and planned features of a city. Spontaneous activities often occur as people find ways to utilize unused or under-utilized spaces: to practice climbing skills on the side of a high railroad viaduct, to have a quick game of handball against a building wall, a pickup football game in an empty field, setting up something to sell under an elevated highway or along a boulevard. Planned elements that play a crucial part include open and built spaces and infrastructure, for example the transportation system which though critical for many people going to and from work or distributing goods further enables individuals to get to the specialized places that as Jane Jacobs has pointed out can only be sustained in a large city with a big population: the rare coin or antiquities shop, the bookseller specializing in detective fiction, the store where toy soldiers are assembled into miniature tin armies to reenact historical battles, shops with an assortment of sexual paraphernalia, or where the society for creative anachronism meets. Or, open spaces are especially flexible for different uses over the course of the day so a *platz* that is a farmer's market in the morning provides room for multiple impromptu ballgames in the afternoon and then the scene for outdoor beer drinking and hanging around at night.

Additional spatial-temporal multiplication occurs as residents shift routines and interests, patterns of behavior, in winter and summer or when an exceptional event presents itself. Many of us shift from what we do during the day to quite other nighttime activities. After a day of selling shoes you can skateboard on office plazas when they have closed for the day. Wearing long sleeves in the course of your day as an accountant in order to conceal your heavily tattooed arms, then changing into a ripped black tee shirt for a long late night in the club scene – much less into Berlin's scenes of decadence – is in itself pleasurable and an exercise of freedoms of choice. In all of these activities we also witness how the city maximizes the ways people can pursue both desired activities and control the degree of social interactions they prefer, ranging from strongly being included in a group where they are known and accepted to strong anonymity with its freedoms. The city's amazing range of places, potential activities, and varying temporal uses promotes the discovery and exercise of one's multiple dimensions as complementary and enriching rather than problematic.

The realistic emphasis on the distance that diverse people in Berlin require and experience is only part of the phenomena. Many of the shared circumstances which lead to a more or less unspoken self-separating also provide occasions for finding solutions to common problems and for developing goals together – as mentioned above concerning generating local political engagement. This often extends into understanding one another, to empathy, whether for a co-worker's health or the depravation suffered by the least well off among us. Berlin is unusually socially sensitive, as seen in part by the amount of continuous spending to provide social services (if not warm personal embrace) through variations in available budget resources as well as by the attention to remembrance of harms past and actively seek reconciliations.

This capacity for community already was seen immediately after WWII when residents, seriously traumatized by the violence inflicted by the factions (including the occupational forces) on each other, nonetheless hoped in the possibility of a self-determined future if social unity could be restored. Thus, in designing his Philharmonic Hall as one of the first major civic projects to be undertaken, Hans Scharoun called on the trust Berliners have in the power of art, explicitly applying Heidegger's thinking to the situation:

> There is a need to find a way to serve and impact the collective effort; to facilitate cooperation – remember and put the arts at the peak of this effort in partnership with other areas of public

life. . . . The task, after the question posed by M. Heidegger, is to consider the meaning or significance for art in our place in the middle [of the city and shattered nation].[10]

The misery shared by everyone after the bombing of the city had a major impact on inter-personal relationships. During the wide-spread chronic disease and deep hunger, endured through four winters without
coal for heating or lights, surely most residents were touched to some degree by a self-centered desperation,
but just as surely many residents came to experience their mutual dependence, (though naturally the feelings dissipated over time and are not shared by the many who have since arrived). As for today, Werner Marx
argues, in our pluralistic societies where we no longer have any shared values or justification for common
practices the only real motivation for positive action would be compassion: we should promote feelings of
compassion for other people in their lifeworlds, the motivation for which could arise from confronting our
own mortality and realizing that we are not self-sufficient but depend on the support of others and our
social constructions.[11]

As the description of Berlin makes clear the diversity of different groups means that from any perspective there are others that don't belong to my group, who may even be at odds with "us." While friction
among individuals and factions is a fundamental characteristic of urban dynamics, perhaps even necessary
for its richness, this also entails that we are called on to help, to give part of what is needed for the well-
being of others.

In terms of the well-being of a city's diverse populations, as "outsiders" arrive their needs and wants
depend not only on what they can do but on what is given to them, or at least offered as possible. For
example, familiarity, empathy, and matter-of-fact re-assessment have led to a shift in the acceptance of
guestworkers by the German government and Berliners. German citizenship had always been a matter of
continuity of bloodline combined with residence, thus excluding a large number of people who wanted to
be accepted as belonging, with citizens' legal status. In 1999 the Federal Refugee Act allowed refugees, those
who had lived in ethnic German settlements, and exiles to apply for citizenship. Yet another re-mixing of
inhabitants and rights. That still left guestworkers on the outside, though many had families who had lived
there for several generations. How to account for the shift? Many factors seem to have combined: explicit
recognition of the increased acceptance that had gradually occurred, the continuous encounters with Turks
and Yugoslavs who spoke fluent German and were fully acculturated because they had been born and raised
there, a vague sense of "well, it's time," opening to the new spirit of globalization, and the need for more
young people to pay into the retirement system which otherwise would run out of funds for the aging
German population.

Other acceptances occur as the result of long advocacy by a minority constituency and an unexpected
shift in public attitudes. Thus while Berlin has long been noted – even envied – for its tolerance of sexual
license, finally the gay and lesbian communities, joined by many others, exuberantly celebrate a new openness in the Christopher Day Parades. Not at all any specter of moral corruption, their mode of living was
recognized and incorporated as another viable pathway for individuals.

The poverty, hunger, cold, and exclusion – once to the point of horror as they unavoidably witnessed,
perhaps supported, the deportation leading to the murder of over 60,000 of their Jewish co-inhabitants –
variously shared over time, have sensitized Berlin's residents to their finitude, to their fragility. The city
has persisted in not turning a blind eye or forgetting, as is witnessed in the deliberately unrepaired bullet
holes pocking buildings, in the high-profile monuments such as the Topology of Terror, Liebskinds' Jewish
Museum, or Eisenmann's Holocaust Memorial (though they may be more focused on visitors from the
rest of Germany or the world), or in the low-key locally experienced Grosse Hamburger Strasse Memorial
sculpture of departing Jews (near the new synagogue) and in the many plaques on buildings and in street
pavement marking the names of former occupants.

We arrive, then, through the diverse people of Berlin at an ordinary way of understanding that is the
same as Heidegger's more poetic articulation of humans as mortals – as those beings who are able to

appreciate their own finitude and anticipate their deaths, who are able to understand the importance of living carefully – caring – in moving toward their end. What more than humans and our concerns could matter in regard to well-being?

Immortals

Here Heidegger provides some guidance by speaking of mortals and immortals together, saying that to speak of one is to speak simultaneously of the other. How so? How in Berlin? Wim Wender's wonderful film, *The Heavens over Berlin* (oddly translated as *Wings of Desire* in the English version) presents life in Berlin after WWII as observed by angels who first appear looking down from the Kaiser Wilhelm Memorial Church, itself in ruins, with neither any mention of God nor, as they say of themselves, of any power whatsoever to intercede in our troubled lives – lives depicted as far from well-being. The sick need to be tended, the psychologically distressed and the dying comforted, the forlorn and abandoned somehow brought in. Our mortality needs be faced, insisted upon. So what about immortals might matter? German gods, pagan or Christian, are all long absent. The helpless angels are able only to witness, to empathize without impact.

No longer looking for all-powerful gods or personifying them as ones who might answer their prayers, the Berliners may have an alternative: in times of desolation, where it certainly seemed that no god dwelt, they have responded by emphasizing the arts as an expression of spiritual impulse. In the troubled time between WWI and WWII a group of artists known as the Blue Riders (*Blau Ritter*) strove to delineate the yearning they and their fellow Germans were experiencing. For example, in his highly influential *Concerning the Spiritual in Art*, which articulated many of the foundational principles of modern art, Kandinsky contended that a spiritual revolution that only could be initiated by art was underway: "That which belongs to the spirit of the future can only be realized in feeling, and to this feeling the talent of the artist is the only road."[12] Once begun, however,

> such a spiritual atmosphere can belong not only to heroes but to any human being.
> . . .
> Every man who steeps himself in the spiritual possibilities of art is a valuable helper in the building of the spiritual pyramid which will someday reach heaven.[13]

Such a project clearly is communal, and is even spoken of in terms of the connection of the human and the heavens, as an attempt to deny the material but to "harmonize the appeal of the material and the non-material," an example of which striving Kandinsky found in Matisse, who "endeavors to reproduce the divine."[14] The master figure of these ideas combines the society of artists and ordinary people, actually making things, in a common movement from the material to the abstract and heavenly in a decidedly urban image:

> Humanity is living in . . . a spiritual city, subject to sudden disturbances for which neither architects nor mathematicians have made allowance.[15]

Nor was Kandinsky alone in deploying this complex of ideas. Some 25 years later, after WWI and when Expressionism had given way to *Neue Sachlichkeit's* commitment to matter of factness, the painter Max Beckmann, explained that he too was "seeking for the bridge which leads from the visible to the invisible" in a healthy facing up to the times:

> I feel the need to be in cities among my fellow men. This is where our place is. We must take part in the whole misery that is to come.[16]

Heavens over Berlin continues the expression of Berliners' impulse to spirituality in the face of the ruin of WWII. Wenders presents a scenario in which both the city's inhabitants and the powerful angels work toward a sober, genuinely existential response to the situation. Importantly the film explores ways to find some positive dimension, without either lapsing into an illusion of a rural or small town utopia or ceasing to face up to human finitude while realistically hoping for well-being.

In taking up the problem of dealing with the urge to spirituality that motivated Kandinsky and his colleagues, *Heavens over Berlin* presents a possible resolution by moving in the opposite direction. Whereas artists in the early 20th century worked to delineate a pathway from the visible to the invisible, Wenders presents an inverse version, affirming the trajectory from the immortal and immaterial to finite embodied existence. Wenders achieves this by having some of the angels come to see the value of embodiment, which entails pleasurable as well as painful experiences. Early in the film, sitting in a BMW showroom, angels Damiel and Cassiel discuss how they wish they could be in the realm of embodied experience and to feel, rather than remain spirits.[17] More and more comes to visibility under the angels' eyes. Pushing itself forward, nothing other than the ordinary – what Heidegger calls "the splendor of the simple" – appears to Damiel; but, in Jean-Luc Marion's terms, in showing itself, what gives itself begins to shine.

Overall, Wenders makes visible the pull exerted on Damiel through a double engagement: by way of the interaction initiated by a former angel, played by Peter Falk, who, even though not able to see Damiel, speaks straightforwardly to him, issuing an invitation, and by the powerful draft that the circus performer Marion exerts upon Damiel even though she can neither see him nor directly call him. The film shows how, in addition to all that is in the world, it is primarily a person who calls out to Damiel, not by addressing him or gazing at him, but by being herself.

One mediation occurs through the character Peter Falk, who lives between the two worlds: though now human, he was an angel and retains the ability to be aware of other angels even though now he no longer can see them. Through this conceit enacting an explicit interchange between the visible and invisible, Falk is able to specifically bid Damiel to come to mortality, to show us an explicit interchange between the visible and invisible. Falk is aware of Damiel's presence and addresses him, extending a hand:

> I wish I could see your face,
> just look into your eyes and tell you how good it is to be here. Just to touch something!
> Here, that's cold! That feels good!
> Here, to smoke, have coffee. And if you do it together it's fantastic. Or to draw: you know, you take a pencil and you make a dark line, then you make a light line and together it's a good line. Of, when your hands are cold, you rub them together, you see, that's good, that feels good! There's so many good things! But you're not here – I'm here. I wish you were here. I wish you could talk to me.
> 'cause I'm a friend.
> *Campañero!*[18]

Here the film intensifies the call of existence and of a now-mortal person. The call calls for response which, Wenders shows us, is evoked by the very character of the things and humans of this world – or, put another way, by "the world itself as psychoanalyst showing us soul, showing us how to be in it soulfully."[19] In the conversation that follows Damiel explains to Cassiel what has come to him and all the earthly things he intends to do now that he is ready to plunge into the flow of time – the history of the world – including what he has just now come to understand from what old men say, that from within time he must engage the moment of fear of time, of death.[20]

In a second, intertwined story, after watching the acrobat Marion and her circus colleagues complete a dress rehearsal (her costume complete with angel's wings, foreshadowing their appropriateness for each other), Damiel reappears next to her in the following scene. Having just learned at the rehearsal that the circus has gone bankrupt, Marion faces the unhappy prospect of returning to being a waitress. She also is fearful about being up on the trapeze and breaking her neck, especially in her forthcoming final performance. She has retreated to her trailer, keenly aware of her condition, which predominantly is one of anxiety and emptiness: "I feel nothing."[21] Yet, out of empathy love emerges. Damiel's urge to comfort Marion turns to affection, passes through an erotic (questionably voyeuristic) phase, to the realization of love – an impulse strong enough for him to give up his angelic existence.

Damiel's "crossing to embodied existence" occurs as an event in which he crashes into himself as well as being thrown to earth at the wall,[22] after which he has the whole range of sensory experience: he feels a cut on his head, and, finding the blood discovers that it has a taste and is red (after which he happily asks a passerby to name colors for him). Subsequently he hears the clanking of the armor he carries under his arm as he walks to a pawnbroker's shop (you need money in Berlin); he smells and tastes coffee and a cigarette.[23] His entry into time is underscored by his proudly acquiring a watch. Now able to actually engage Marion at a dance club, the beginning of the actual mutual relationship is accomplished. The tension between the two realms remains however; indeed, with Cassiel still an angel the film highlights the power of existential possibilities in the project of coming into one's own (which includes relationships to others and all there is on this earth).

Specifically presented by way of events in Berlin, the thoughtful, passionate choice for mortality rather than immortality reaffirms a much older story of decision and identity, as is underscored by the film's device of naming the character embodying memory and a sense of Berlin's history Homer. Damiel's choice then echoes Odysseus's where the latter declined the possibility of remaining on Circe's island forever, enjoying being alive and the pleasures of Circe's bed; instead he cast his lot as a mortal, continuing his trying journey home and heading toward dreaded death, all for the sake of being able to carry on living out his identity as a husband, father, and king – because only thus could he be who he really was.

The scope of a broad well-being opens up here. Not only a matter of adequate material-economic support and health in a narrow sense of absence of illness (since the acceptance of death brings the many hurts and diseases along with it), but in terms of one's lifeworld. As we learn from the angels' becoming mortal both individuality and openness are crucial aspects of our finitude and thus of genuine health. As philosophical anthropologists have convincingly argued, where health is understood properly in terms of our capacities to move ourselves or alter our world with a measure of control – without being incapacitated by disorders or diseases – it needs to be interpreted in terms of each unique individual, in terms of "the general equilibrium of the life in which [we are normally] active and able to be" ourselves, "involved in the world and being together with one's fellow human beings, in active and rewarding engagement in one's everyday tasks."[24] Thus, relieving the suffering of the patient at hand, even working to restore or maintain a patient's normal condition (given the actual changing limitations of existential possibilities) refers to their particularity, not to a general category.[25] Further, the variety of viable human lifeworlds is not accidentally related to our flexibility and resilience since the possibilities generated by our symbolic transformations eventually play out as the openness critical for our well-being.[26]

> Especially in humans, health is precisely a certain latitude, a certain play in the norms of life and behavior. What characterizes health is a capacity to tolerate variations in norms. . . . Humans are truly healthy only when capable of several norms, when they are more than normal. The measure of health is a certain capacity to overcome organic crises and to establish a new physiological order, different from the old.[27]

Taking ourselves to be mortals in this way, accepting our lifeworld and life's phases in terms of openness, mobility, and dwelling[28] affirms that though there may be no gods (obviously) operative in one's own place and time (though traditional believers would take another path, as would those in the new fundamentalisms) the immortals are always in play. They provide the measure; or, perhaps it is the unresolvable gap between immortals and mortals that does so. In having neither envy nor sadness at not being immortal, many people maturely, necessarily courageously, accept the fact and focus on their existential conditions so that the question becomes "How shall I move?" into and through my own mortality. Though each individual remains such, we come into our own only when open to and given much by others and the earth, and even by the immortals and heavens insofar as their "possibilities" play a part in deliberate decisions. In reflecting on the way Berliners may exercise their mortality, by way of *Heavens over Berlin*'s depiction of angels looking down upon the earth and its history from the heavens we find ourselves in fact, as Heidegger said, speaking of mortals, immortals, heavens, and earth all at the same time. We find ourselves already in the midst of the dynamic gathering of the four which are all given together as World.

Heavens

Still, to speak concretely of the existential decision to reaffirm our lives on earth requires corresponding attention to the actual heavens over Berlin. How does the city stand in regard to the sky and its rhythms such that they directly bear on well-being? The historically important film already considered, *Berlin: Symphony of a City*, provides a clue. The powerfully presented urban dynamic of the city shows the striving and achievements, the technology and poetic dimensions so that through the vivid images of the diverse, often contending, groups, places, and activities with which we began this essay, we experience the rhythm of the city, the palpable movement through time, of time. As a giant agglomeration of activities, clearly never ceasing, always robustly pulsing and generating centrifugal force that propels itself along, Berlin shows itself as an enormous dynamo.

Berlin's industrial and commercial force has achieved a technological velocity that dramatically removes it from any direct relationship to "natural" rhythms. Though factory workers' hours now are shorter than the cruel 12–16 hour shifts of earlier times many people still work long hours, many work through the night not only delivering and replenishing stock, repairing the infrastructure, cleaning and maintaining buildings and open spaces, but coordinating their activities as stockbrokers, currency exchangers, and investors to constantly changing markets around the globe. These un-natural rhythms of the city which operate 24 hours a day all year around have effectively become independent from the patterns of the heavens, as Heidegger explains it:

> the vaulting path of the sun, the course of the changing moon, the wandering glitter of the stars, the year's seasons and their changes, the light and dusk of the day, the gloom and glow of night, the clemency and inclemency of the weather, the drifting of the clouds and the blue depth of the ether.[29]

With electrical lighting we are no longer bound to the sun's orchestrating our waking and sleeping, or periods for work and rest. There is a loss of connection with the ancient patterns of behavior, which many experience as a loss because it drives us past the point at which we should rest, because it puts us out of joint with the cosmos, because it leaves us open to exploitation by our employers or professions, even to the point where the greatest success seems to come when we are not driven by a supervisor but when we have internalized the drive, pushing ourselves as long as the computer works, data and news on a planetary scale flows, or demand for reaction and adjustment continues – which is to say, always, unceasingly. We know that this is not healthy, not good for us. One related biochemical-physiological-psychological problem is the disturbance of our circadian rhythms, that is our internal biological rhythms for many bio-functions such as blood pressure and metabolic processes that operate on a regular 24-hour cycle (other rhythms are monthly or seasonal), providing a consistent response to regular environmental changes. Those triggered by the light-darkness cycle include sleep-wake rhythms which when disturbed enough to become disorders can cause significant problems for behavioral competence or hormone balance (e.g. of cortisol which operates on a diurnal rhythms and is critical in protecting against hypoglycemia). The loss of coordination of our bodily rhythms with those of sunlight and darkness seriously troubles nurses and medical staff working night shifts, air traffic controllers and pilots, police and fire personnel, and data processers.[30]

At the same time the artificial milieu of the city gives us great freedoms, open to otherwise unavailable possibilities. We can work at different times of day and week, not always because we are forced to but often at a shift that we prefer or at times that are convenient and preferable. If the most interesting part of my life occurs from midnight to dawn because I need the money, thrive on the contact with others like myself, and want to able to listen to the music without paying the cover, I can mix work with pleasure by being a bartender or bouncer at a club during those hours. If I have kids that need to be seen off to and picked up from school, and played with before bedtime, I can be home from 7 am to 9 pm and work a night shift at the hospital. Or, I can work at home anytime in tele-commuting on a-synchronic projects where all that matters is that the work be done by a certain deadline. If an exciting project spurs me on I don't have to quit because it becomes dark, leaving off likely to lose the thread of an idea or the momentum of a discovery. We can ice skate on an indoor rink in August, grow hydroponic vegetables in the interior of a converted factory or high-rise with grow-bulb light 24 hours a day all year long, or on a smaller scale grow marijuana at home in the basement.

Earth

It has been a recent "discovery" in the last decade that nature is not equivalent to wilderness, but also exists in the city. Of course. Perhaps exceptionally, Berlin has long considered nature as part of the urban. Originally settled in the early 13th century in the Spree valley, in the midst of glaciated plains and plains vegetated respectively with indigenous oak-hornbeam woods and pinewoods, and with a high water table with numerous bogs, in the modern era Berlin was transformed into a powerful national capital with the creation of the Prussian nation state. The Prussian kings created grand boulevards and squares; the Royal hunting grounds already opened to the public in 1740 (such as the large *Große Tiergarten*) were developed into landscape parks; and beautification projects touted ornamental green areas.[31] After the mid-19th century public health and planning factions pushed for *Volksgarten* (people's gardens), including planting trees for fresh air and landscaping to facilitate pleasure strolls. At the turn of the century, in order to focus more on urban health, planners and social reformers generated the *Volkspark* (people's park) intended as recreational-exercise grounds for sports and children's playgrounds for the working class, especially in the areas of overly dense tenements.

Nature conservation in the first third of the 20th century set aside reserves to affirm and display landscape elements considered exemplary of national or regional identity. This was a key factor in establishing the Grünewald as a "permanent forest" in 1915, following 11 years of "public protests mounted against projected city extensions and clearing measures and against the effect of urban water use on the forest's ground water level."[32] The timing for such action was critical for by then the Prussian state was already selling the forests surrounding the city to private real-estate developers who were busily creating suburbs. With the establishment of Greater Berlin as an administrative municipality in 1920 new parks and greenbelts were created, allotment associations and plots multiplied, and continued attention was given to preserving natural spaces, especially forests, at the city's edges. The ideas of conservation as preserving the natural heritage in Berlin in the 1920s focused on sites considered particularly representative of the glacier-formed landscape of the Brandenburg region: fens, creeks, ponds, and a few sand dunes scattered around the metropolis.

Significant activities studying and planning the landscape and the call for an "urban ecology" persisted through WWII among ecological groups and neighborhood activists concerned with residents' well-being. A large, diverse set of amateur and professional naturalists conducted field work; gardeners, hikers, interested nature lovers, and city planners had become especially accomplished at close studies of local features, appreciating and affirming that there was not a separation, but a continuum of biotic and cultural realms since the urban environment had clearly impacted the vegetation regimes for a long time. In the late 1940s, with the intention of reaffirming Berlin's identity, plans for the Tiergarten were "not intended simply to reestablish the prewar situation; they were intended to restore features of the alder swamp and the riparian forest that once had covered the area in which the park was *located*." From 1949–1952 the policy and practices of "greening," for example with open spaces and playing fields, functioned as a mode of restoring a sense of urban order in the midst of the ruined city; also deploying many of the unemployed, it provided a means to look to better times ahead.

The broad community interested in local biotopes advocated for features historically acknowledged as characteristic of and crucial to the then-enclosed city (such as the substantial 32 square km Grünewald and its lakes, Tiergarten, and Botanical Garden in Dahlem) and also promoted appreciation of significant areas that had been abandoned and, from the viewpoint of ecology, protected, especially the abandoned Potsdamer Güterbahnhof and Personenbahnhof and Tempelhofer Rangierbahnhof railroad yards and facilities, where diverse flora and fauna were observed onward from the 1950s. Similarly, ruderal areas resulting from the shaping of rubble from the bombings into waste heaps then left unattended to quickly become wooded, were not only appreciated by botanists, but used by the homeless and by children as favorite play spaces. Overall, a great many Berliners gained an increased self-understanding that their finite urban area was distinctive and important insofar as it was uniquely constituted by the interaction of political and biological environmental processes which were worth nurturing for their own sake as well as central to delineating the identity of the city.

The contemporary phase has dramatically developed through the strong and innovative green movements of the 1980s in which the theory and practical application of eco-urbanism became well-established. The green roofs, sophisticated water retention and purification techniques workable for greening urban courtyards, and urban agriculture projects as well as alternative practices such as advocated by bicycle activists made vivid the ordinary, everyday difference that a green urban way of living could make in Berlin's relations to earth and well-being.[33]

At times alternative planners were tensed with other ecological groups if the latter argued too vehemently for non-development at the cost of possible socially oriented projects, but coordinated with them in opposing projects that would destroy the local bio-cultural character of neighborhoods (such as the highways). There was interest by all parties in more open green spaces given the still overly dense built fabric and lack of recreational spaces, in more positive forms of vibrant community- and eco-oriented courtyards in buildings that retained the traditional Berlin scale and interior spaces rather than modernist high-rises.[34] The open space forms, urban connections, and attendant experiential affordances that emerged are a valuable contribution to urban design and life: the open courtyards not only are central to the semi-public life of the dwelling units (as is traditional in Berlin's morphology) but differentiate a central communal space from the areas more closely associated with the individual surrounding units, then additionally provide access to the street and nearby *plätze*. There appears to be significant benefit from and appreciation of the non-industrial, non-commercial character of these and other courtyard elements such as the play spaces, vegetable and flower gardens, and often greened walls. Connecting the social housing units to the urban neighborhood is a critical accomplishment "designed to accommodate the everyday reality of work, shopping, relaxing, traveling and knowing Berlin's weather" encouraging the "inherent desire of the Berliner for public life," indeed allowing for ordinary Berlin residents' well-being.[35]

Bio-ecologists and political activists agree that ecological care directly promotes the health of residents (as well as that of earth itself) and well-being of the city. In pragmatic terms it is critical to continuing an adequate material basis for living; the political struggle to maintain open spaces, vegetation, and accessible riverfronts is again a key in many dimensions of mental and physical health as well as a lively site in which public debate and choice is maintained.

Thus, the interest in the earth all along has been simultaneously ecological and political. The political charge continues in the urban ecologists' projects of the 1990s and following to conserve and protect small pockets of flora and fauna in the form of "urban nature parks" such as Südgelände railroad area and in the recent referendum about how to use the former Tegel airport, the closing of which offered a rare resource of open space in the dense city. The vote affirmed that loose social uses "on the grass" as it were, were valued more than merely pragmatic and economic development.

Even where economic interests dominate over local preferences Berlin is in the avant-garde of environmental innovation in design and construction. For example, part of the excitement of Potsdamer Platz is due to its advanced eco-design. Specifically, the touted "green skyscrapers" were among the first to demonstrate the viability of ecologically positive buildings. The three towers comprising the Daimler Benz Offices by Richard Rogers Partnership use natural ventilation and daylighting to manage air exchange through great vertical rises and technological devices: by orienting the building to use prevailing breezes and by employing operative windows, large atriums, air inlets and outlets, an air plenum, external vertical shading devices, and solar shading provided by variable glazing. These features, along with passive solar energy, cut the facilities' energy usage and carbon dioxide emissions by more than 30 per cent.[36] There also is an elaborate underground collection system of cisterns in which stormwater is purified and reused, providing a retention pond for enjoyment by humans and birds and an agreeable running-water feature (emulating a stream) along the shops within the site's dense urban fabric.[37] This new regime ecology does not focus on local biotopes or neighborhood green spaces, but operationalizes non-linear engineering resilience, a new approach to environmental well-being,[38] though to the chagrin of advocates of everyday neighborhoods and alternative or deeply ecological localism.

Without a doubt, Berlin is "not all one." It regularly has been described as always having been constituted variously by ecological bio-patches and politically by diverse players. It has been seen as an assemblage not a unity; "as a city of fragments"; and by Sukopp, who in arguing for an urban ecology of biotopes, noted the heterogeneity of human influences on the city's environment:

> In spite of the fact that some features are shared by the entire space of the city, it is not possible to conceive of the city as a single location. In contrast, it is a living space that resembles a mosaic, composed of many different locations.[39]

How do these distinctive manifestations of the earth in Berlin bear on well-being? The well-being of what and whom, for how long, especially insofar as there is no one thing that is Berlin? The core insistence on the importance of open space contributes to residents' mental health, political freedom both in the multiplicity of uses (emphasizing the value of play and thus the connection of the earth and art) and in the decision-making processes themselves. Correlate, for all its significance as part of the city's political dynamic it needs to be remembered that another important dimension of public art is the sheer pleasure it gives to those who create it and to many who take joy it in during their everyday experiences in the city.[40]

The care of the city's water, air, and still-fertile soil all bear directly on the inhabitants' health in several ways. Disciplined use to conserve natural resources is critical to continuing the material basis of urban life (both in regard to materials in the literal sense and to the economics of production and consumption as well the growth of new sectors providing employment and profit that range from a) environmental technologies to b) real estate development and the attraction of global capital to c) amenities for enjoyment and tourism, such as occur when the city repurchases riverfront for public use or when business owners bring in sand to create artificial beaches along the Spree. The people who gather there on an afternoon to drink a Berliner Weisse (a light, effervescent ale, by law brewed only in Berlin) made from the pure water that results from the natural processes of evaporation and precipitation, as do the grains and hops (not to mention the Spree itself), are enjoying what is brought forth from the gathering of the heavens and the earth – or should they drink a beer brewed by a monastery, at least the monks involved would hold that all this is a gift from God. So at least three, perhaps even all, of the fourfold would be gathered together.

In any case, throughout the often contending positions and activities two major features of the relation Berlin to the earth persist: first, nature and the urban are seen together – nature is taken to be an inherent urban dimension and, second, the earth as an integrated aspect of the city is experienced in the course of everyday life (neither as an abstract idea nor as a merely symbolic dimension, but existentially). What is the same throughout all these variations is that the well-being of the earth remains related to the heavens in ecological processes and that what occurs in the city's relation to the earth speaks at the same time, as Heidegger puts it, of mortals and their well-being and of political action as a catalyst in the gathering of the fourfold.

Conclusion

In looking at what happens in Berlin a common sense description of what we seek and do in relation to each other as persons, to the presence or absence of an urge toward any spiritual dimension, to the rhythms of our lives in the great artifact of the city that we have made, and to the natural environment generates a complex of factors that at least begin to articulate what might be meant by well-being and how we succeed or fail at attaining it to a greater or lesser degree. It turns out that these features present the same central characteristics and relationships as Heidegger's more "poetic" view that the four dimensions of mortals and immortals, heavens and earth gather together to constitute a meaningful World. At the same time, the figure of World provides a more sophisticated and powerful means to explore the subtleties of well-being, both in terms of avoiding a reduction to one aspect (such as economic prosperity or health) and by giving a fuller interpretation of their mutual inter-determination into historical-concrete meaningful realms.

Though a "summary" of the findings is not possible since they are woven into the case itself and complexly interlinked with each other, we can at least remember that through describing Berlin it becomes clear that health is far more than the absence of illness; that it is a matter of the capacity of a specific individual to carry on in her own lifeworld as she would choose, and more than that, to be open to develop capabilities she may not have had before a sickness; that though a matter (which also creates the Spree itself) of her own life as an individual it also is a matter of relationship to other people, what they give and whether what they do creates stress or empathetically provides support, of what sorts of institutional care and service is available to her, of whether the group is at war or at peace. It is a matter of her relation to the earth and its resources, remembering that as embodied she is humus, made of the earth (and that our relation to nature is also inextricably political); it is a matter of her relations to the rhythms of the heavens. (The tangle in just that small, partial review of health shows that a summary is not possible.) The city showed how individuality is a matter of the multiplicity that a person is (in different places and times, in differing activities and uses of the cities affordances, in plural relationships); that choice and freedom (exemplified in art and politics) are fundamental to what it means to be a person; that openness to what we might become is crucial (since what that might be that itself is entirely open); that it also is a matter of one's own particularity being possible only as being-with-others-in-a-shared world (especially but not only in one's local neighborhood or scene, making do within the frictions of the heterogeneous city), which means being able to participate politically in the contested struggle for decent jobs, adequate goods and services such as health care and education, and affordable housing. Which connects with the importance of reflection, of deliberately choosing mortality, as Wenders' angels showed us echoing Odysseus, but that this not only entails accepting our coming death but embracing the openness to our existential possibilities. Given all this, it is clear that well-being is not simply "one thing," but instead a dynamic emergent state to which we aspire, toward which we journey if we are able to move away from impoverishment in regard to the mutually interactive features – where the heterogeneity of the city provides an exceptional site and means for such a state to emerge and be maintained.

In fact, then, this approach is able a) to include all the significant aspects that more limited theories of well-being propose as important, but now in their dynamic co-constitution through reciprocal positive feedbacks so that we are able to discern far more nuances of each element and the whole – to use the vocabulary of complexity theory rather than Heidegger's terms that say "all four dimensions occur in a gathering within which, simultaneously, each comes to its own" – and b) to complement the valuable findings of other approaches ranging from philosophical anthropology, psychotherapy, and health care to complexity theory and ecology (as with the *Millennium Ecosystem Assessment*).

Notes

1 This is the list of the fundamental features necessary for well-being identified in the United Nation's *Millennium Ecosystem Assessment*, one of the most comprehensive and sophisticated considerations of the topic.

2 Important work that advocates and practices a reduction of well-being include those that focus on the economics of time use, goods, and utility (Krueger, 2009), on utilitarian approaches with a focus on measurement (Griffin, 1986), and on the Bradburn Affect Balance Scale (Smith, 1995); significant broader approaches include Nussbaum's on developing capabilities (2011), the focus on psychological wellness and community change (Prilleltensky and Prilleltensky (2006), as well as the older hedonic approach (Kahneman et al., 1999).

3 In Heidegger's ontological terms the city would be a "thing" that gathers the fourfold; in the complementary ontic terms the same is said with greater sensitivity and in concrete detail by James Hillman who appreciates the importance of the built environment and things, as well as of conflicting forces, to the well-being of the soul (2006). For a short, focused account of thing and fourfold see Mugerauer, 1995.

4 Thus, this essay does not yet again rehearse the ideas in the vast literature on the city (ranging from Simmel to Sennett and Hillman) important though that task is. Nor do I directly enter the debates about the contested meaning of well-being, systematically covering all the major factors and their possible combinations. Rather, the goal is to carry out a more fundamental case study through which concrete empirical findings can emerge and be reasonably interpreted.

5 Lutes, 2001, pp. 10, 16.

6 James Baldwin, *The Price of the Ticket*, 1985, cited in Sennett, 1990, p. 142.

7 Kemper, 1998.

8 Hämer and Krätke, 1983, p. 28.

9 Hämer, 1987, pp. 243, 249.

10 Cited in Balfour, 1990, pp. 214–215.

11 Marx, 1987.

12 Kandinsky, 1977, p. 12.

13 Ibid., pp. 16, 20.

14 Ibid., pp. 32, 18.

15 Ibid., p. 12.

16 Cited in Gay, 2001, p. 109.

17 [1048–1069] – references in brackets are to numbered shots in *Der Himmel Uber Berlin,* nd.

18 [5038–5044].

19 Hillman, 2006, p. 75.

20 [5046–5052].

21 [2050].

22 Cf. Heidegger, 1962, on Thrownness [*Geworfenheit*] into being-in-the-world, p. 135 and section 38, "Falling and Thrownness."

23 [5068–5076].

24 Gadamer, 1996, pp. 43, 112–115.

25 Canguilhem, 2008, p. 132; Goldstein, 2000, pp. 128–129, 131.

26 Heidegger, 1995; Plessner, 1980.

27 Canguilhem, 2008, p. 132.

28 See Galvin and Todres, 2014.

29 Heidegger, 1975, p. 149.

30 Silverthorn, D. 2001. *Human Physiology* (New York: Prentice Hall, 2001).

31 AD Architectural Design Profile, 1984, p. 33.

32 Lachmund, 2013, 30. In the section on 20th-century Berlin ecological movements I draw substantially from Lachmund as well as Lekan, 2004. For more on the relationships among contending groups and the real estate, speculative market since the wall came down, see Mugerauer, 2015.

33 Kennedy, 1984.

34 Kleihues, 1987.

35 Clelland, 1983, p. 104.

36 Toy, 1997.

37 Mugerauer, 2011.
38 Mugerauer and Liao, 2012.
39 Lachmund, 2013, pp. 17–18; Gregotti, 1983, p. 70; Sukopp, 1973, p. 93 cited in Lachmund, 2013, p. 74.
40 Carver, 2018.

References

Balfour, Alan. 1990. *Berlin: The Politics of Order*. (New York: Rizzoli).

Canguilhem, Georges. 2008. *Knowledge of Life*. (New York: Fordham University Press).

Carver, Evan. 2018. *Public Art in Berlin: Open Space and Unproductive Play*. (Seattle: University of Washington, Ph.D. Dissertation, in progress).

Clelland, Doug, Phillips, M., Stiff, M., Tavernor, R., Cumming, J., Dudek, M., Evans, D., Sutton, P., Trevillion, A. 1983. Wilhelmstrasse, Block 19. In AD Architecture Design Profile. *Architecture in Progress International Bauausstellung Berlin 1984*, 103–108. Frank Russell, editor. (London: London AD).

Der Himmel Uber Berlin: Ein Filmbuch von Wim Wenders und Peter Handke (Frankfurt am Main: Suhrkamp Verlag).

Gadamer, Hans-Georg. 1996. *The Enigma of Health: The Art of Healing in a Scientific Age*. (San Francisco: Stanford University Press).

Galvin, Kathleen and Les Todres. 2014. *Caring and Well-Being: A Lifeworld Approach*. (New York: Routledge).

Gay, Peter. 2001. *Weimar Culture: The Outsider as Insider*. (New York: W.W. Norton).

Goldstein, Kurt. 2000. *The Organism*. (New York: Zone Books).

Gregotti, Vittorio. 1983. Lutzowstrasse. In AD Architecture Design Profile. *Architecture in Progress International Bauausstellung Berlin 1984*, 70–71. Frank Russell, editor. (London: London AD).

Griffin, James. 1986. *Well-Being: Its Meaning, Measurement, and Moral Importance*. (Oxford: Clarendon Press).

Hämer, Hardt-Waltherr. 1987. Careful Urban Renewal: An Experiment and an Example. In *International Building Exhibition Berlin 1987*. A + U E8705, 243–252. Toshio Nakamura, editor. (Tokyo: A + U Publishing Co).

Hämer, Hardt-Waltherr and Stefan Krätke. 1983. Urban Renewal without Displacement: Assessing an Experiment in Charlottenburg: The Prelude to IBA's Activities in SO 36. In AD Architecture Design Profile. *Architecture in Progress International Bauausstellung Berlin 1984*, 27–30. Frank Russell, editor. (London: London AD).

Heidegger, Martin. 1962. *Being and Time*. (New York: Harper & Row).

Heidegger, Martin. 1975. Building Dwelling Thinking. In *Poetry, Language, Thought*. (New York: Harper and Row), p. 149.

Heidegger, Martin. 1995. *Country Path Conversations*. (Bloomington: University of Indiana Press). Hillman, James. 2006. *City and Soul*. (Putnam, CT: Spring Publications).

Kahneman, Daniel, Ed Diener and Norbert Schwarz, editors. 1999. *Well-Being: The Foundations of Hedonic Psychology*. (New York: Russell Sage Foundation).

Kandinsky, Wassily. 1977. *Concerning the Spiritual in Art*. (New York: Dover Publications).

Kemper, Franz-Josef. 1998. Restructuring of housing and ethnic segregation: Recent developments in Berlin. *Urban Studies* 35.10 (October): 1765–1789.

Kennedy, Margrit, editor. 1984. *Öko-Stadt: Prinzipien eier Stadtökologie, Band 1 Materialien zur Internationalen Bauausstellung Berlin (IBA,) Band 2 Mit der Natur die Stadt planen*. (Frankfurt am Main: Fischer Alternativ).

Kleihues, Josef Paul, editor. 1987. *750 Jahre Architektur und Städtebau in Berlin: Die Internationale Bauausstellung im Kontext der Baugeschichte Berlins*. (Stuttgart: Verlag Gerd Hatje).

Krueger, Alan. 2009. *Measuring the Subjective Well-Being of Nations: National Accounts of Time Use and Well-Being*. (Chicago: University of Chicago Press).

Lachmund, Jens. 2013. *Greening Berlin: The Co-Production of Science, Politics, and Urban Nature*. (Cambridge, MA: MIT Press).

Lekan, Thomas. 2004. *Imagining the Nation in Nature: Landscape Preservation and German Identity 1885–1945*. (Cambridge, MA: Harvard University Press).

Lutes, Jason. 2001. *Berlin: City of Stones*. (Montreal: Drawn and Quarterly).

Marx, Werner. 1987. *Is There a Measure on Earth: Foundations for a Non-Metaphysical Ethics*. (Chicago: University of Chicago Press).

Millennium Ecosystem Assessment. 2003. *Ecosystems and Human Well-Being: A Framework for Assessment*. (Washington, DC: Island Press).

Mugerauer, Robert. 1995. *Interpretations on Behalf of Place*. (Albany: SUNY Press).

Mugerauer, Robert. 2011. The City: A Legacy of Organism-Environment Interaction at Every Scale. In *The Natural City: Revisioning the Built Environment*, 257–294. I. Stefanovic & S. Scharper, editors. (Toronto: University of Toronto Press).

Mugerauer, Robert. 2015. Berlin: Resilience through Transformation. In *Transforming Distressed Global Communities into Healthy & Humane Places*, Fritz Wagner, editor. (London: Ashgate).

Mugerauer, Robert and Kuei-Hsien Liao. 2012. Ecological design for dynamic systems: Landscape architecture's conjunction with complexity theory. *Journal of BioUrbanism* II: 29–49.

Nussbaum, Martha C. 2011. *Creating Capabilities: The Human Development Approach.* (Cambridge, MA: Harvard University Press).

Plessner, Helmuth. 1980. *Die Stufen des Organischen und der Mensch: Gesammelte Schriften,* Vol. IV, Günter Dux, Odo Marquard and Elisabeth Stoker, editors. (Frankfurt am Main: Suhrkamp).

Prilleltensky, Isaac and Ora Prilleltensky. 2006. *Promoting Well-Being: Linking Personal, Organizational, and Community Change.* (New York: Wiley & Sons).

Sennett, Richard. 1990. *The Conscience of the Eye: The Design and Social Life of Cities.* (New York: Alfred Knopf).

Silverthorn, Dee. 2001. *Human Physiology.* (New York: Prentice Hall).

Smith, Jennifer. 1995. *Well-Being: Results of the Bradburn Affect Balance Scale.* (Ottawa: Health Canada).

Sukopp, Herbert. 1973. Die Großstadt als Gegenstand ökologischer Forschung. *Schriften z. Verbreitung naturwissenschaftlicher Kenntnisse* 113: 90–140.

Toy, Maggie, editor. 1997. *The Architecture of Ecology.* (London: Architectural Design Profile No. 125).

4

DWELLING IN THE WORLD WITH OTHERS AS MORTAL BEINGS

"Well-being" in post-disaster Japanese society

Hirobumi Takenouchi

On March 11, 2011 Japan was struck by the largest earthquake ever recorded in history, the "Great East Japan Earthquake". The 9.0 magnitude earthquake caused subsidence and liquefaction of land and collapse and submergence of buildings. Subsequently a tsunami hit the Pacific coast areas of the Tohoku region (northeastern Japan). Core meltdowns occurred at three reactors of Fukushima No. 1 nuclear power plant because of loss of power and emergency cooling functionability.

The complex disaster caused 15,893 fatalities and 2,565 missing people, most of whom were never recovered and assumed drowned (National Police Agency, 2016). Numbers of "disaster-related deaths", caused not directly by the earthquake or tsunami but by later indirect events (exclusive of the large number of suicides), reached 3,472 in total, 2,038 in Fukushima Prefecture (Reconstruction Agency, 2016a). Internally displaced people still number 140,988, though this has significantly decreased from the approximately 470,000 in the peak period (Reconstruction Agency, 2016b).

The disaster now historically marked as "3.11" is not a past but present event. While a large number of people have already migrated from disaster-hit areas, many still live in temporary housing, in both cases detached from their own homes. A great number of people live on, deprived of their livelihoods, such as in agriculture and fishery, faced with disintegration of family and local community, while many others went to their deaths. We find numerous sufferers who have lost their "ordinary" everyday lives and remain unable to retrieve them.

Though the disaster was frequently described as "unprecedented", this exoneration or vindication has the effect of concealing valuable lessons. What have we learned from the bitter experiences? How can we put them to use for the future society?

We have learned, in the first place, the meaning of "home" as the foundation of a basic human activity "dwelling". Living in the shadow of death, we have been also faced with a question: how to form or reform connections with the dead. Furthermore, the disaster also revealed problems concerning the understanding of "welfare" in Japanese society.

After focusing on the learned lessons, we will review Tokuzo Fukuda's concept of "human reconstruction" in contrast to the "reconstruction" policy in progress, and find some basic ideas of "well-being". Then led by the philosophical ideas of "being-at-home" and "being-in-the-world", our concept "dwelling in the world with others as mortal beings" ("Mit-wohnen in der Welt als die Sterbliche" in German) will be framed as the fundamental way of human being (das fundamentale menschliche Seinsweise in German), which would contribute to founding human "well-being" at least in post-disaster society.

Lessons concerning well-being: home and welfare

A great number of reports have pointed out the "slow" or "delayed" progress of reconstruction. Why is this so? It seems not because of a deficiency in budget. In "the concentrated rebuilding period" until fiscal 2015 approximately 25 trillion yen had been budgeted for reconstruction efforts by the Japanese government (The Asahi Shimbun, 2015). Neither is it attributable to the fact that the concerned people, including public officials, have made strenuous efforts. Most have worked extremely hard. It rather results from inappropriate "reconstruction schemes" or "recovery programs" (Oguma, 2014, 84). "Reconstruction" has missed the point of respect for individual choices and decisions, and has lost sight of the original object, namely each sufferer's life, for which various projects and programs were drawn up at the outset.

In the face of the "unprecedented" disaster, the Japanese government and bureaucracy aimed to restore a "normal" state, i.e. "restoration of order", rather than to ensure the well-being of each disaster survivor. To achieve this, they tried to hide information and cover up the truth. A desire for a "normal" state also took the form of a de facto forced "resettlement policy" in the contaminated areas in Fukushima, creating a myth of a return to normalcy. The idea of "reconstruction" policy was thus misled by a false sense of "normal", instead of "crisis". In contrast, a Chinese researcher points out the significance of a crisis.

Although a crisis is something not favorably received, it is the only way for human beings to reflect on the true colors of self and society. It was a crisis of calamity on March 11, 2011 that revealed the true colors of Japanese society (Sun, 2013, 157).

In the following we will focus on the lessons learned in the face of a crisis, with reference to "well-being", not "happiness". Individuals pursuing an ego-centered "happiness" could be easily satisfied with the made-up "normal" state that covers up a common crisis, in particular when it is driven by an obsession of "normal" not based on a realistic assessment of the situation, to say, "normal paranoia" dominant in modern society (ibid., 162).

Meaning of "home"

As is poignantly learned in life, we first recognize the significance of something when it is lost. In the case of the victims of the disaster, they first realized the importance of "home" after the earthquake, tsunami, or nuclear accident. Especially in nuclear disaster areas, it is quite difficult to open up the prospect of restoring "home" in the near future. A Japanese sociologist, based on dialogues with the evacuees from nuclear disaster areas, gives an insightful description of what "home" means for them.

It is the place where one feels safe or secure, being convinced to say "I am OK" (Yamashita, Ichimura and Sato, 2013, 114).

Hearing a call "get away from here!", they immediately left the dwelling place. Then they became aware that they had lost home, families, human relationships, jobs, schools, family albums, presents from loved ones, familiar landscape and favorite places; everything connected with family history, life history and ordinary everyday life (ibid., 222).

A sense of security and presence of family are essential elements of "home", as pointed out in an OECD report on "well-being".

Everyone has the right to adequate housing, which means more than just four walls and a roof over one's head. Housing is essential to meet basic needs, such as being sheltered from extreme weather and climate conditions. Housing should offer people a suitable place to sleep and rest, where they are free of risks and hazards. In addition, housing should give a sense of personal security, privacy and personal space. Finally, housing is important to satisfy other essential needs, such as having a family. All these elements make a "house" a "home" and are intrinsically valuable to people (OECD, 2011, 82).

But "home" carries connotations of land and therefore literally exceeds "just four walls", as was the case with many refugees from nuclear disaster, expressing the will to go "home". "Home" is grounded in land, which the present generation inherited from precedent generations and will hand over to following generations. In this sense a community the living belong to potentially includes both the dead and the unborn as its members, insofar as it is based upon the land. Actually in a rural community in Japan, you will see a cemetery on a rise of land, which recalls the people who built and molded the community by deforesting and developing the land. This seems why many people are resolved to sacrifice their own health and lives not to abandon their contaminated land.

What was lost by the nuclear accident includes values peculiar to the land, such as ancestral farmland and mountain forests, land history and culture, and human relations and social structure (Yamashita, Ichimura and Sato, 2013, 149).

As described here, everything valuable for one's life is connected to the land, which is the basis of "dwelling" as fundamental human activity. This is precisely what the disaster endangered, so that great numbers of people are still struggling for well-being.

"Welfare" in Japanese society

The Japan Federation of Bar Associations (JFBA) reports that the ratio of the elderly among the dead due to the disaster was approximately 65 percent, while the rate of the disabled was twice as high (JFBA, 2014, 1).

The prior confirmation of the elderly and the disabled was quite insufficient. Both systems of safety confirmation and evacuation assistance failed to function properly because of the disaster-affected local municipalities. Loss of power forced the elderly and the disabled to forgo the assistance of artificial respirators and additional life-saving equipment. Welfare services at home were interrupted because of the disaster-affected welfare centers. Furthermore, online communications were shut off. A fuel shortage cut off transportation. This is how many of the elderly and the disabled became faced with major challenges to their survival.

Based upon this investigation JFBA points out that housing is important to honor the dignity of individuals and that it is necessary for the elderly and the disabled to have "home" to lead a life of security and prevent isolation and solitary death (ibid., 3).

These are the lessons already learned from the preceding disasters, such as the Great Hanshin Earthquake (1995) and The Mid Niigata prefecture Earthquake (2004). Several national guidelines were provided, which focused on caring for and supporting those with special needs in times of disaster. Nevertheless most local municipalities were unprepared to implement these guidelines. As a result many of the elderly and disabled were both physically and mentally severely debilitated when they were brought not to special evacuation centers but to general evacuation centers that were not equipped to assist those with special needs.

The disaster revealed the "lack of welfare service continuity" as well as the missing perspective on "life" in Japanese society, which is inseparably linked to lack of interaction between "medicine" and "welfare" and the fractionalization of "welfare" in specific areas. The "Disaster Relief Act" in Japan, for instance, refers to "medicine" but makes no reference to "welfare".

Japanese society is challenged to construct basic principles and conceptual framework of welfare in full view of "dwelling" and "medical access" for individual life, in particular for the elderly and the disabled. This leads us to introduce an integrating conception of "well-being" into the society.

"Human reconstruction" and "well-being": in search of a basic philosophy of reconstruction

A basic philosophy is essential to reconstruction, not only because it leads the government to work out a scheme and devise a program, but to integrate a variety of movements and activities for "reconstruction" by clarifying the goal. Conversely, if such philosophy is inappropriate or missing, then reconstruction will be misled or unsuccessful, as Tokuzo Fukuda, a pioneering liberal economist in Japan sounded the alarm at the time of the Great Kanto earthquake in 1923.

As Fukuda described, "in the aftermath of the disaster people cared for each other to the full extent" and "sympathetic voices were raised around the globe" (Fukuda, 2014, 64). But afterward the policy distortion made all the difference so that "gratitude changed into resentment and compassion turned into envy" (ibid., 65).

This reminds us of the situation after the disaster in 2011. Harmonization and composure of the affected people drew world-wide praise. Relief money from home and abroad reached 335,903,477,714 yen as of September 11, 2015 (Japanese Red Cross Society). Moreover, led by the spirits of "solidarity" and "cooperation" advocated in the "Basic Act on Great East Japan Earthquake Reconstruction", the "Act on Special Measures for Securing Financial Resources Necessary for Reconstruction from the Great East Japan Earthquake" (December 2, 2011) was promulgated, which set forth imposing "special income tax for reconstruction" (2.1 percent) on all the withholding agents from January 1, 2013 to December 31, 2037.

Reconstruction-related budgets have been used, however, for unrelated projects on the basis that they could boost national economic revival. It has been also reported that in some areas little reconstruction work has been carried out and questions have been raised about the reconstruction effort. Under the circumstances it seems quite difficult to maintain public support for the special income tax for 25 long years. We may well encounter the same difficulty as the Great Kanto earthquake in the near future. This is why we are led to examine the philosophy of reconstruction.

From this perspective it is noteworthy that Japan-wide economic revitalization is adopted as an objective in the aforementioned acts. The "Seven Principles for the Reconstruction Framework" drew up, for instance, a blueprint of reconstruction as follows: "if no reconstruction of disaster-affected areas, then no economic revitalization of Japan, and if no economic revitalization of Japan, then no true reconstruction of disaster-affected areas" (Cabinet Secretariat, 2011). In the same manner "Basic Guidelines for Reconstruction in response to the Great East Japan Earthquake" declares that they will succeed the "basic philosophy" set forth in the preceding acts and principles.

The reconstruction of the disaster-afflicted areas plays a leading role in the revitalization of vibrant Japan, and the disaster areas cannot be truly rebuilt unless Japan's whole economy is revitalized (Reconstruction Agency, 2011).

Upon reconstruction, bonds ("kizuna" in Japanese) with the international community would be reinforced and the government aims for reconstruction open to the world, incorporating various types of vigor from foreign countries (ibid.).

The guidelines confirm and stress the connection between reconstruction of disaster-affected areas and economic revitalization of all Japan, making no distinction between disaster-affected people and disaster-affected areas and thereby losing sight of the original object. It is a possible outcome that with the loosened regulations in the name of "open" reconstruction, some major companies and multinational corporations will make forays into disaster-hit areas, changing them into fields of exploitation. This is the common maneuver of "disaster capitalism", which is defined as "the orchestrated raids on the public sphere in the wake of catastrophic events, combined with the treatment of disasters as exciting market opportunities" (Klein, 2007, 6).

What is required is to address a question overlooked in the guidelines. It is nothing other than well-being of disaster-affected people, which gives the substance to the words "true reconstruction". It is what Oda Makoto, a Japanese novelist, struggled to express as a survivor of the Great Hanshin Earthquake, stressing the compelling need for a basic philosophy of reconstruction that focuses on life of the disaster-affected individual from the viewpoint of well-being (Oda, 1998, 11–13).

In the face of the Great Kanto earthquake in 1923, Fukuda advocated "human reconstruction" as "true reconstruction".

What is of prime importance for reconstruction project is human reconstruction. It means restoration of opportunities for subsistence lost by disaster. Today for subsistence human beings have to make a living by business and labor. Therefore restoration of opportunities for subsistence will be achieved through business and labor, collectively termed making a living (Erwerbs-gelegenheit). Roads and buildings are merely means to maintain and protect these opportunities. There is no point in restoring roads and buildings without opportunities for making a living (Fukuda, 2014, 133).

Despite lost tangible properties by the disaster, each person is bestowed with intangible properties such as skills, aptitude, expertise and habits suitable to occupational life. With all these properties, a self-reliant person resolved to live independently will be the driving force for "true reconstruction". For this reason Fukuda regards it as government's primary responsibility to guarantee everyone the right to opportunities for making a living.

The word "subsistence" has a negative connotation that evokes a situation close to the edge of survival, such as poverty and hard labor, as is the case with such idiomatic phrases as "subsistence wage" and "subsistence level". In contrast, Fukuda finds a positive meaning to the same word, as not merely living dependently on charity but living well by independently earning one's living. Maria Mies pursues this direction further, giving a new perspective on subsistence as joy in life, happiness and abundance (Bennholdt-Thomsen and Mies, 1999, 5).

Fukuda's concept of "subsistence" or "making a living" carries a positive connotation leading to "living well" ("eu zēn") in ancient philosophy as well as "well-being" in modern society. In this regard Fukuda also seems to take into consideration "home" as the stronghold of making a life and dwelling as a fundamental living form, when referring to both destruction of virtue and an affirmative attitude towards subsistence and impairment of will to live a human life caused by collective living in barracks (Fukuda, 2014, 62).

Disaster reconstruction must include the basic philosophy of "human reconstruction", which aims at opportunities for a good human life or human well-being for the affected individual. Since well-being is largely affected by where, how and with whom we live, we will next explore well-being in connection with dwelling, illustrating the key roles of home and world alike.

Dwelling in the world with others as mortal beings

Nel Noddings, a feminist philosopher known for her work on ethics of caring, stresses the significance of "home". It is not only the place where "basic needs" of food, sleep and security are provided, one's belongings and cherished objects are stored, but also the place where the habit of response is learned and directed at people, animals, plants, objects and ideas (Noddings, 2002, 175, 249).

At home we begin our lives, learning to care for others and ourselves. At home, sheltered, we can be ourselves. Home is "a place from which, and in which, one claims an identity", to say, "place-based identity" (ibid., 249, 263). When the time comes, we step out of "four walls" and move about in the greater world, guided by what we acquired at home. Home provides us with the stronghold of life in the world.

In this manner home meets not only the basic needs of food, shelter and personal security, but also other human needs of caring relationship, privacy, mutual recognition and sense of identity, every one of which is essential to human life. If it is possible to make a new home or move home, for instance, on the occasion of a marriage, it remains difficult to suppose a human life without home. We could then say that "home" has an ontological significance which concerns being or becoming human, whether one settles down in a specific place or changes the dwelling place. This fundamental form of the human beings could be named "being-at-home".

The concept "being-at-home" leads us to the German philosopher, Martin Heidegger's concept "being-in-the-world" ("In-der-Welt-Sein" in German), which concerns the way in which human beings dwell in the world. It seems possible to connect both concepts, so far as home is the foundation of dwelling in the world. To get the picture, let us draw a rough sketch of his idea.

The concept "being-in-the-world" signifies a unitary phenomenon with various dimensions concerning "being-there" ("Dasein" in German), which is defined as the entity "which we ourselves in each case are and which includes inquiry among the possibilities of its being" (Heidegger, 1979, 7). It is, nonetheless, possible to divide this into two components, namely "being-in" ("In-Sein") and "world" ("Welt").

What deserves close attention here is that the term "being-in" designates the way of being of human beings, not a spatial relation of two things (e.g. a glass and water in it) objectively present (ibid., 54). From this viewpoint Heidegger introduces the etymology of "in", as below.

"In" stems from *innan-*, to live, *habitare*, to dwell. "An" means I am used to, familiar with, I take care of something. It has the meaning of *colo* in the sense of *habito* and *diligo*. . . . The expression "bin" is connected with "bei". "Ich bin" (I am) means I dwell, I stay near . . . of the world as something familiar in such and such a way. Being as the infinitive of "I am" . . . means to dwell near. . . , to be familiar with. . . . (ibid.).

According to this explanation in *Being and Time*, "being-in-the-world" means dwelling in the world I am familiar with, that I take care of. That is to say, "being-in-the-world" corresponds to the human way of dwelling in the world I am at home with and in. "Being-at-home" provides the basis of "being-in-the-world; and the sense of identity, "who I am", is formed by both ways of being.

The "world" designates the context or network of meanings given in our everyday lives, widely shared with other members, supporting our concerns and practices with other members and objects (ibid., 65). As with "home", the "world" is that which we already belong to even without being aware at first. Realizing the fact then, we will participate in reforming and reshaping the "world" (ibid., 87). Learning to care for other members and objects, acquiring the specific social manners, cultural customs and a language at home, we prepare ourselves for becoming a member of the "world".

On the one hand the world is that which is already there, even before we enter it. It is that which endures even after we leave it. On the other hand the world has been molded, is now being formed and will be reformed in the future. This is because every member of the world is mortal. The world is the public sphere, which includes both the dead and the unborn as its intergenerational members, in which we learn that we are all mortals. We dwell in the world with other members as mortal beings.

Conclusion

Noddings stresses the significance of "a social policy driven by care theory", which will "make finding homes for those now homeless its first priority" (Noddings, 2002, 249). This resembles in appearance the "resettlement policy" in the contaminated areas and the "collective relocation policy" in tsunami-affected areas. But Nodding's social policy differs sharply from that of the Japanese government in two important respects.

First, the former is led by the recognition that home is essential to human life. A state of "homeless" makes a life deprived and challenged, far from attaining well-being. Home has the function of integrating basic human needs. This turns our eyes back to the suffering of those who have lost homes by disaster. Together with home, they have lost the place to eat as a family, to sleep and rest, free of risks and hazards, and to keep security and privacy, as well as caring relationships, mutual recognition and place-based identity. Moreover, they have lost houses, fields, forests, which they inherited from the precedent generations and expected to hand over to following generations. To put it briefly, the world to which they belong has been impaired or at least endangered.

Second, Nodding's social policy grasps the importance of individual freedom. In contrast, both "resettlement policy" and "collective relocation policy" are characterized as de facto forced, and therefore lack respect for individual freedom, though it "may have intrinsic importance for the person's well-being achievement", as the Indian economist and philosopher Amartya Sen points out (Sen, 1993, 39). He also states that "the well-being achievement of a person can be seen as an evaluation of the wellness of the person's state of being", which we have tried to shape so far, led by the concept "dwelling in the world with others as mortal beings".

What is required in the first place in post-disaster Japanese society is not restoration of roads and buildings. Rather it means to accomplish "human reconstruction", which aims at affording opportunities for making a good life. This philosophy, with the perspective on well-being, not only contributes to "true reconstruction" but also is promising enough to bridge the gap between "medicine" and "welfare" and to integrate the compartmentalized caring practices and theories in post-disaster society. Caring always means caring for specific individuals, and we are all challenged to reflect on well-being. For we all need to learn to care for others and ourselves to make a good human life.

References

Act on Special Measures for Securing Financial Resources Necessary for Reconstruction from the Great East Japan Earthquake (2011), December 2 (Japanese), *Official Website of Ministry of Finance*. [online] Available at: www.mof. go.jp/about_mof/bills/179diet/20111028 houritsu.pdf [Accessed October 14, 2016].

The Asahi Shimbun (2015), *Three Years after the Great East Japan Earthquake in Terms of Money*, *Official Website of the Asahi Shinbun*. [online] Available at: www.asahi.com/shinsai-fukkou/3nen/en/ [Accessed October 14, 2016].

Basic Act on Great East Japan Earthquake Reconstruction (2011), June 24 (Japanese), *Official Website of Reconstruction Agency*. [online] Available at: www.reconstruction.go.jp/ english/topics/Basic_Act_on_Reconstruction.pdf [Accessed October 14, 2016].

Bennholdt-Thomsen, V. and Mies, M. (1999), *The Subsistence Perspective, beyond the Globalised Economy*, Zed Books Ltd, London and New York, Spinifex Press.

Cabinet Secretariat (2011), Seven Principles for the Reconstruction Framework, May 10 (Japanese), *Official Website of Cabinet Secretariat*. [online] Available at: www.cas.go.jp/jp/fukkou/pdf/kousou4/7gensoku.pdf [Accessed October 14, 2016].

Fukuda, T. (2014), *Principles of Reconstructing Economy and Some Problems* (Japanese), edited by Yamanaka S. and Inoue T., Japan, Kwansei Gakuin University Press, reprint edition, original 1924, Dobunbkan, Tokyo.

Heidegger, M. (1979), *Sein und Zeit*, Tübingen, Max Niemeyer Verlag, 15. Auflage.

Japan Federation of Bar Associations (2014), A Report on Support for the Elderly and Disabled at the Time of Disaster, a Year after the Great East Japan Earthquake, April 12 (Japanese), *Official Website of Japan Federation of Bar Associations*. [online] Available at: www.nichibenren.or.jp/library/ja/committee/list/data/sien_houkoku.pdf [Accessed October 14, 2016].

Japanese Red Cross Society (2015), *Official Website of Japanese Red Cross Society*. [online] Available at: www.jrc.or.jp/ english/ [Accessed December 16, 2015].

Klein, N. (2007), *The Shock Doctrine, The Rise of Disaster Capitalism*, A Metropolitan Book, New York, Henry Holt and Company.

National Police Agency (2016), Damage Situation of Great East Japan Earthquake and Police Measures, September 9 (Japanese), *Official Website of National Police Agency*. [online] Available at: www.npa.go.jp/archive/keibi/biki/higaijo kyo.pdf [Accessed October 14, 2016].

Noddings, N. (2002), *Starting at Home, Caring and Social Policy*, Berkeley, CA, University of California Press.

Oda, M. (1998), *Do We Live in "Human Country"? An Objection from a Westward* (Japanese), Tokyo, Chikumashobo.

OECD (2011), *How's Life? Measuring Well-Being*, Paris, OECD Publishing.

Oguma, E. (2014), No Death from a Ghost Town, Path Dependence of Post-Disaster Reconstruction in Japan (Japanese), *Sekai, no. 855*, Tokyo, Iwanami Shoten, pp. 84–96.

Reconstruction Agency (2011), Basic Guidelines for Reconstruction in Response to the Great East Japan Earthquake, August 11, *Official Website of Reconstruction Agency*. [online] Available at: www.reconstruction.go.jp/topics/0810basic-guidelines-reconstruction-20110729.pdf [Accessed October 14, 2016].

Reconstruction Agency (2016a), Earthquake-Related Death Toll Linked to Great East Japan Earthquake, March 31 (Japanese), *Official Website of Reconstruction Agency*. [online] Available at: www.reconstruction.go.jp/topics/main-cat2/ sub-cat2-6/20160630_kanrenshi. pdf [Accessed October 14, 2016].

Reconstruction Agency (2016b), Numbers of Evacuees in Japan, September 12 (Japanese), *Official Website of Reconstruction Agency*. [online] Available at: www. reconstruction. go.jp/ topics/main-cat2/sub-cat2–1/20160930_hinansha. pdf [Accessed October 14, 2016].

Sen, A. (1993), Capability and Well-Being. *The Quality of Life*, edited by Martha C. Nussbaum and Amartya Sen, Oxford, Oxford University Press.

Sun, G. (2013), "Normal Paranoia" and Modern Society (Japanese), *Sekai, no. 842*, Tokyo, Iwanami Shoten, pp. 153–164.

Yamashita, Y., Ichimura, T. and Sato, K. (2013), *Inhumane Reconstruction, Nuclear Power Plant Evacuation and "Un-Understanding" of an Ordinary Japanese Citizen* (Japanese), Tokyo, Akashi Shoten.

5

WELL-BEING AND BEING-WELL

A Merleau-Pontian perspective on psychosomatic health

Jennifer Bullington

As a shift occurs in our understanding of health and well-being from evaluating measurements of on-going material processes in the body towards more holistic conceptualizations, it is important to have theoretical frameworks which enable us to articulate this new understanding. The coming chapter will provide such a framework by drawing upon the work of Maurice Merleau-Ponty in order to conceptualize health as a mind-body-world phenomenon. The dualism between mind and body is circumvented by his concept of "the lived body" and the dichotomy between the experiencing human being (as a mind-body presence to the world) and the experienced world is overcome in a new way of understanding the human way of being-in-the-world. This new understanding is particularly helpful in the area of psychosomatic pathology. The phenomenon of psychosomatic ill health presents a challenge to the classical dualistic biomedical paradigm, where health problems are either in the mind or in the body. Many of the enigmas surrounding psychosomatics can be solved by re-thinking our ideas about bodies and minds and how human beings exist in the world. The case of psychosomatic ill health will be used in order to show how insights on the lived body provide a fruitful grounding of health and well-being as a multi-dimensional phenomenon.

The psychosomatic anomaly

International research points to the increasing prevalence of patients with psychosomatic health-related issues seeking health care within primary health care (Barsky, Orav & Bates, 2005; Fink, Rosendal & Olesen, 2005; Kirmayer *et al.*, 2004; Wileman, May & Chew-Graham, 2002). A variety of problems are associated with this form of ill health, both for the patients as well as the clinicians. These symptoms are often medically unexplainable, meaning that there are no underlying somatic reasons for the symptoms.[1] The patient is convinced that there is something wrong with their body, yet all somatic treatment strategies fail, leaving the patient with an increasing sense of panic about the symptoms and a determination to find a somatic solution to their health problem. This situation results in a vicious circle, where the patient who has amplified somatic sensations (the presenting symptoms), becomes anxious and fearful about their bodies as vulnerable and inexplicably ill, giving rise to cognitions and behaviors which lead to further contact with health care professions, who once again cannot offer an explanation or cure, leading to further amplification of sensations and anxiety and so on. This "somatic fixation" can readily become a way of life, incapacitating the patient and leading to unnecessary dependence on medical care. Patients with this type of ill health have a poor prognosis for recovery (Arnold *et al.*, 2006; Jackson & Passamonti, 2005). As a result, they have social dysfunction, occupational difficulties and a high consumption of health care, as well as dissatisfaction with the health care provided. Some studies show that up to a third of the physical symptoms that cause patients to seek primary health care are medically unexplainable (Kirmayer *et al.*, 2004; Steinbrecher *et al.*, 2011; Toft *et al.*, 2005).

There are controversies surrounding the diagnosis of psychosomatic disorders (Wessely & White, 2004) although some common characteristics have been found, such as overrepresentation of females, a history of negative early experiences, sudden onset, waxing and waning of the symptom, altered stress response (altered nervous system functioning during stressful periods) and resistance to therapeutic approaches (Buffington, 2009). There is some evidence in the international literature that immigrants (non-natives) are overrepresented in this patient group. Some older studies show up to 50% of the immigrant population suffered from physical symptoms related to psychosocial stress (Pang & Lee, 1994; Pincelli & Simon, 1997). A recent large Italian study of 3015 immigrant patients (Europeans, Asians, South Americans and Africans with 16 subgroups based on nationality) attending a first visit to primary care showed that approximately one-fourth of the immigrants who accessed primary care used somatization to express their distress (Aragona *et al.*, 2012). In a German study, persons with migrant backgrounds were less successful in psychosomatic rehabilitation programs than native Germans (Gruner *et al.*, 2012). It has also been found that somatization among immigrants seeking health care in primary care is significantly related to traumatic events and posttraumatic symptoms (PTSD) (Aragona *et al.*, 2010).

Persons who seek excessive medical attention, the so-called "frequent attenders" have traditionally been found to be female, older, less well-educated, living with their spouses and/or children (Ferrai *et al.*, 2008). However, another study found that medically unexplained symptoms were over represented in younger females with employment (Nimnuan, Hotopf & Wessely, 2001). There is thus no clear cut picture of who will develop psychosomatic symptoms although female overrepresentation and the failure of traditional treatments seem to be consistently found in the literature. A further difficulty is that this condition can be "hidden" in other diagnostic categories, such as psychological/psychiatric conditions as well as musculoskeletal disorders. Treatment and rehabilitation programs are often based on single diagnoses, and as such are inadequate for capturing complex health problems, like medically unexplained symptoms (Hanel *et al.*, 2009; Maeland *et al.*, 2012). Attempts have been made to construct questionnaires in order to identify these patients in primary care (Körber *et al.*, 2011; Morriss *et al.*, 2012; Smith *et al.*, 2009) although screening procedures for psychosomatic health care problems are not widespread. Despite the lack of diagnostic precision, it is beyond a doubt that patients who seek health care for somatic symptoms that cannot be properly handled with traditional somatic treatments present a clinical problem for primary health care professionals and incur substantial health care costs (Barsky, Orav & Bates, 2005; Burton *et al.*, 2012; Konnopka *et al.*, 2012).

Clinicians in primary care are seldom prepared for these patients in terms of expertise, treatment strategies or communication skills. This results in unsatisfying clinical encounters for an increasing number of patients with this type of health complaint (Salmon *et al.*, 2004; Werner & Malterud, 2003). It has been shown that health care professionals do not feel comfortable with these patients because they do not respond to somatically based treatment, thus constituting a challenge to the competence and professional identity of the health care worker (Aiarzaguena *et al.*, 2008; Wileman, May & Chew-Graham, 2002; Woivalin *et al.*, 2004). The inability of the clinician to help the patient understand the nature of a psychosomatic reaction (symptom formation) is one of the main reasons that these patients do not find adequate help (Morriss *et al.*, 2010). Interventions such as psychological and traditional psychiatric treatment (non-specific to psychosomatics) have not been shown to be of any use for treating frequent attenders in a systematic literature review of RTC studies (Smits *et al.*, 2008). Although it is recognized within specialist care that patients with psychosomatic problems need specialized communication and a good relationship with the care giver, these elements are scarce in primary care settings (Heijmans *et al.*, 2011). Clinicians often view psychosomatic health issues as illegitimate medical problems, finding the patients to be "difficult" (Reid *et al.*, 2001; Steinmetz & Tabenkin, 2001). Efficacious treatment strategies are lacking, although the most prominent symptoms accounting for consultation in primary care (chest pain, fatigue, dizziness, headache, swelling, back pain, shortness of breath, insomnia, abdominal pain and numbness) often cannot be related to any biological causes.

There are only a few systematic treatment strategies available, despite the prevalence of this kind of health care problem. One of these is a structured, cognitively based therapy aimed at helping patients see links between symptoms and psychosocial issues, the so-called "reattribution theory" (Gask *et al.*, 1989; Morriss *et al.*, 2007; Morriss & Gask, 2002; Rosendal *et al.*, 2005). Another is the STreSS model (Specialized Treatment for Severe Bodily Distress Syndromes) proposed by the Research Clinic for Functional Disorders and Psychosomatics at the Århus University Hospital in Denmark (Schröder *et al.*, 2012). The theoretical basis for the STreSS model is an extension of the reattribution theory-based therapy, taught to clinicians in the so-called TERM program, The Extended Reattribution and Management Model (Fink, Rosendal & Toft, 2002). The literature is divided on how effective this cognitive form of treatment actually is for this group of patients (Aiarzaguena *et al.*, 2007; Blankenstein, 2001; Gask *et al.*, 2011; Larisch *et al.*, 2004; Morriss & Gask, 2002; Morriss *et al.*, 2007; Peters *et al.*, 2008; Rosendal *et al.*, 2005). Some studies have found that the approach seems to be positive for the clinicians, giving them some confidence in the face of these exasperating health problems (Dowrick *et al.*, 2008; Rosendal *et al.*, 2005), although there is no solid evidence in terms of randomized controlled studies that reattribution theory-based treatment actually helps the patients (Morriss & Gask, 2002; Larisch *et al.*, 2004). Even the leading proponents of reattribution theory maintain that the reattribution model as it stands today is too simplistic (Blankenstein *et al.*, 2002; Gask *et al.*, 2011). According to a systematic review of the literature (Konnopka *et al.*, 2012) there is no unequivocal evidence that cognitively based treatments reduce the costs of health care for this patient group. Given the widespread prevalence of this form of ill health and the lack of well-functioning treatment, we need to widen the perspective from cognitive strategies to more comprehensive strategies in order to help this group of patients. Phenomenology can provide the philosophical grounding for such a perspective.

Phenomenology and the lived body

The problems associated with psychosomatic health issues illustrate the need for an alternative way of conceptualizing mind, body and world (i.e. the experienced lifeworld of the patient). The psychosomatic condition is neither "in the mind" (in a conscious thematic sense) nor "in the body" (with demonstrable somatic causes). Psychosomatic ill health is "in" the being-in-the-world of the person. These persons find themselves in a no-man's land in the health care system, since they are not amenable to psychological treatment nor can somatic care provide any long-lasting solutions to their suffering. The answer to this problematic condition can be found in an understanding of "the lived body" and how this lived, subjective body is involved in meaning-constitution in both health and ill health. The notion of the lived body comes from the phenomenology of Maurice Merleau-Ponty, whose inspiring work provides a relevant point of departure for a new understanding of psychosomatics.[2] But first, a word about phenomenology is needed in order to understand the point of departure for Merleau-Ponty's thinking.

Phenomenology is the philosophical movement in Continental philosophy arising from the philosophical works of Edmund Husserl (1913/1962, 1954/1970). The term "phenomenology" means literally the *logos* (or inherent meaning or order) of phenomena, that is to say, the meaning of that which appears or "shows itself" to man. How human beings perceive, understand and live in the world is the subject matter of phenomenology. Subjectivity, that "wonder of all wonders" as Husserl put it, is the focus of interest for phenomenological studies. Husserl's life-long project was to establish phenomenology as a rigorous science, on a par with the natural sciences that so successfully studied nature (the world of things). However, since the subject matter for phenomenology differed in kind from the subject matter of the natural sciences, Husserl had to create a methodology and concepts that would be suitable for the study of human "meaning-constitution", to use another phenomenological term. He understood that the methodologies of natural science would not do justice to the realm of the subjective. The study of "appearances", i.e. the way in which the world is revealed to and understood by human beings, would need a new scientific approach. This approach was worked out in by Husserl's phenomenological works and gave inspiration to an entire phenomenological movement.[3]

Merleau-Ponty was one of the French existentialists who became inspired by Husserl's phenomenology. He had already at the age of 25 formulated two research proposals that contained the themes he would address in his first two major philosophical texts, *The Structure of Behavior* from 1942 and *Phenomenology of Perception* from 1945. The subject matter of these two seminal works was a phenomenological analysis of the nature of perception and human embodiment. Later on in his career he treated a variety of other topics, such as language acquisition (1964/1973), expression and meaning (1960/1964) and literature and art (1948/1964, 1969/1973), but his interest in perception and the role of the body in human experience remained with him throughout his career. In this chapter, his early work on "the lived body" will be the main focus.

In order to understand the subject matter of phenomenology, one must first implement the phenomenological reduction, which means putting into brackets (or suspension) all ideas, hypotheses and pre-understandings one has concerning the object of inquiry. These pre-conceived, everyday notions prevent us from being able to reflect upon and discover how the phenomenon under study reveals itself on its own terms. In this case, the way in which we think about and conceptualize our bodies, as "objective" bodies (natural scientific descriptions of the body) stands in the way of understanding our bodies as they are lived in the world. According to Merleau-Ponty, many of our ideas about the human body and the nature of perception are conditioned by notions and concepts from natural science. These ideas prevent us from being able to reflect upon and discover how we experience our bodies in the world, and how we experience the world through our bodies. To take a common example, we typically understand visual perception in the terms of stimuli-response. Although we never experience a visual stimulus *as such*, we are convinced that sight is "really" all about light waves hitting the occipital lobe in the brain. This is a perfectly legitimate way to describe vision from within a certain perspective, but it is not the way we *live* seeing the world. If we merely focus upon chemical, neurological processes in the brain, we miss the way in which the experience and meaning of the world unfolds for us through sight.[4] All human experience is the result of a unique relation between the embodied subject with his/her perceptual possibilities and socio-cultural understanding and that which shows itself to him/her at every instant. The subject and the world are "born together" (the word for knowledge in French is *conaissance*, which means literally, born together) in a movement that has been poorly understood by both science and philosophy.[5] We need to bracket our everyday notions about the objective body and natural scientific notions about the nature of perception in order to elucidate the "dialogue" between the subject and his/her world.

If the body is not merely a thing in the world like other material objects, and the world is not a fixed set of pre-determined stimuli causally invoking responses, how can we understand the relationship between man and world, or between body and mind? Merleau-Ponty's answer is the realm of the "in-between" which he sometimes calls "the third term". For example, body and mind are indeed two distinct realms of human existence, yet they are not as separate as Cartesian dualism has led us to believe. There is mind in the body and body in the mind. This is not something to be confused by; it is rather a *given* of experience, a primordial ground of our existence as human beings, which our ways of thinking have obscured with ideas about an "objective" material body separated from mind and person. We should not concern ourselves with trying to solve a mystery (mind-body relations) which is simply the result of our faulty conceptualizations. Rather, we should, as good phenomenologists, lend our reflection to our way of being mind and body in the world:

> In so far as it sees or touches the world, my body can therefore be neither seen nor touched. What prevents its ever being an object ... is that it is that by which there are objects. It is neither tangible

nor visible in so far as it is that which sees and touches. The body therefore is not one more among external objects, with the peculiarity of always being there. If it is permanent, the permanence is absolute and is the ground for the relative permanence of disappearing objects.

(1945/1962, p. 92)

True reflection presents me to myself not as an idle and inaccessible subjectivity, but as identical with my presence in the world and to others, as I am now realizing it: I am all that I see, I am an intersubjective field, not despite my body and historical situation, but on the contrary, by being this body and this situation, and through them, all the rest.

(*ibid.*, p. 452)

The psycho-physical event can no longer be conceived after the model of Cartesian physiology and as the juxtaposition of a process in itself [the body] and a *cogitatio* [the mind]. The union of soul and body is not an amalgamation between two mutually external terms, subject and object, brought about by arbitrary degree. It is enacted at every instant in the movement of existence.

(*ibid.*, p. 88–89)

In a similar way, our conceptualizations about our access to the world in terms of physiological natural scientific descriptions have led us astray.[6] According to Merleau-Ponty, there is indeed something outside of ourselves which we are born into, a physical psychosocial world not of our making. This "something" is present to us in ways that we experience through our senses. But this world outside ourselves is not imprinted upon us like a photograph, but taken up in an active moment of meaning-constitution. Merleau-Ponty describes this meeting in the following way:

Thus a sensible datum which is on the point of being felt sets a kind of muddled problem for my body to solve. I must find the attitude which *will* provide it with the means of becoming determinate, of showing up as blue; I must reply to a question which is obscurely expressed. And yet I do so only when I am invited by it, my attitude is never sufficient to make me really see blue or really touch a hard surface. . . . As I contemplate the blue of the sky I am not over and against it as an a-cosmic subject; I do not possess it in thought, or spread out towards it some idea of blue such as might reveal the secret of it, I abandon myself to it and plunge into this mystery, it "thinks itself within me".

(1945/1962, p. 214, italics in original)

And, "Apart from the probing of my eye or my hand, and before my body synchronizes with it, the sensible is nothing but a vague beckoning" (*ibid.*). Merleau-Ponty's calls this description of the lived unity of the mind-body-world system "the lived body".[7] The body understood as a lived body is necessarily ambiguous, since it is both material and self-conscious. These realms are to be understood as levels, intertwined with each other, constituting a unified field. The self, the body and the world of things and others are neither separated from each other nor to be confused with each other, but rather can be seen as three sectors or levels of a unique field. The lived body is always oriented towards the world outside itself (otherness) in a constant flow. The human being cannot be understood apart from the system "mind – body – world". Where there is a body, there is a personal world, an opening upon the world which is unique. This uniqueness has to do with our life as mind, as persons, with the fact that we have language, history and culture and can ask questions about our own existence. Likewise, there is no personal life or mind without a body. Finally, this intertwined mind-body-presence is always embedded in a concrete situation. There is no world (as perceived) without a human to experience it, and there is no human experience that is not of the world.

Thus, we cannot discuss the body as if it were something cut off from both mind and world. This is an important insight when working with patients who express their problem somatically.

Psychosomatic health and well-being as a
multi-dimensional phenomenon

Let us return to the person who experiences psychosomatic ill health. In terms of the lived body, they experience what could be called a dis-articulation of the field.[8] We find here a disturbance in the mind-body-world unity. Instead of the automatic flow of attention from self-awareness to the world and back again, the object of focus has become the painful/disturbing/recalcitrant body. Instead of allowing situations (i.e. the mind – body – world "dialogue") to arise, be sustained and develop, the meaning constitution of the person with this type of ill health has broken down. All situations are reduced to problems (related to the body), effacing the beckoning of the world in terms of projects and things of interest to be pursued. Things and situations receive their meaning in terms of negotiating the body, e.g. "can I make it up these stairs?" "Can I sit that long in a chair?" "I will never be able to be away from home that long" and so on. There is no longer anything "there" that pulls the person out of the body focus. This process can be understood as the collapse in meaning constitution at the appropriate level, where all meaning is reduced to the mute signaling of the psychosomatic body symptom. Where the person in health can respond to the world in terms of mind (the level of the self), the person with psychosomatic symptoms has fastened in the web of their own bodies. Challenges which should be handled at the level of "mind" become responded to at the level of the body, resulting in the psychosomatic symptom. Until meaning constitution is reinstated at the proper level, this body meaning will continue in the attempt to respond to the challenge at the psychosocial level.

Following Merleau-Ponty, we find when we reflect upon our being-in-the-world a constant contact between the self, as a mind-body presence to the world, and a variety of concrete situations that unfold in time. We are always at grips with the world in one way or another. As mind-body entities, that is, beings who are self-aware, we engage our environment at various levels on a mind-body continuum. At times, we allow the "habit body" to navigate us through a situation, like the habile cab driver weaving in and out of traffic. At other times, our mental, personal levels of existence are in the fore, like giving a lecture or arguing for political views. We are always both mind and body, although situations bring forth the "level" which corresponds to the situation, so that it may unfold and be fulfilled. In health, it is not difficult to maintain this correspondence, as we automatically bring forth that meaning constitution (at the level of mind or body) which successfully meets the call of the situation. The person with a psychosomatic way of being-in-the-world no longer has access to this well-functioning dialogue between man and world. In order to regain psychosomatic health and well-being, the fixation on the body must be broken as well as the insistence upon somatic solutions to their suffering.

In the first section of this chapter, we saw that purely cognitive therapies have little impact on these patients. This is because the reason for the psychosomatic problem is precisely their inability to engage the world at the level of thoughts, feelings and actions. For meaning constitution to be reinstated at levels other than body meaning (symptoms), one must first help the patient experience something other than the body. Their fixation with body sensations has reduced the world to a place of problems, the body to an obtrusive thing and the person to a slave of the body. The treatment aims at transforming body meaning to personal meaning, which means uncovering those areas of life which the person cannot at the moment constitute in terms of thoughts and feelings. To jar them out of their habitual dis-articulation, one works in treatment with opening up perceptions. For example, can the body be experienced as something other than painful, cumbersome and irritating? Is the entire body involved in the distress, or are there parts of the body which feel "normal"? The process of articulation moves from perception of one's own body as differentiated towards the articulation of their environment. They are instructed to carry a notebook with them at all times, to record smells, sounds and sights which they notice when they are in various situations.

This exercise of focusing upon the qualities of the world allows the patient to gradually be able to focus upon the situation around them. The more one looks, the more one sees. And the more one sees, the more one wants to look. In this way, the dominance of the body is gradually replaced by an articulated field that can eventually become meaningful situations, to be responded to as a person (not body).

One should also work in therapy with the articulation of affect.[9] Often, strong feelings are somatized into symptoms instead of being contained, reflected upon and perhaps acted upon. To enable the patient to function with others, basic emotional skills need to be developed, such as knowing what one is feeling, why one is feeling it and how to respond to a particular feeling in concrete situations. When patients can experience a variety of situations in terms of nuanced perceptions, cognitions and emotions, there is no longer any need for the body to express meaning in terms of psychosomatic symptoms.

When psychosomatic health and well-being is (re) established, one's way of being-in-the-world is characterized by the seamless flow of the lived body. The ability to allow different "poles" of this mind-body-world unity to dominate is reinstated. At times the situation (the world pole) will be in focus, at times the level of mind, and in other situations the body will be most prominent in experience. Meaning constitution at the appropriate level is reinstated so that the body is no longer the main avenue of expression. Psychosomatic health allows for the experience of being-in-the world as a mind-body presence in a meaningful world.

Notes

1 The abbreviation MUS (medically unexplainable symptoms) is just one of many terms for this form of ill health. Other terms are "frequent attenders", "functional somatic disorders", "severe bodily distress syndromes", "somatic symptom disorders", "multi somatoform disorders" and "somatoform syndromes".
2 See Bullington (2013) for a more detailed account of this topic.
3 See Spiegelberg (1982) for a comprehensive overview of the phenomenological movement.
4 Merleau-Ponty on the nature of sight:

> Visual contents are taken up, utilized and sublimated to the level of thought by a symbolical power which transcends them, but it is on the basis of sight that this power can be constituted. The relationship between matter and form is called in phenomenological terminology a relationship of *Fundeirung:* the symbolic function rests on the visual as on a ground: not that vision is its cause, but because it is that gift of nature which Mind was called upon to make use of

(1945/1962, p. 127)

And from the later Merleau-Ponty:

> We see the things themselves, the world is what we see: formulae of this kind express a faith common to the natural man and the philosopher – the moment he opens his eyes; they refer to a deep-seated set of mute 'opinions' implicated in our lives. But what is so strange about this faith is that if we seek to articulate it into theses or statements, if we ask ourselves what is this *we*, what *seeing* is, and what *thing* or *world* is, we enter into a labyrinth of difficulties and contradictions.

(1964/1968, p. 3)

5 "We must rediscover, as anterior to the ideas of subject and object, the fact of my subjectivity and the nascent object, that primordial layer at which both things and ideas come into being" (Merleau-Ponty, 1945/1962, p. 219).
6 See the late Merleau-Ponty (1964/1968) for his radically new ontology of "the flesh" which formulates an alternative to the dualistic conceptualization of the relations between man and world.
7 Translated from the French *le corps propre,* which means literally one's own body, the actual body, the pure/clean body. Sometimes the term *le corps vivant* is used as well, which translates as "the living body". The distinction between the objective and lived body was described in Husserl as a differentiation between the body's thing-like aspects (*körper*) from the intentional, living aspects (*Leib*).
8 See Bullington (2009).
9 There are a variety of techniques available to work with affect, both body-oriented (affect-focused body psychotherapy) and psychotherapeutic. See Downing (1994), Monsen and Monsen (1999, 2000) and Tomkins's affect imagery consciousness (AIC) (1962, 1963).

References

Aiarzaguena, J.M., Grandes, G., Gaminde, I., Salazar, A., Sanchez, A., & Arino, J. (2007) A randomized controlled clinical trial of a psychosocial and communication intervention carried out by GPs for patients with medically unexplained symptoms. *Psychological Medicine*, 37: 283–294.

Aiarzaguena, J.M., Grandes, G., Salazar, A., Gaminde, I., & Sanchez, A. (2008) The diagnostic challenges presented by patients with medically unexplained symptoms in general practice. *Scandinavian Journal of Primary Health Care*, 26: 99–105.

Argona, M., Catino, E., Pucci, D., Carrer, S., Colosimo, F., LaFuente, M., Mazetti, M., Maisano, B., & Geraci, S. (2010) The relationship between somatization and posttraumatic symptoms among immigrants receiving primary care services. *Journal of Traumatic Stress*, 23 (5): 615–622.

Argona, M., Rovetta, E., Pucci, D., Spoto, J., & Villa, A.M. (2012) Somatization in primary care service for immigrants. *Ethnicity & Health*, 17 (5): 477–491.

Arnold, I.A., De Waal, I.M.W.M., Eekhof, J.A.H., & Van Hermert, A.M. (2006) Somatoform disorder in primary care: Course and the need for cognitive-behavioral treatment. *Psychosomatics*, 47: 498–503.

Barsky, A.J., Orav, E.J., & Bates, D.W. (2005) Somatization increases medical utilization and costs independent of psychiatric and medical comorbidity. *Archives of General Psychiatry*, 62: 903–910.

Blankenstein, A.H. (2001) *Somatizing patients in general practice reattribution, a promising approach*. PhD thesis. The Netherlands: Vrije University.

Blankenstein, A.H., van der Horst, H.E., Schilte, A.F., de Vries, D., Zaat, J.O.M., Knottnerus, J.A., van Eijk, J.T.M., & de Haan, M. (2002) Development and feasibility of a modified reattribution model for somatising patients, applied by their own general practitioners. *Patient Education and Counseling*, 47: 229–235.

Buffington, C.A.T. (2009) Developmental influences on medically unexplained symptoms. *Psychotherapy and Psychosomatics*, 78: 139–144.

Bullington, J. (2009) Embodiment and chronic pain: Implications for rehabilitation practice. *Health Care Analysis*, 17 (2) (June): 100–109.

Bullington, J. (2013) *The Expression of the Psychosomatic Body from a Phenomenological Perspective*. Dordrecht: Springer.

Bullington, J. & Cronqvist, A. (2017) Group Supervision for healthcare professionals within primary care for patients with psychosomatic health problems: a pilot intervention study, *Scandinavian Journal of Caring Sciences*, doi: 10.1111/scs.12436.

Burton, C., McGorm, K., Richardson, G., Weller, D., & Sharpe, M. (2012) Healthcare costs incurred by patients repeatedly referred to secondary medical care with medically unexplained symptoms: A cost of illness study. *Journal of Psychosomatic Research*, 72 (3): 242–247.

Downing, G. (1994). *The Body and the Word*. New York: Routledge.

Dowrick, C., Gask, L., Hughes, J.G., Charles-Jones, H., Hogg, J.A., Peters, S., Salmon, P., Rogers, A.R., & Morriss, R. (2008) General practitioners' views on reattribution for patients with medically unexplained symptoms: A questionnaire and qualitative study. *BMC Family Practice*, 9: 46 (open access).

Ferrai, S., Galeazzi, G.M., Mackinnon, A., & Rigatelli, M. (2008) Frequent attenders in primary care: Impact of medical, psychiatric and psychosomatic diagnoses. *Psychotherapy and Psychosomtics*, 77: 306–314. Fink, P., Rosendal, M., & Olesen, F. (2005) Classification of somatization and functional somatic symptoms in primary care. *Australian and New Zealand Journal of Psychiatry*, 39: 772–781.

Fink, R., Rosendal, M., & Toft, T. (2002) Assessment and treatment of functional disorders in general practice: The extended reattribution and management model – an advanced educational program for nonpsychiatric doctors. *Psychosomatics*, 43 (2): 93–98.

Gask, L., Dowrick, C., Salmon, P., Peters, S., & Morriss, R. (2011) Reattribution reconsidered: Narrative review and reflections on an educational intervention for medically unexplained symptoms in primary care settings. *Journal of Psychosomatic Research*, 71: 325–334.

Gask, L., Goldberg, D., Porter, R., & Creed, F. (1989) The treatment of somatization: evaluation of a teaching package with general practice trainees. *Journal of Psychosomatic Research*, 33: 697–703.

Gruner, A., Oster, J., Müller, G., & von Wietersheim, J. (2012) Symptoms, disease models and treatment experiences of patients in psychosomatic rehabilitation with and without a history of migration. *Zeitschrift für Psychosomatische Medizin und Psychoterapie*, 58 (4): 385–393.

Hanel, G., Henningsen, P., Herzog, W., Sauer, N., Schaefert, R., Szecsenyi, J., & Löew, B. (2009) Depression, anxiety, and somatoform disorders: Vague or distinct categories in primary care? Results from a large cross-sectional study. *Journal of Psychosomatic Research*, 67 (3) (September): 189–197.

Heijmans, M., Olde Hartman, T.C., van Weel-Baumgarten, E., Dowrick, C., Lucassen, P.L.B.J., & van Weel, C. (2011) Expert's opinions on the management of medically unexplained symptoms in primary care: A qualitative analysis of narrative reviews and scientific editorials. *Family Practice*, 28: 444–455.

Husserl, E. (1913/1962) *Ideas: General Introduction to Pure Phenomenology*, Vol. 1. New York: Collier Books.

Husserl, E. (1954/1970) *Crisis of European Sciences and Transcendental Phenomenology*. Evanston, IL: Northwestern University Press.

Jackson, J.L. & Passamonti, M. (2005) The outcomes among presenting in primary care with a physical symptom at 5 years. *Journal of General Internal Medicine*, 20: 1032–1037.

Kirmayer, L.J., Groleau, D., Looper, K.J., & Dominicé, M. (2004) Explaining medically unexplained symptoms. *The Canadian Journal of Psychiatry/La Revue Canadienne de Psychiatrie*, 49 (10): 663–672.

Konnopka, A., Schaefert, R., Heinrich, S., Kaufmann, C., Luppa, M., Herzon, W., & König, H.H. (2012) Economics of medically unexplained symptoms: A systematic review of the Literature. *Psychother Psychosom*, 81: 265–275.

Körber, S., Frieser, D., Steinbrecher, N., & Hiller, W. (2011) Classification characteristics of the Patient Health Questionnaire – 15 for screening somatoform disorders in a primary care setting. *Journal of Psychosomatic Research*, 71 (3) (September): 142–147.

Larisch, A., Schweickhardt, A., Wirsching, M., & Fritzsche, K. (2004) Psychosocial interventions for somatizing patients by the general practitioner: A randomized controlled trial. *Journal of Psychosomatic Research*, 57: 507–514.

Maeland, S., Werner, E.L., Rosendal, M., Jonsdottir, I.H., Magnussen, L.H., Ursin, H., & Eriksen, R. (2012) Diagnoses of patients with severe subjective health complaints in Scandinavia: A cross sectional study. *International Scholarly Research Notices Public Health*, 2012, doi.org/10.5402/2012/851097

Merleau-Ponty, M. (1942/1963) *The Structure of Behavior*. Boston: Beacon Press.

Merleau-Ponty, M. (1945/1962) *Phenomenology of Perception*. London: Routledge & Kegan Paul.

Merleau-Ponty, M. (1948/1964) *Sense and Non-Sense*. Evanston, IL: Northwestern University Press.

Merleau-Ponty, M. (1960/1964) *Signs*. Evanston, IL: Northwestern University Press.

Merleau-Ponty, M. (1964/1968) *The Visible and the Invisible*. Evanston, IL: Northwestern University Press.

Merleau-Ponty, M. (1964/1973) *Consciousness and the Acquisition of Language*. Evanston, IL: Northwestern University Press.

Merleau-Ponty, M. (1969/1973) *The Prose of the World*. Evanston, IL: Northwestern University Press.

Monsen, J.T. & Monsen, K. (1999) Affects and affect consciousness: A psychotherapy model integrating Silvan Tomkin's affect and script theory within the framework of self psychology. In A. Goldberg (Ed.), *Pluralism in Self Psychology: Progress in Self Psychology*, Vol. 15 (pp. 287–306). Hillsdale: Analytic Press.

Monsen, K. & Monsen, T.J. (2000) Chronic pain and psychodynamic body therapy. *Psychotherapy*, 37: 257–269.

Morriss, R., Dowrick, C., Salmon P., Peters, S., Dunn, G., Rogers, A., Lewis, B., Charles-Jones, H., Hogg, J., Clifford, R., Rigby, C., & Gask, L. (2007) Exploratory randomized controlled trail of training practices and general practitioners in reattribution to manage patients with medically unexplained symptoms. *British Journal of Psychiatry*, 191: 536–542.

Morriss, R. & Gask, L. (2002) Treatment of patients with somatized mental disorder: Effects of reattribution training on outcomes under the direct control of the family doctor. *Psychosomatics*, 43: 394–399.

Morriss, R., Gask, L., Dowrick, C., Peters, S., Ring, A., Davies, J., & Salmon, P. (2010) Randomized trial of reattribution on psychosocial talk between doctors and patients with medically unexplained symptoms. *Psychological Medicine*, 40 (2) (February): 325–533.

Morriss, R., Lindson, N., Coupland, G., Dex, G., & Avery, A. (2012) Estimating the prevalence of medically unexplained symptoms from primary care records. *Public Health*, 126 (10) (October): 846–854.

Nimnuan, C., Hotopf, M., & Wessely, S. (2001) Medically unexplained symptoms: An epidemiological study in seven specialities. *Journal of Psychosomatic Research*, 51 (1): 361–367.

Pang, K.Y. & Lee, M.H. (1994) Prevalence of depression and somatic symptoms among Korean elderly immigrants. *Yonsie Medical Journal*, 35 (2): 155–161.

Peters, S., Rogers, A., Salmon, P., Gask, L., Dowrick, C., Towey, M., Clifford, R., & Morriss, R. (2008) What do patients choose to tell their doctors? Qualitative analysis of potential barriers to reattributing medically unexplained symptoms. *Journal of General Internal Medicine*, 24 (4): 443–449.

Pincelli, M. & Simon, G. (1997) Gender and cross-cultural differences in somatic symptoms associated with emotional distress: An international study in primary care. *Psychological Medicine*, 27 (2): 433–444.

Reid, S., Whooley, D., Caryford, T., & Hotopf M. (2001) Medically unexplained symptoms: GPs' attitudes towards their cause and management. *Family Practice*, 18: 519–523.

Rosendal, M., Bro, F., Sokolowski, I., Fink, P., Toft, T., & Olesen, F. (2005) A randomized controlled trail of brief training in assessment and treatment of somatization: Effects on GPs attitudes. *Family Practice*, 22: 419–427.

Salmon, P., Dowrick, C.F., Ring, A., & Humphris, G.M. (2004) Voiced but unheard agendas: Qualitative analysis of the psychosocial cues that patients with unexplained symptoms present to general practitioners. *British Journal of General Practice*, 54: 171–176.

Schröder, A., Rehfeld, E., Örnböl, E., Sharpe, M., Licht, R.W., & Fink, P. (2012) Cognitive-behavioral group treatment for a range of functional somatic syndromes: A randomized trial. *British Journal of Psychiatry*, (April 26). doi:10.1192/bjp.bp. 111.098681

Smith, B.J., McGorm, K.J., Weller, D., Burton, C., & Sharpe, M. (2009) The identification in primary care of patients who have been repeatedly referred to hospital for medically unexplained symptoms: A pilot study. *Journal of Psychosomatic Research*, 67 (3): 207–211.

Smits, F., Smits, K.A., Wittkampf, K.A., Schene, A.H., Bindels, P., & Van Weert, H. (2008) Interventions on frequent attenders in primary care. *Scandinavian Journal of Primary Health Care*, 26: 111–116.

Spiegelberg, H. (1982) *The Phenomenological Movement.* The Hague: Martinus Nijhoff Publishers.

Steinbrecher, N., Koerber, S., Frieser, D., & Hiller, W. (2011) The prevalence of medically unexplained symptoms in primary care. *Psychosomatics*, 52 (3) (May–June): 263–271.

Steinmetz, D. & Tabenkin, H. (2001) The "difficult" patient as perceived by family physicians. *Family Practice*, 18 (5): 459–500.

Toft, T., Find, P., Oernboel, E., Christensen, K., Frostholm, L., & Olesen, F. (2005) Mental disorders in primary care: Prevalence and co-morbidity among disorders. Results from the Functional Illness in Primary care (FIP) study. *Psychological Medicine*, 35 (8): 1175–1184.

Tomkins, S. (1962). *Affect, Imagery, Consciousness, The Positive Affects,* Vol. 1. New York: Springer.

Tomkins, S. (1963). *Affect, Imagery, Consciousness, The Negative Affects,* Vol. 2. New York: Springer.

Werner, A. & Malterud, K. (2003) It is hard work behaving as a credible patient: Encounters between women with chronic pain and their doctors. *Social Science & Medicine*, 57: 1409–1419.

Wessely, S. & White, P.D. (2004) There is only one functional somatic syndrome. *British Journal of Psychiatry*, 185: 95–96.

Wileman, L., May, C., & Chew-Graham, C.A. (2002) Medically unexplained symptoms and the problem of power in the primary care consultation: A qualitative study. *Family Practice*, 19: 178–182.

Woivalin, T., Krantz, G., Mantyranta, T., & Ringsberg, K.C. (2004) Medically unexplained symptoms: Perceptions of physicians in primary health care. *Family Practice*, 21: 199–203.

6

FEMINIST PERSPECTIVES ON WELL-BEING

Charlotte Knowles

The question of well-being is fundamentally bound up with the question of who we are. In the *Nicomachean Ethics* Aristotle approaches the question of the good life, *eudaimonia*, via an account of the human function.[1] From a feminist perspective, we can approach the question of well-being in a similar way: we can ask what it will be to live well for woman, by examining what is distinctive about being a woman.[2] The insight we get, however, is rather different from Aristotle's. Whereas he identified the human function with rationality, and thus living well with reasoning well;[3] when we turn to ask what is distinctive about women's existence, we find that one of the most common answers is 'oppression'.[4] Simone de Beauvoir's *The Second Sex* argues that the general situation of woman is one of oppression, an idea which crystallises in the notion of woman as 'Other'.[5] Woman is not an autonomous being, but is seen as passive and objectified.[6] More recently, Sally Haslanger has argued that, in general, women can be defined as agents who are, in some way, socially subordinated on the basis of presumed female sex.[7] From a feminist perspective, we are therefore furnished with a different starting point from which to theorise well-being, a starting point that not only alters how we approach this notion, but that also alters how we come to understand it.

In this chapter I shall argue that from a feminist perspective well-being is most productively defined in relation to freedom, and it is with regard to questions of freedom that well-being should be pursued. Pursuing well-being from a starting point of oppression and working towards an ideal of freedom involves two things: a reconception of the self as fundamentally relational and an emphasis on the importance of self-understanding for well-being. The former is something that has been widely acknowledged in the feminist literature, where relational conceptions of the self figure centrally, and the notion of a socially situated self has been identified as one of the key contributions to living well from a feminist perspective. Self-understanding, however, has been largely ignored in feminist accounts of well-being, where the social aspects of well-being are often emphasised to the detriment of individual considerations. I shall argue that this can cause problems for well-being as the pursuit of freedom, but that such problems can be overcome by supplementing the relational account of the self with an emphasis on self-understanding and highlighting the interrelation between them in the pursuit of well-being *qua* freedom from oppression.

Oppression as an alternative starting point: reorienting accounts of well-being

Ruth Ginzberg argues that canonical accounts of well-being are organised around a hierarchy of needs, where the lower levels must be satisfied in order for the higher levels of need to arise. She characterises the hierarchy thus:

(1) individual bodily well-being,
(2) community well-being,
(3) psychological and spiritual well-being,
(4) intellectual and aesthetic well-being.[8]

On this account, well-being in its highest or most complete form – what we might call 'flourishing' – is truly realised only at the fourth level, through intellectual pursuits such as contemplation. This is an idea we find endorsed in Aristotle's account. Although he recognises that some 'external goods', such as food, shelter and relations with others are needed in order for us to live well, these goods are not seen as constitutive of flourishing,[9] since flourishing is identified with the contemplative life: a life of intellectual well-being that can be pursued largely independently of others and of external goods.[10]

Ginzberg rejects models of well-being such as this, which identify the full realisation of well-being *qua* flourishing with individual and intellectual pursuits such as 'personal happiness . . . leisure. . . [and] reflection',[11] arguing that they are androcentric.[12] In mainstream accounts of well-being, she argues, 'survival' – that which is identified with the lower levels of the hierarchy and is necessary before flourishing can emerge as a need – is simply assumed. For women, however, whose existence is primarily determined by oppression, 'survival' cannot be so easily assumed:

> For women, survival is a fundamental issue. . . . Women must constantly concern ourselves with
> how to survive batterings, rapes, wars and other violence . . . depression, mother-blaming, poverty,
> hatred, isolation, silencing, rupturing of our communities, exhaustion, spiritual co-optation . . .
> trivialization of our knowledge. . . . None of these things is of our own doing. They are the results
> and the evidence of our oppression. . . . No level of the posited survival hierarchy is assured: not
> our individual bodily well-being, or our community well-being, or our psychological well-being,
> or our intellectual or aesthetic well-being.[13]

Ginzberg argues that traditional conceptions of well-being *qua* flourishing implicitly exclude women from attaining the idea of living well, since '"flourishing" is applicable only to those who've moved beyond "mere" survival'.[14] Rather than defining well-being in terms of flourishing then, Ginzberg argues that from a feminist perspective we should reconceive well-being in terms of survival. According to Ginzberg, survival should not be seen as a precondition for well-being *qua* flourishing, but as that in terms of which well-being is fundamentally defined. Ginzberg argues that this shifts our orientation in analyses of well-being from a narrow focus on flourishing achieved via individual pursuits such as happiness, contemplation and reasoning, to an account where well-being means achieving freedom by rejecting domination and overcoming oppression in all its forms, and in all aspects of our lives. For Ginzberg, 'any form of domination inhibits some sort of well-being and therefore is antithetical to survival in its fullest meaning'.[15] This reconfiguration of well-being in terms of freedom from oppression and domination has consequences, not only for how we conceive of well-being, but also for how we conceive of the self that lives well. In what follows I shall explore how notions of freedom can be related to two key ways in which feminists have encouraged us to reconceive the self of well-being. First in terms of the idea of relationality, and second through an emphasis on the importance of self-respect and self-understanding. Whilst the former has gained extensive ground in feminist circles, the latter has been less widely embraced. Nevertheless, I shall attempt to show that the two are interlinked in the pursuit of well-being *qua* freedom from domination and oppression and thus must be thought together.

Well-being and the relational conception of the self

In canonical accounts of well-being, such as Aristotle's, we find that well-being is conceived primarily as an individual pursuit. Moreover, the self-sufficiency of the contemplative life (that in which human flourishing will be most fully realised) is valued *because* of its self-sufficiency and the fact that it can be pursued independently of others.[16] From a feminist perspective, however, where survival *qua* freedom from oppression and domination pervade every consideration of well-being, such an independent notion of the self is inadequate for theorising well-being.

The independent account of the self that we find in mainstream theories of well-being and in moral and political philosophy more generally, has been criticised by feminists on the grounds that it portrays the self as 'a mushroom [that] has neither mother nor father, nor childhood education'.[17] In other words, the self as it is conceived in mainstream moral and political theories from Aristotle to Hobbes and up to the present day in the work of liberal theorists like John Rawls, have posited a self that, like a mushroom, springs up independently of others and is totally self-sufficient and self-created. Feminists have objected to this view on the basis that it ignores the necessary relations and the hidden labour that enable such 'independent' human subjects to exist.[18]

In place of this independent self-supporting subject, feminists have substituted a relational model of the self. This is a picture of the self that involves a recognition of its socially embedded nature and the way others can both inhibit and enhance what we can do, who we can be and how we can live our lives. We see this relational notion of the self embedded in feminist accounts of well-being, such as Ginzberg's, that take freedom from oppression as their guiding principle, in the simple fact that oppression implies a relation between two or more people.[19] To say that to achieve well-being we must resist domination in every aspect of our lives, will mean being constantly attentive to the way in which others can enhance our well-being *qua* freedom or can diminish it. If I am in an emotionally abusive relationship; if I am subject to sexual harassment; if I am undermined at work or not valued as an equal member of the team; I am subject to forms of domination and oppression that inhibit my ability to live well.

However, this is not to say that the relational notion of the self suggests that to achieve well-being we must seek to separate ourselves from others. The relational notion of the self is not simply the idea that others can affect us negatively; it is also the recognition that positive relations with others are necessary in order for us to live well.[20] As Cheshire Calhoun has argued, in the conception of the self deployed in mainstream moral theory, the positive relations we have with others, whether in our moral education, the general support and guidance offered to us by our friends, family and community, the enabling friendships or the positive learning experiences we draw from our encounters with others, remain invisible.[21] The relational conception of the self highlights both the enabling and disabling relations we have with others and holds that these relations are existentially relevant. To say that the self is fundamentally relational is thus to acknowledge, as Lauren Freeman argues that 'others not only help to constitute what we know, they also help to constitute an essential part of who we are, who we were and who we can become'.[22] From the perspective of well-being, this account tells us that we must take seriously our relations with others in our understanding of what it is to live well, but at a more practical level what does it tell us about the pursuit of well-being?

The practical implications of the relation model: well-being as a communal pursuit

The idea that we must recognise that others can both enhance and diminish our ability to live well implies that the pursuit of well-being cannot be a purely individual one. This idea is brought out in Ginzberg's survival-based account of well-being when she argues that from a feminist perspective, I should be 'as committed to your survival as I am to my own'.[23] One way of interpreting this is by returning to the situation of gender oppression with which our analysis of well-being began. If living well is defined in terms of overcoming oppression and resisting domination in all its forms, then we will be better able to realise such freedom from oppression if we work together.

Much of the oppression that characterises women's situation does not articulate itself on an agential level – a particular person or group using their power to harm another – but instead plays out at a structural level.[24] There is not any one particular individual or group that can be identified as responsible for the oppression, rather the oppression persists and is perpetuated through social structures and institutions. Therefore, in order to make well-being possible, we will need to work together as a society to correct the social injustices and unfree states of affairs that constitute women's oppression, perpetuate domination and bar the way to well-being. This may be achieved via practical means such as eradicating the glass ceiling, instituting affordable child care and shared paternity leave, closing the pay gap and eliminating sexual harassment. It might also involve bringing about more diffuse social change by challenging sexist attitudes in our interpersonal relationships, workplaces and communities, questioning restrictive gender norms and educating people about gender oppression. These will be things that will be best achieved collectively, as they involve societal change, but they also entail being committed to survival and freedom from oppression for all women, since these societal changes will not only benefit us as individuals, but will enhance the well-being of women as members of an oppressed social group.[25] On this account, in order to attain well-being I must not simply see myself as a 'lone wolf' seeking the good life; I must understand myself as part of a community working together with others to bring about a better way of life for us all by eradicating domination in all its forms.[26]

We can see, then, that from a feminist perspective achieving well-being will be a collaborative, social project, but is it also an independent one? Feminist theorists have often tended to shy away from an emphasis on the individual, seeing the orientation towards independent agents as a mark of an androcentric theory that obscures relational conceptions of the self and the socially embedded nature of human agents. However, in thinking about well-being it seems essential to recognise that we must bear in mind the well-being of us as individuals, lest relationality come to manifest as another form of oppression. We can see this danger more clearly if we turn to an account of well-being where relationality is put firmly at the centre: care ethics.

Noddings's care ethics: a cautionary tale of relationality

Nell Noddings is one of the key proponents of an ethic of care, a form of practical virtue theory that suggests well-being is grounded in caring relations. In contrast to traditional virtue theories, such as Aristotle's, the virtue of care cannot be practiced in isolation from others.[27] Care ethics thus takes seriously the relational conception of the self and places it at the core of its theory. The centrality of caring relations in matters of well-being converges with an account of well-being primarily focussed on survival rather than flourishing, since care ethicists emphasise that human existence and human societies are dependent upon relations of care and could not survive without them.[28] This cements the notion of relationality at the heart of what it is to live, and what it is to live well. Moreover, it is arguably in an ethic of care that we get the most robust account of well-being as a communal, rather than an individual pursuit.[29]

Noddings argues that my well-being is not only achieved through working together with others on shared projects to, for example, combat structural oppression. Rather, she suggests that, owing to the relational nature of the self, the other's well-being *is* my well-being.[30] Noddings implies that the essentially relational nature of human beings means that to distinguish oneself from the other and see our ends as distinct is somehow misleading. If the self is truly relational, then your ends are also my ends and thus I achieve my own well-being in helping you to realise yours. For Noddings, then, the relational conception of the self makes the pursuit of well-being as an individual project nonsensical, and suggests instead that achieving well-being is necessarily a communal activity, realised in and through caring relations with others.

However, as Sarah Hoagland has argued, taking relationality to its logical conclusion in this way and reconceiving well-being as a *solely* communal activity may in fact diminish well-being by helping to perpetuate gendered forms of oppression that are inimical to living well. Hoagland suggests that in Noddings's account of care there is so much emphasis on the other, that the self gets lost. Since care is conceived as unidirectional,[31] the caring agent is a model of self-sacrifice,[32] subordinated to the needs and well-being of others. The result being that the caring practice that was supposed to aid well-being in fact generates a state of affairs 'not significantly different from the situation of exploitation'.[33] Hoagland further criticises care ethics and its emphasis on 'feminine virtues', such as care,[34] by identifying them as 'virtues of subservience'.[35] Far from being a radical feminist challenge to traditional moral theories and mainstream assumptions about the metaphysical structure of moral agents, the extreme emphasis on relationality *qua* relations of care for achieving well-being, ends up reifying oppressive views of what it is to be a woman and thus diminishes well-being by perpetuating oppression and domination.

While Noddings's interpretation of the relational conception of the self and its consequences for well-being is an extreme one, it does draw our attention to the fact that it is important to say something about the realisation of well-being in more individual terms, and not only as a communal pursuit, in order to guard against possible situations of self-sacrifice and self-loss if relationality is pushed to its logical conclusion. This does not mean forsaking an emphasis on the relational nature of our existence, but it does mean considering well-being at both an individual and a social level.[36]

Valuing oneself: self-respect as a necessary precondition for achieving well-being

We began by arguing that the basic situation of woman was one of oppression and thus, from a feminist perspective, well-being should be oriented towards resisting and overcoming oppression. We have seen how this can be achieved at the level of the social, underpinned by a recognition of the fundamentally relational nature of the self. But if we return to Beauvoir, we find that oppression is not only articulated in terms of external, social and interpersonal relations, but also manifests itself in terms of something internal at the level of the oppressed agent. Beauvoir argues that women are not only oppressed by men, but are in some way complicit in their own oppression.[37] Women do not only have oppression imposed upon them, but can often help to perpetuate their own unfree ways of life by embracing, rather than resisting, oppression. If this is the case, it is not clear that combatting oppression solely at a structural or interpersonal level will ensure well-being will be achieved.[38] Rather, we also need to stipulate something about the agent themselves in order to secure well-being *qua* freedom from oppression.

Why might an agent embrace rather than resist oppression? One answer we find in the literature is a lack of self-respect.[39] In general, self-respect is viewed as important for well-being,[40] but it is arguably even more important in feminist accounts where well-being is defined in terms of resisting oppression and domination. To lack self-respect is to fail to value oneself as an equal member of the human community. Without valuing oneself and viewing oneself as worthy of respect, agents will be more likely to accept oppression, since they will not see themselves as deserving of anything else. Self-respect can therefore be seen as a prerequisite for resisting oppression and domination, and thus central to feminist accounts of well-being. A lack of self-respect can help to explain why an abused wife stays with her violent husband, or why a working woman accepts less pay for doing the same job as her male counterpart. The agents in question lack an appropriate regard for themselves 'as . . . intrinsically valuable human being[s]'[41] and so cannot be said to live well because they accept, rather than resist, domination and oppression.[42] As these gendered examples suggest, and as Robin Dillon has argued, 'developing and maintaining self-respect is particularly difficult for women',[43] therefore making it even more essential to emphasise self-respect in feminist accounts of well-being.

Moreover, an appeal to self-respect can also help guard against the tendency toward self-subordination in an ethic of care. Recognising that I am a valuable human being in my own right means that I must practice self-care, not only so I can care better for others,[44] but because I myself am worthy of care.[45] Supplementing the emphasis on the relational and interdependent nature of our existence with an emphasis on self-respect can thus also be seen to help ensure that the unidirectional nature of care does not lead to a situation of exploitation.

Self-understanding and the relational conception of the self: ensuring well-being as freedom from oppression

It seems clear, then, that self-respect is essential for well-being and can help in resisting domination by ensuring we reject rather than accept oppression, not only for others but also for ourselves. But how can such self-respect be achieved?

One of the key underpinnings of self-respect is self-understanding.[46] One might be concerned about this claim from a feminist perspective, as it may appear to be androcentric in its emphasis on the self, abstracting from the relational and socially embedded nature of our existence. However, taken together with the emphasis on the fundamentally relational conception of the self, self-respect *qua* self-understanding need not be grasped in this way. As Robin Dillon argues, from a feminist perspective, to understand oneself is to grasp oneself in one's concrete specificity.[47] In a feminist context where the self is thought to be essentially relational, self-understanding is not an abstraction from relationality. Rather, it reinforces the importance of understanding ourselves in an honest and accurate way, which includes a recognition of the relational nature of our existence.[48] Self-understanding and the relational conception of the self are thus necessarily intertwined.

However, this is not to say that self-understanding simply reiterates the fact that we are bound up with others at an existential level. Rather, what an emphasis on self-understanding brings into focus is myself as a unique and intrinsically valuable human being resulting from the relations that constitute me existentially. Whereas a focus on relationality draws our perspective outwards to our interpersonal relationships and our socially embedded nature, an emphasis on self-understanding draws our focus back on to the specific self constituted by those relations. As Jean Baker Miller has argued 'subordinates often know more about the dominants than they know about themselves'.[49] Thus rather than simply concentrating on the relations of domination in which we exist and the distorted and unjust social settings in which we find ourselves, self-understanding encourages us to attend to ourselves. This brings us back to the question with which we began our analysis, but casts it in a new light. Self-understanding encourages us to ask who we are, but it demands a more detailed answer than that initially given. It demands an answer that takes in our concrete particularity as unique and valuable individuals, deserving of respect and capable of living well.[50] To think about and come to understand oneself in this way is, in itself, an act of resistance against oppression and domination. As Dillon argues, 'striving to understand oneself is reclaiming oneself from oppression through one's own insistence that one is worthy of being known'.[51] Self-understanding is thus not a way of acceding to the male domain of androcentric theory; it is a way of resisting the real oppression and domination that women face in their day-to-day lives by asserting ourselves as unique, concrete and valuable subjects. By focussing on oneself, one can develop the understanding necessary for self-respect, since taking the time to focus on myself suggests that I have begun to regard myself as valuable.[52] Thus by being attentive to ourselves, coming to understand and value ourselves, we will be in a better position to secure our own well-being than if our gaze is solely fixed in an outward direction towards others.

Through this analysis I have highlighted three key contributions to accounts of well-being from a feminist perspective. First, well-being should be thought not in terms of narrow conceptions of flourishing, but in relation to the wider notion of survival. Achieving well-being thus becomes framed in terms of resisting domination and oppression in all its forms. Second, we are led to revise the notion of the self in accounts of well-being, replacing ideas of independence with ideas of relationality. To live well we must recognise the way in which we are fundamentally bound up with others at both a practical and an existential level. The relational conception of the self suggests that well-being is a social, collective pursuit. To live well is to work together to resist oppression and domination. However, to think well-being only in this social and relational context may not secure well-being. In addition to an emphasis on others and our relations with them, we must also emphasise a third key factor: the self, specifically in terms of self-respect and self-knowledge. Without this we may miss oppression as it articulates itself 'internally' in the form of complicity. Only by taking both this outward-looking relational perspective, and tempering it with an inward-looking emphasis on self-knowledge will well-being be achieved in its feminist form as freedom from oppression.

Notes

1 He seeks to discover what is distinctive about human beings in order to discern what it will be to live well as a human being. Aristotle 350BC/2009: 1.7; 1097b: 22–28.

2 This does not mean presupposing an essentialist account of sex and gender, but rather, approaching the question from a phenomenological perspective. It might therefore be better phrased as: what is it like to be a woman or what is distinctive about the situation of women.

3 Aristotle 350BC/2009: 1.13; 1102a: 5–6.

4 There is not an exact parallel with the Aristotelian approach, as he seeks to identify a distinctive, abstract essence for human beings. My approach appeals to theorists who seek to say something general about the historical situation of woman and what it is like to be a woman in contemporary society. Such accounts reject the idea of a universal, eternal and unchanging 'feminine essence'.

5 Beauvoir [1949] 1953: 5–6.

6 Beauvoir [1949] 1953: 9.

7 Haslanger 2000: 31–55.

8 Ginzberg 1991: 126–127.

9 Aristotle 350 BC/2009: 10.8; 1178b: 33–35.

10 Ibid.: 10.7–8.

11 Ginzberg 1991: 128.

12 Ibid.

13 Ibid.: 130.

14 Ginzberg 1991: 129.

15 The full passage reads:

> [W]hen survival is reconceived as *not* "that which is a precondition for the emergence of culture" but rather as "that which infuses every aspect of well-being," it is going to turn out that any form of domination inhibits some sort of well-being and therefore is antithetical to survival in its fullest meaning. Thus a philosophical system in which survival is central necessarily will be one in which domination holds the position of an inconsistency.
>
> (ibid.: 133)

16 Aristotle 350BC/2009: 10.7; 1177a: 27–34.

17 Calhoun 1988/2013: 71.6 citing Benhabib 1987.

18 See Benhabib 1987: 77–96.

19 Sally Haslanger argues that 'the most familiar notion of oppression is one that implies an agent or agents misusing their power to harm another' (Haslanger 2004: 98).

20 This idea is articulated most robustly in care ethics, as we shall see in the section 'Noddings's care ethics: a cautionary tale of relationality'.

21 Calhoun 1988/2013: 716.

22 Freeman 2011: 370.

23 Ginzberg 1991: 134.

24 Haslanger 2004.

25 I focus on gender oppression here, but Ginzberg implies that reconceiving well-being in terms of survival will mean rejecting domination in all its forms, whether that be gender oppression, racial or class discrimination, ageism or ableism.

26 This also suggests that the pursuit of well-being will be an ongoing process and that well-being should be conceived on a scale, rather than as a matter of either/or. My well-being is increased when domination and oppression are decreased.

27 Noddings 1984/2013: 700.

28 Ibid.: 707.

29 Noddings 1984/2013: 5.

30 Since I am defined in relation, I do not sacrifice myself when I move towards the other as one-caring. Caring is, thus, both self-serving and other-serving ... if one's frame of reference focusses on the individual, caring seems self-sacrificing. But if the focus is on the group, on the species, it is the ultimate self-serving device – the sine qua non of survival (Noddings 1984/2013: 709).

31 Hoagland 1991: 253.

32 Despite what Noddings claims (Noddings 1984/2013: 709).

33 Hoagland 1991: 255.

34 See for example Gilligan (1982) who identifies care as a female moral orientation. Noddings (1984/2013) also endorses the idea of care as a feminine virtue.

35 Hoagland 1988: 82.
36 Care ethics, especially in Noddings's formulation does stress the importance of care as a relation between particular individuals. The problem in Noddings's case is that this relation is unidirectional, thus generating the problems of self-sacrifice and self-loss Hoagland identifies.
37 Beauvoir argues that woman 'chooses to desire her enslavement [*son esclavage*] so ardently that it will seem to her the expression of her liberty [*liberté*]' ([1949] 1953: 653) and that 'males find in woman more complicity than the oppressor [*l'oppresseur*] usually finds in the oppressed [*l'opprimé*]' (ibid.: 730).
38 Ann Levey makes this argument with regard to adaptive preferences, i.e. preferences formed in response to an unjust social setting, which reflect the injustice of the situation. E.g. women living under patriarchy expressing preferences that prop-up rather than challenge oppressive patriarchal norms. These preferences may have come to form such a central part of a person's life or their conception of the good, that simply correcting the social injustices will not guarantee that the adaptive preferences will be lost (Levey 2005: 131).
39 See for example Dillon (1992); Superson (2005) and Charles (2010).
40 Dillon 1992: 52.
41 Superson 2005: 111.
42 Beauvoir's own explanation for complicity is a little more complex, but it does root explanations for complicity in a kind of distorted self-understanding.
43 Dillon 1992: 52.
44 This is how Noddings explains the necessity of self-care.
45 Dillon also makes this point (1992: 62).
46 Dillon also makes this point (1992: 63).
47 Ibid.: 64.
48 Ibid.: 64.
49 Miller 1976: 11.
50 Dillon stresses that in feminist accounts of self-respect the idea of the relational nature of the self brings with it an emphasis on people as particular individuals, rather than generalised ones (Dillon 1992: 61).
51 Dillon 1992: 64–65.
52 Dillon identifies other conditions for self-respect such as patience and acceptance, but these must be practiced in the context of self-understanding if self-respect is to be achieved.

References

Aristotle. (350BC/2009), *Nicomachean Ethics*, trans. Ross, D. Oxford: Oxford University Press.
Beauvoir, S. D. ([1949] 1953), *The Second Sex*, trans. Parshley, H.M. London: Vintage.
Benhabib, S. (1987), 'The Generalized and the Concrete Other: The Kholberg-Gilligan Controversy and Feminist Theory', in Benhabib, S. and Cornell, D. (eds.) *Feminism as Critique: Essays on the Politics of Gender in Late-Capitalist Societies*. Cambridge: Polity Press, 77–96.
Calhoun, C. (1988/2013), 'Justice, Care and Gender Bias', *The Journal of Philosophy*, 85, 451–463. Reprinted in Shafer-Landau, R. (ed.) *Ethical Theory: An Anthology*, 2nd edn. Chichester: Wiley-Blackwell.
Charles, S. (2010), 'How Should Feminist Autonomy Theorists Respond to the Problem of Internalized Oppression?' *Social Theory and Practice*, 36, 3: 409–428.
Dillon, R. (1992), 'Toward a Feminist Conception of Self-Respect', *Hypatia*, 7, 1: 52–69.
Freeman, L. (2011), 'Reconsidering Relational Autonomy: A Feminist Approach to Selfhood and the Other in the Thinking of Martin Heidegger', *Inquiry*, 54, 4: 361–383.
Gilligan, C. (1982), *In a Different Voice: Psychological Theory and Women's Development*. Cambridge, MA: Harvard University Press.
Ginzberg, R. (1991), 'Philosophy is not a Luxury', in Card, C. (ed.) *Feminist Ethics*. Kansas: University Press of Kansas.
Haslanger, S. (2000), 'Gender and Race (What) Are They? (What) Do We Want Them to Be?' *Nous*, 4, 31: 31–55.
———. (2004), 'Oppressions Racial and Other', in Levine, M. and Pataki, T. (eds.) *Racism in Mind*. Ithaca: Cornell University Press.
Hoagland, S. (1988), *Lesbian Ethics: Toward New Value*. Palo Alto, California: Institute of Lesbian Studies.
———. (1991), 'Some Thoughts about "Caring"', in Card, C. (ed.) *Feminist Ethics*. Kansas: University Press of Kansas.
Levey, A. (2005), 'Liberalism, Adaptive Preferences, and Gender Equality', *Hypatia*, 20, 4: 127–143.
Miller, J.B. (1976), *Toward a New Psychology of Women*. Boston: Beacon Press.
Noddings, N. (1984/2013), 'An Ethic of Caring', in *Caring: A Feminine Approach to Ethics and Moral Education*. Berkeley, CA: University of California Press. Reprinted in Shafer-Landau, R. (ed.) *Ethical Theory: An Anthology*, 2nd edn. Chichester: Wiley-Blackwell.
Superson, A. (2005), 'Deformed Desires and Informed Desire Tests', *Hypatia*, 20, 4: 109–126.

7

PHILOSOPHICAL TAXONOMIES OF WELL-BEING

Samuel Clark

Introduction

The philosopher's question about well-being is 'what is it for someone's life as a whole to go best for her?'. This isn't the same question as 'what does she need if her life is to go best?' or 'what would help or harm her?'. The philosopher's question is about what well-being *is* rather than about what are its *conditions* or *causes*. Compare the difference between 'what is health?' and 'is smoking bad for your health?'. The question about well-being also isn't the same question as 'what is it to be a good person?' or 'what is moral righteousness?': compare the difference between being healthy and being a saint.[1]

We might think that we already know the answer to this question, even if we can't articulate it right now; and indeed the correct answer couldn't be completely unrecognizable or alien to human experience. But our imagination of what well-being could be is typically too narrow and simple. I make my case for widening and complicating the range of answers we should consider in two stages: I first set out a widely used taxonomy of theories of well-being which picks out some important possibilities, and argue that it is nonetheless inadequate; I then offer a different and more expansive way to map the territory, and consider some of the many distinctions and connections among theories and families of theories of well-being it suggests.

Against Parfit's taxonomy

In *Reasons & Persons*, Derek Parfit offered a now-standard taxonomy of theories of well-being (Parfit 1984: Appendix I, used by Crisp 2006: chapter 4, Crisp 2015; Griffin 1986; Hooker 2000: §2.3; Hurka 2006; Kagan 1992; Scanlon 1998: chapter 3; Sumner 1996: chapters 3–5, etc.).

Parfit divides theories of well-being into three main types:

> On *Hedonistic Theories*, what would be best for someone is what would make his life happiest. On *Desire-Fulfilment Theories*, what would be best for someone is what, throughout his life, would best fulfil his desires. On *Objective List Theories*, certain things are good or bad for us, whether or not we want to have the good things, or to avoid the bad things.
>
> (Parfit 1984: 493)

All three families have well-known exemplars: hedonists include Jeremy Bentham (1996) and Fred Feldman (2004); desire-fulfilment theorists, Thomas Hobbes (1994) and John Rawls (1999: Part III); objective list theorists, Aristotle (1999) and Martha Nussbaum (2011). But there are three things wrong with Parfit's taxonomy.

First, it is incomplete: it doesn't include all of the major extant theories. For example, it leaves out the *Authentic Happiness Theory* (Sumner 1996) on which happiness is *life-satisfaction* – you are happy if you judge that your life is going well or find it satisfying – and well-being is happiness which is not based on fundamental errors about your life (so someone whose happiness is based on falsely believing that her husband adores her does not have well-being, even though she does have happiness). More generally, Parfit's taxonomy leaves out *Reflexive Theories* (see below), on which well-being is some relation of oneself to oneself or to one's life – of satisfaction, endorsement, narration – as the class of which *Authentic Happiness* is a member.

Second, Parfit's taxa are too broad: they fail to make significant internal distinctions. *Hedonism* conflates distinct theories of happiness: is it tranquility (Epicurus 1964), a high balance of pleasure over pain (Bentham 1996), life-satisfaction (Sumner 1996), or a stable emotional condition (Haybron 2008)? Worse, *Objective List* is an incoherent 'everything else bin': it is miscellaneous and uninformative, offered only to catch accounts which don't fit into the other two categories. It conflates distinct meanings of 'objective' as *not up to its subject, not a mental state, knowable by others*, and *a proper matter for interference by others* (see below for more on these distinctions). It conflates objectivity in all these senses with *pluralism*, the idea that there are multiple distinct goods. It fails to distinguish *explanatory* from merely *enumerative* lists (Crisp 2006: 102–103).[2]

Third, Parfit's boundaries are poorly drawn: some significant views are in more than one taxon; some important distinctions cut across taxon-boundaries, making new and potentially interesting groupings and contrasts. On the first point: Parfit himself recognizes the possibility of *Composite Theories* on which desiring or taking pleasure in goods, *and* these goods being on the objective list of goods, are both necessary but neither individually sufficient for well-being (defenses of such 'enjoying the good' theories include Adams 1999: chapter 3; Kagan 2009; Wolf 2010). But this possibility mostly gets lost when his taxonomy is wheeled out. John Stuart Mill is usually forced into *Hedonism*, but his view also has important affinities with Aristotelian *Objective List* theories (Clark 2010, 2012). The second point is my focus in the rest of this chapter.

There are more adequate but less influential attempts at taxonomy in Parfit's style: they add extra taxa, clarify internal distinctions, and move boundaries (for example Haybron 2008: chapter 2; Heathwood 2010; Woodard 2013). But the root of the problem, which these better attempts share, is an assumption that taxa must neatly nest and exclude one another. This biological style of taxonomy is appropriate to the realm of living creatures where speciation derives from selection of random variations in descent. But there's no a priori reason to think that *theories* speciate by such errors, and when we go and look they turn out not to nest or to exclude in the way that would imply.

I therefore propose that instead of elaborating Parfit-style taxonomies, we should make interesting distinctions among theories and families of theories of well-being, without concern that they should be organized into a cladistic tree diagram, and accepting that they will cross-cut – that there will be multiple boundaries between families of theories, which won't mark out unique territories – and that many of them will be scales not either/or. We should think of these distinctions as usefully various ways of looking, rather than as attempts to cut theory-space at its joints, and should pursue possible combinations, exclusions, and derivations between the contrastive features they pick out.

Better taxonomic distinctions

In the rest of this chapter I offer some interesting distinctions among (families of) theories of well-being, and consider some of the contrasts, relations, and degrees of freedom or constraint on theorizing which they allow us to see.

Empirical vs. normative theories

Empirical Theories of well-being pick out something in the world which we can measure, represent, compare across people and across time, and intervene to change. Self-reported life-satisfaction perhaps works well here (unless such reports turn out to be situational or otherwise unstable: Tiberius & Plakias 2010), and is certainly widely used in empirical studies of well-being and popularizations of their results (e.g. Diener 2009; Layard 2005).

Normative Theories, in contrast, offer something it makes sense to aim at, which is not a completely alien goal and could motivate ordinary human beings: a standard of correctness, or at least a guide, for human action. Life-satisfaction is a poor attempt at this, because it's essentially a by-product (Elster 1983), and aiming directly at it is therefore self-defeating: to gain life-satisfaction – perhaps to gain happiness on any plausible definition – one needs to have other goals than being satisfied or being happy. More generally: there is no guarantee that what seems best to aim at will be intersubjectively measurable, nor amenable to the kinds of (numerical?) representations and (statistical?) calculations we might like to make, nor such that we can change things to make it easier to get. But this might pull us in the direction of revision rather than description (see below), given our practical interests in such measurement and intervention.

Descriptive vs. revisionary theories

Descriptive Theories leave everything unchanged, merely regularizing and making explicit what we already thought. They are the typical ambition of analytic philosophy of well-being.

Revisionary Theories come as a surprise, offering to change our lives. They are the ambition of much ancient philosophy, of Buddhist and other religious traditions, and of contemporary self-help books: all hope to reveal that our efforts at well-being have been misdirected because we have misidentified it.

We might have at least two different reasons for revision: either that our current thinking on well-being is *unhelpful* because it is unable to support our interests in measurement and intervention, as suggested above; or that our thinking on well-being is *wrong*. In the latter case, perhaps we have been tricked by a corrupt culture into chasing status, wealth, and power, when all we need is a few good friends and enough to eat (Epicurus 1964; Nussbaum 1994). Perhaps that revelation should lead us to abandon our current lives for something very different.

Reflexive vs. non-reflexive theories

Reflexive Theories make well-being depend on some relation of oneself to oneself or to one's life. Life-satisfaction theories appeal to a relation of *positive judgement about* or *positive feeling about*: one has well-being when she judges that her life is going well, or experiences it as satisfying. As noted above, other such theories appeal to other reflexive relations. *Narrative Theories*, in particular, make well-being depend on having an autobiographical relation of *self-narration* to one's own life: one's life goes best, or even has a determinate value at all, only when she tells it as a story which makes sense of it (MacIntyre 1981; Rosati 2013). Not to self-narrate is to have a life which is bad for you, because it is fragmentary, incoherent, or meaningless for you.

Non-Reflexive Theories deny this condition: *Desire-Fulfilment Theories*, for one example, typically say that one's life goes well when what one desires to happen does happen, whatever reflexive relation one has to those desires or to their fulfilment. But some desire-based theories build in a reflexive condition: well-being is the fulfilment not of one's actual desires, but of the desires one would want to have if one were fully rational and informed, that is of hypothetical desires about one's own desires (Railton 2003). So, for example, the alcoholic wants a drink, but if she were thinking clearly she would want not to want it, and her life would therefore be made better by not having it.

Compositional vs. additive theories

The distinction between *Compositional Theories* and *Additive Theories* of well-being is about the relation between the goodness of a life as a whole and the goods and bads in that life (pleasures and pains felt, desires fulfilled or unfulfilled, ambitions achieved or thwarted, capacities brought to full expression or stunted, or whatever else one's preferred theory identifies as good and bad). *Additive Theories* take that relation to be simple addition: to weigh the whole, sum the weights of its parts (putting bad parts on the other side of the scale).

Compositional Theories (Slote 1983; Velleman 2000; Wollheim 1984; I take the term 'compositional' from Brännmark 2001) claim that the overall temporal order, shape, or structure of the life also matters for the goodness of a whole. The standard intuition pump for that conclusion is a comparison between two lives which contain the exact same good and bad parts, but in one, the goods are towards the start and the bads towards the end, and in the other, vice versa. So, for example, in one life early success and happiness give way to loss and failure; in the other, hard beginnings of loss and failure are overcome and crowned with late success and happiness. Compositionalists claim that we can see that the second, improving life goes better than the first, declining one.

But why, even if so? *What* shape or structure is making the difference here? One popular answer is the *narrative* structure of the life (MacIntyre 1981; Velleman 2000), but that idea is doing different work here than in my discussion of reflexive theories above: there what's important is the relation of self-narration; here, the narrative relations – ironic contrast, aesthetic balance, etc. – of individual goods and bads to one another and to the whole story. Narrative is not the only available structure here: Michael Slote (1983), for example, takes the important shape of a life to be the biological arc from childhood to 'prime of life' to old age, and argues that goods and bads in the prime of life are far more weighty than in other stages.

Multiple distinctions between subjective and objective

We should stop using a distinction between subjective and objective theories, because those terms mean too many different things.

Subjective can mean that well-being is a mental state, a quality of experience; that it has no standard of correctness other than first-personal assertion; that it is in some sense a matter of choice for its subject; that no interference by others in one's well-being state is legitimate (and *objective* then means these claims' respective denials). But these come apart in several ways: *belief* is a mental state, and has a standard of correctness, the state of the world (my grandmother's belief that smoking was good for her asthma was *false*); *seeing something as red* is a quality of experience, and has a standard of correctness, what the thing is actually like (my colourblind grandfather often *mistook* green strawberries for ripe red ones). Plenty of such states – most obviously *pain* – are not up to their subjects. There's at least no *obvious* connection between the claim that well-being is a mental state and the claim that a political community should not intervene to change it – consider pain again. However there is a tempting but mistaken tendency to connect epistemic with political authority, which I now examine in more detail.

One subjective/objective distinction is about *epistemic authority*: well-being's subjectivity or objectivity is about whether well-being is *transparent* to its subject, in the sense that she knows her own well-being. The limit of transparency is that well-being is first-person incorrigible, like being in pain (there is no illusory pain, and no illusory well-being either), and the limit of non-transparency – call it *opacity* – is that only *others* can know my well-being (as though well-being were like a paint spot on my forehead). Many positions on the distribution of epistemic authority between self and others are available between these extremes.

A separate distinction is about *political authority*: whether what we *do* about someone's well-being should or should not be up to her. But this is a question about the *right*, not about the *good*: about what we should do not what's best. Even if we know the latter, should we maximize good, bring everyone up to a minimum, pursue good only as constrained by rights and duties, or what?

To get from a claim about what's best to a claim about what we should do, we would need to add, first, an account of any *other* values apart from well-being at stake in the decision; and second, a theory of the *relation* between the right and the good. For example, direct act utilitarianism: well-being is the only intrinsic value; the right action is always the action which maximizes expected intrinsic value. But there is no simple or automatic or theory-free route from the good to the right: no direct way from claims about well-being to claims about what it would be right or rational to do, or about what anyone should or may or must do.

I now want to explore an important application of this general point to the collective case, as when we wonder what our national education or health policy should be. Talk of well-being is sometimes mistakenly understood as troublingly *paternalistic* or politically *perfectionist* – as failing to respect liberal constraints on state action, which require neutrality about citizens' conceptions of the good (Rawls 1999; Rawls 2005)[3] – especially when the talk is of well-being as opaque enough that someone's evaluation of her own well-being can be mistaken.

But the question of the legitimacy of an action or policy is a question about what's right, and as already argued, no account of well-being on its own entails a result about that. It's worth digging more deeply into why there is no such entailment, either in that or in the opposite direction, in the case of political perfectionism.

First, it would be a mistake to deduce the legitimacy or illegitimacy of perfectionist policy directly from any account of well-being, including strongly opaque accounts (in support of perfectionism) or strongly transparent accounts (against it).

Suppose one is trying to legitimate some perfectionist policy with an account of well-being on which someone can be wrong about her own well-being: on which first-personal well-being judgements are like first-personal health judgements in being opaque and therefore corrigible. Perhaps: I can wrongly think I have lung cancer and be corrected by a doctor who explains my symptoms; I can wrongly think that my life of easy pleasure is good for me and be corrected by an Aristotelian philosopher who explains that the life of pleasure is fit for cattle, not humans.

Even from here, to make the move to perfectionist policy we would, first, need to add and defend an account of the right – with what *authority* do the government house perfectionists act? What *rights* against them have those they treat as children? Or are these concerns all subordinate to a requirement to maximize the good, as in utilitarianism? Second, we would need either an account of what other values are at stake – individual autonomy, for example – and how they are outweighed; or a defence of the welfarist claim that there are no other intrinsic values (Sumner 1996: chapter 6). Third, we would need an account of how the perfectionist policy succeeds in maximizing value compared to the other policy options. The path from a theory of well-being as opaque to a perfectionist policy about it is, at best, long and winding; that there is such a path at all depends on some highly controversial theoretical claims.

Second, it would equally be a mistake to move from the assumed illegitimacy of political perfectionism to any particular account of well-being – for example, a strongly *transparent* account on which first-personal well-being judgements are incorrigible, and each of us is the *sole and infallible epistemic authority* on our own well-being. Perhaps: if you want to find out how well someone's life is going, just ask her – she and no one else really knows.

But in the first place, consider the parallel argument for health: that I ought not to steal your cigarettes doesn't tell us anything about whether cigarettes are bad for your health, or give you authority to decide that question. Political and legal authority are not epistemic authority.

In the second place, such 'sole and infallible authority' accounts of well-being are false: consider a small child's desire to explore the electrical sockets as an obvious counter-example. If the response is that we're talking about competent adults, then that just further reveals the failure of this argument, because the question here is *human* well-being, not competent adult well-being, and many humans whose lives can go better or worse are not competent adults. Indeed if 'competent adult' means 'someone who is entirely independent, completely knows her own good, and needs no help from others to get it', then *no* human is a competent adult. Only Epicurean gods could be.

Even an account of well-being which is more plausible than such extreme transparency views, but which still limits others' epistemic authority about my well-being, is not a guarantee against the legitimacy of political perfectionism. Weakness of will is still possible, and one might justify perfectionist policy to keep me doing what I authoritatively judge is for my own good: consider, for example, the aid given to people trying to give up cigarettes by a ban on smoking in public places.

What makes these mistaken moves tempting is an equivocation between *epistemic* and *political* authority. Even if we (wrongly) think that each individual has total *epistemic* authority about her well-being – that is, even if no one could possibly know my well-being better than I do, your well-being better than you do, etc. – it is confused to take that in itself as assigning to each of us sole *political* authority to *manage* our own well-being. It might be a pragmatic reason to make that assignment: people often know and care about themselves, and vulnerable things tend to do better in the charge of those who know and care about them. But there are other pragmatic reasons which pull in different directions and which also need to be taken into account: collective action problems, for example.

In the opposite direction, even if we think that each individual has sole *political* authority to manage and pursue her own well-being, it is confused to take that in itself to reveal anyone's degree of *epistemic* authority about her well-being, or therefore as constraining our accounts of well-being in general. Compare the fact that I do have *political* authority to manage my own pension (within legal and other constraints), but that I don't *know* very much – I certainly have far less epistemic authority than a professional financial advisor – about pension fund management. The epistemic and the political come apart here as elsewhere.

An account of well-being is therefore the wrong place to rest political perfectionism or challenges to it, and particular accounts of well-being should neither worry anti-perfectionists nor comfort perfectionists. Subjective/objective is not a useful distinction, but attention to some of the contrasts it conflates allows us to see something about the degrees of freedom between different theories and claims: in particular, to see that our answers to the question, to what extent am I an authority on my own well-being?, leaves open the question of political authority.

There are many other lines of enquiry into relations between different kinds of theory which this non-cladistic perspective opens. For example, and as briefly discussed above, *Reflexive Theories* and *Compositional Theories* can be linked by ideas of narrative; and our interests in measurement and intervention may push us in the direction of *Revisionary* rather than *Descriptive Theories*.

Concluding summary

I have argued for an expansion in imagination about what well-being could be, in two stages. I set out and rejected Parfit's influential triad of *Hedonist*, *Desire-Fulfilment*, and *Objective List Theories* of well-being, and further suggested that we shouldn't elaborate Parfit-style cladistic taxonomies, but should instead make multiple, cross-cutting distinctions between (families of) theories of well-being, and consider their interactions. I then put that suggestion into practice by distinguishing between *Empirical* and *Normative*, *Descriptive* and *Revisionary*, *Reflexive* and *Non-Reflexive*, and *Compositional* and *Additive Theories*, and by breaking up the much-used but incoherent subjective/objective distinction into various distinctions, out of which I focused mostly on questions of *Epistemic Authority*, *Political Authority*, and political perfectionism.

I have not argued for or against any particular theory of well-being. My aim has rather been to display some of the wide variety of theories, and of distinctions between theories, available to thinking about well-being.

Notes

1 We have a tendency to confuse ill health with lack of righteousness – Sontag (1991) – which suggests that we should be particularly careful to mark this distinction.
2 Parfit says much more about the internal distinctions of the desire-fulfilment taxon. I don't have space here to follow him through these complexities, but they don't refute my general point.
3 This is actually too simple, because there are perfectionist as well as neutralist liberals (e.g. Raz 1986, and see further Wall 2012), but this complication doesn't interfere with what follows.

References

Adams, R. M. 1999. *Finite and Infinite Goods: a framework for ethics* (Oxford: Oxford University Press).

Aristotle. 1999. *Nicomachean Ethics*, Terrence Irwin trans. (2nd edn, Indianapolis: Hackett).

Bentham, J. 1996. *Introduction to the Principles of Morals and Legislation*, J. H. Burns & H. L. A. Hart eds. (Oxford: Clarendon Press).

Brännmark, J. 2001. 'Good Lives: Parts and Wholes'. *American Philosophical Quarterly* 38: 221–231.

Clark, S. 2010. 'Love, Poetry, and the Good Life: Mill's *Autobiography* & Perfectionist Ethics'. *Inquiry* 53: 565–578.

Clark, S. 2012. 'Pleasure as Self-Discovery'. *Ratio* 25: 260–276.

Crisp, R. 2006. *Reasons and the Good* (Oxford: Clarendon Press).

Crisp, R. 2015. 'Well-Being'. *The Stanford Encyclopedia of Philosophy* (Summer 2015 edn), Edward N. Zalta ed. http://plato.stanford.edu/archives/sum2015/entries/well-being/

Diener, E. 2009. 'Satisfaction With Life Scale'. http://internal.psychology.illinois.edu/~ediener/SWLS.html (accessed 12 November 15).

Elster, J. 1983. *Sour Grapes: studies in the subversion of rationality* (Cambridge: Cambridge University Press).

Epicurus. 1964. *Letters, Principal Doctrines, and Vatican Sayings*, Russel M. Geer trans. (Indianapolis: Bobbs-Merrill).

Feldman, F. 2004. *Pleasure and the Good Life: concerning the nature, varieties, and plausibility of hedonism* (Oxford: Clarendon Press).

Griffin, J. 1986. *Well-Being: its meaning, measurement & moral importance* (Oxford: Clarendon Press).

Haybron, D. M. 2008. *The Pursuit of Unhappiness: the elusive psychology of well-being* (Oxford: Oxford University Press).

Heathwood, C. 2010. 'Welfare' in *The Routledge Companion to Ethics*, John Skorupski ed. (London: Routledge): 645–655.

Hobbes, T. 1994. *Leviathan*, Edwin Curley ed. (Indianapolis: Hackett).

Hooker, B. 2000. *Ideal Code, Real World: a rule-consequentialist theory of morality* (Oxford: Clarendon Press).

Hurka, T. 2006. 'Value Theory' in *The Oxford Handbook of Ethical Theory*, David Copp ed. (Oxford: Oxford University Press): 357–379.

Kagan, S. 1992. 'The Limits of Well-Being'. *Social Philosophy & Policy* 9: 169–189.

Kagan, S. 2009. 'Well-Being as Enjoying the Good'. *Philosophical Perspectives* 23: 253–272.

Layard, R. 2005. *Happiness: lessons from a new science* (New York: Penguin).

MacIntyre, A. 1981. *After Virtue: a study in moral theory* (London: Duckworth).

Nussbaum, M. C. 1994. *The Therapy of Desire: theory and practice in Hellenistic ethics* (Princeton: Princeton University Press).

Nussbaum, M. C. 2011. *Creating Capabilities: the human development approach* (Cambridge, MA: Belknap).

Parfit, D. 1984. *Reasons and Persons* (Oxford: Clarendon Press).

Railton, P. 2003. 'Moral Realism' in *Facts, Values, and Norms: essays towards a morality of consequence* (Cambridge: Cambridge University Press): 3–42.

Rawls, J. 1999. *A Theory of Justice* (revised edn, Oxford: Oxford University Press).

Rawls, J. 2005. *Political Liberalism* (expanded edn, New York: Columbia University Press).

Raz, J. 1986. *The Morality of Freedom* (Oxford: Clarendon Press).

Rosati, C. 2013. 'The Story of a Life'. *Social Philosophy and Policy* 30: 21–50.

Scanlon, T. M. 1998. *What We Owe to Each Other* (Cambridge, MA: Harvard University Press).

Slote, M. 1983. *Goods and Virtues* (Oxford: Clarendon Press).

Sontag, S. 1991. *Illness as Metaphor and AIDS and Its Metaphors* (London: Penguin).

Sumner, L. W. 1996. *Welfare, Happiness, & Ethics* (Oxford: Oxford University Press).

Tiberius, V. & Plakias, A. 2010. 'Well-Being' in *The Moral Psychology Handbook*, John Doris ed. (Oxford: Oxford University Press): 402–432.

Velleman, J. D. 2000. 'Well-Being and Time' in *The Possibility of Practical Reason* (Oxford: Oxford University Press): 56–84.

Wall, S. 2012. 'Perfectionism in Moral and Political Philosophy'. *The Stanford Encyclopedia of Philosophy* (Winter 2012 edn), Edward N. Zalta ed. http://plato.stanford.edu/archives/win2012/entries/perfectionism-moral/

Wolf, S., Macedo, S., Koethe, J., Adams, R. M., Arpaly, N., & Haidt, J. 2010. *Meaning in Life and Why it Matters* (Princeton: Princeton University Press).

Wollheim, R. 1984. *The Thread of Life* (Cambridge, MA: Harvard University Press).

Woodard, C. 2013. 'Classifying Theories of Welfare'. *Philosophical Studies* 165: 787–803.

8

DWELLING-MOBILITY

An existential theory of well-being

Les Todres and Kathleen T. Galvin

Introduction

The proper dwelling plight lies in this, that mortals ever search anew for the essence of dwelling, that they *ever learn to dwell*.

Heidegger, 1993: 363

In this chapter we offer a theory of well-being that has been centrally informed by Heidegger's notion of 'homecoming'. We do not systematically present Heidegger's scholarly exposition and refer readers to other relevant texts (Heidegger, 1962, 1966, 1971, 1973, 1993a/b). Rather, we will draw on a particular aspect of Heidegger's later works in relation to homecoming and a particular development of this that he calls 'Gegnet'. We pursue the implications that these aspects of his work provide for an existential theory of well-being. The theory includes the notion of 'dwelling', the notion of 'mobility' and the unity of these two dimensions (Gegnet as 'abiding expanse'). More than providing a philosophical description of 'abiding expanse' we are particularly interested in how this possibility can be experienced by human beings as a great resource and possible direction.

Heidegger's task is philosophical and ontological. In relation to issues relevant to everyday human experience he provides an ontological context; that is, he concerns himself with what it is about being – as such that makes various kinds of human experiences possible. In other words, with reference to the phenomenon of human well-being, he provides a framework to approach the question: what is it about Being that gives to human beings the possibility of well-being? In drawing on Heidegger's later works we want to note the difference between his task as a philosopher and our task of trying to understand the implications of this ontological concern for well-being as a possibility in human life.

The specific trajectory of Heidegger's ontological writings that we wish to draw on concerns how his notion of homecoming can be usefully extended towards a more ontic understanding of the nature of well-being in our daily lives. We do this by building on a previous paper (Dahlberg et al., 2009) in which we articulated well-being as the intertwining of 'peace' and 'movement', at metaphorical, existential and literal levels. In articulating the essence of well-being, we also expressed these notions of peace and movement more metaphorically as 'home' and 'adventure'. In this current chapter we wish to expand our earlier notion of peace towards the more encompassing term 'dwelling' and expand our earlier notion of movement towards the more encompassing term 'mobility'. More than this, we will consider how Heidegger's notion of 'Gegnet' can open up an understanding of how 'dwelling' and 'mobility' are both implicit in the deepest experience of well-being. We are substantially guided in this trajectory by Mugerauer's (2008) book *Heidegger and Homecoming*, but wish to use his analysis in a way that can throw some light on the phenomenon of human well-being. Mugerauer helped us to see how a rather obscure idea in Heidegger's work, namely 'Gegnet', could be highly productive when trying to integrate the experiences of movement and stillness.

The discourse that is especially relevant to well-being occurs in a number of Heidegger's later works (1966, 1971, 1973, 1993). In some of these texts he describes the 'togetherness' of things in an interrelated horizon that gives space for things and their movement ('the fourfold' of sky, earth, mortals and Gods). This 'together' fourfold is the source for the possibility of dwelling with things as they are, and moving with things as they become what they can. It is this ontological 'togetherness', with its 'horizon' of room-making (einraumen), that provides the template within which human beings' experience of 'dwelling with', and 'moving with', can be credibly understood.

The ontological possibility of well-being: the harmony of dwelling and mobility

Heidegger's (1993) introduction of the fourfold, sky, earth, mortals and divinities is his way of indicating an alternative ontological context for the relationship between Being and beings, an alternative to the technological perspective of the Western metaphysical tradition. The Western metaphysical tradition posits neutral space within which one can 'put' beings and things, and time is the neutral context in which all things happen sequentially. But Heidegger was concerned that this metaphysical framework missed a 'cosmos' in which Being was not just space and time (merely a neutral context), but a wholeness that was more intimately implicated in the way beings are related to one another and Being-as-a-whole. This relatedness is both a relatedness of movement and a relatedness of kinship and is indicated in Heidegger's notion of Gegnet (Heidegger, 1966).

Gegnet gives both a continuity between Being and beings, as well as a rupture, so that beings can become figural and stand out of their ground. Gegnet means open expanse/abiding expanse, but it is at the same time also a gathering. "The gathering is a multidimensional letting" (Mugerauer, 2008: 467).

Human beings are intimately implicated in Gegnet by being the 'there' of being, the 'place' where there is a clearing for the gatherings of beings and things; in this way being-as-such does not happen without human being.

Heidegger then also offers a consideration of how this ontological context above can be relevant for the ontic everyday lives of human beings. Can a human being remember his or her own dwelling in Being while also sojourning in the 'mobility-current' of being, thus called into a novel future? We would like to leave this ontological analysis for now, and consider how this framework may play out in relation to the human experience of well-being.

Delineating the phenomenon of human well-being

In his book *The Hermeneutics of Medicine and the Phenomenology of Health*, Svenaeus (2000) draws on Heidegger's *Being and Time* (Heidegger, 1962) and the *Zollikon Seminars* (Heidegger, 2001) to progress a view of health as 'homelike being-in-the world': "Health is to be understood as a being-at-home that keeps the not-being-at-home in the world from becoming apparent" (Svenaeus, 2000: 93). In this present chapter we cannot do justice to all the ways that Svenaeus insightfully elaborates this theme. However, building on some of these insights we would like to concentrate more on how the phenomenon of 'homelessness', although never fully eradicated, can become reframed within a more encompassing possibility of homecoming: the possibility of finding home within the homeless.

The journey through homelessness before authentic homecoming

In *Being and Time* Heidegger refers to a form of being-at-home (zuhause) that is inauthentic in that human beings can take excessive refuge in 'das man' or 'the man-in-general'. Such taken-for-granted familiarity constitutes a kind of 'at homeness' but at great cost to what he sees as the possibility of taking on a life of one's own. The numbing comfort of this taken-for-granted familiarity is in Heidegger's view not sustainable as human finitude and vulnerability inevitably announce themselves in many ways. In his analysis of the journey towards authenticity he emphasises the importance of anxiety as a form of attunement that opens up a certain aloneness in facing the uncertain cares of one's personal life that is always in the shadow of its potential falling away. Heidegger uses the term 'uncanniness' (unheimleich) to indicate this kind of existential homelessness that is faced when one is able to embrace the 'resolute' responsibility of moving away from the 'taken for granted' securities of the familiar 'at-homeness'. Within this perspective, ill health can be one of the ways in which human vulnerability reminds us of an existential homelessness that cannot be denied. Illness then can be 'a wake up call' to face existential tasks that may have been avoided. If Heidegger just left us here he would leave us in quite a nihilistic position in which we have to stoically come to terms with our homelessness. But later, in what Mugerauer (2008) calls 'the homey papers' Heidegger articulates another kind of homecoming which is authentically possible for human beings: a movement from the inauthenticity of a familiar being-at-home (zuhause) through a more authentic embrace of existential homelessness to the possibility of an authentic homecoming. Facing this 'not being at home', although an anxiety-provoking experience, can also open up a path of movement; and this can provide an energising potential that can itself be felt as well-being. Homelessness paradoxically provides an important motivation for the quest to seek the experience of homecoming. Our theory of well-being thus wishes to incorporate the value of experiences of homelessness as well as experiences of homecoming. As will be shown, homelessness gives mobility to life as a positive potential, while homecoming gives peace to life as a positive potential.

An existential theory of well-being as 'dwelling-mobility'

The following exposition of our existential theory of well-being first articulates existential mobility and existential dwelling as distinct dimensions before considering them together, and dialectically, as the unity of dwelling-mobility.

Existential mobility

In many different ways Heidegger conveyed how homelessness does not just bring insecurity but also provides the ontological possibilities of authentic movement or what we call 'existential mobility'. Homelessness carries with it a sense of unfinishedness that seeks future possibilities, people and projects. It is a creative restlessness in which we are called into our future possibilities. We could say that it is a kind of 'eros' or energy which can give a feeling of flow, aliveness and vibrant movement. When called in this way we may feel connected to our life's desires. We can also metaphorise this movement as a 'sense of adventure'. Therefore such existential mobility forms one of the dimensions of our theory of well-being.

Although they do not use this term, it could be said that the writings of Gadamer (1996), Boss (1979) and Toombs (1993) emphasise this notion of existential mobility in their considerations of well-being. In this view, well-being is about the access to one's existential possibilities in time and space, with one's body and with others. In emphasising the notion of possibilities, we are also emphasising the 'forward moving' quality of living towards the future and finding meaningful projects there. For Boss (1979), well-being is understood as all the ways in which we are able to have access to and actualise a full range of experiential and behavioural possibilities as articulated by Heidegger in *Being and Time*. These possibilities which

Heidegger called 'existentiale' include spatiality, temporality, intersubjectivity, embodiment and mood. For Boss, to restore well-being is to restore one's potential to be connected in all of these ways. Thus for example, to help restore a depressed person's temporal range, the psychotherapist becomes interested in the ways in which the future has become uninviting to the person; to help restore well-being for a person whose physical movement is very limited, a helper may focus on the well-being possibilities of facilitating contact with greater spatial horizons through accessing beautiful and expansive sights, smells and sounds; to help restore well-being in an ill person isolated in intensive care, a mere human touch or voice may be the inter-subjective welcome that is needed to invite the person out of their sense of isolation. In his writings on health and well-being, Gadamer (1996) indicates how healthy people are embodied in such a way that they are unpreoccupied with their physical condition, thus free to participate in all the powers that their bodies afford. Also, Toombs (1993) provides a number of descriptions of ill health as the truncation of, or deficit in, healthy existential possibilities of spatiality, temporality, intersubjectivity, embodiment and mood. Both Heidegger and Boss have emphasised how these different existential possibilities are equi-primordial, that is, that they are all implicated in one another without privileging any one of them in a way that sets up any particular existential dimension as primary. Our theory of well-being, in its emphasis on 'existential mobility', is thus interested in all of the ways one can experience existential mobility with different emphases. However, this dimension of 'existential mobility' alone is at risk of obscuring another equally important but distinctive dimension of well-being: the dimension that we call 'existential dwelling'.

Existential dwelling

In his later work Heidegger became more focused on a kind of existential homecoming that authentically grounds the human potentiality for a peaceful attunement to existence. In his writings on 'letting-be-ness' (Gelassenheit), and 'making a space for', Heidegger articulated the possibility of a human relationship to Being that was characterised by acceptance and the possibility of peace. Already in *Being and Time* there was a concern to face and come to terms with finitude and the existential vulnerabilities of existence. There is some question here about the extent to which such 'coming to terms' was a true acceptance rather than a resolute form of courage to bear one's aloneness and responsibility. After what has been called the 'turning' (Kehre), Heidegger concerns himself much more directly with the kind of comportment required that allows Being and beings 'to be'. He believed that this had great import for a philosophical project that tries to think of Being in a fresh way that is more original than traditional Western metaphysical frameworks. However, implicit in this we also find some important clues for a more peaceful attunement to life's everyday vicissitudes. In the comportment of 'Gelassenheit' or 'letting-be-ness' there is an openness to allow whatever is there to simply be present in the manner that it is present, before one rushes in to try to change it. We would like to express the essence of this quality in the term 'existential dwelling'. To dwell is to come home to one's situation, to hear what is there, to abide, to linger and to be gathered there with what belongs there. When such dwelling is able to be fully supported, there may be a mood of peacefulness. But peacefulness is only one possible attunement within dwelling. The essence of dwelling is simply the willingness to be there, whatever this 'being there' is like. One can come to dwelling in many ways such as sadness, suffering, concern, attentiveness, acceptance, relaxation or patience. Dwelling is intentional in its attunement in that it allows the world, the body, things, others and the flow of time to be what it is. It is a form of being grounded in the present moment, supported by a past that is arriving and the openness of a future that is calling. Dwelling makes room for all this. Although peacefulness and 'being at one' with 'what is there' is its deepest calling and possibility, such homecoming is invariably through homelessness if it is to be authentic. To dwell is to 'come home' to what is there with oneself and the world, whatever the qualities of that may be.

There is a paradox to existential dwelling. In coming home to what 'is there', there is not necessarily an eradication of suffering, pain and the existential vicissitudes of life. So how can such dwelling constitute a core dimension of well-being? What is it about this dwelling that can be called well-being? Just this: that there is a felt quality to 'making room for' and 'letting-be-ness' that constitutes a kind of peace, in spite of everything, that is different from the kind of peace that depends on the eradication of limiting conditions. If we were to follow Heidegger's project to speak the possibility of possibilities, we would say that, in existential dwelling, human being is inhering in Being; that is, that such dwelling is not just a psychological state but a description of a relationship of belonging between human being and her/his ground.

Conceptually it is possible to distinguish the two dimensions of mobility and dwelling: mobility emphasises the call of the future and the energetic feeling of possibility; dwelling emphasises a settling into the present moment with its acceptance of things as they are. In his later work however, Heidegger opened up the term 'Gegnet', and offers a way to speak of how dwelling and mobility can come together as an integrated unified experience that forms the deepest possibility of well-being. We thus now turn to Gegnet and what we have called 'dwelling-mobility'.

Dwelling-mobility: Gegnet

In this section we wish to consider how Heidegger's notion of Gegnet may help us to think about the ultimate essential unity of mobility and dwelling in the context of well-being.

Heidegger never eradicates the givenness of homelessness, but what he does open up at various levels and stages is a space in which homelessness does not exclude the possibility of well-being. This kind of well-being has to be inclusive enough in order to hold open the possibility of homecoming within homelessness. He thus had to find a language and a way of thinking that could express this paradox. Because the words 'dwelling' and 'mobility', 'home' and 'homelessness' divert attention from each other, it is difficult to imagine how both these dimensions can live together as a source of well-being. But we can do this by unfolding some of the implications of Heidegger's use of the term Gegnet in an ontological context. Mugerauer (2008) provides a useful summary of what is meant by the term:

> Gegnet is the opening that lets the horizon come forth as horizon, permits all to shelter, and lets everything come back home to its ownness, which is, at one and the same time, in/as their belonging together. *To the already potent figure of homecoming in 'return to itself', Heidegger adds the long-anticipated, long held off final possibility of completion: opening gathers and returns everything 'to rest in its own abiding' to rest, to stay at home in itself and to that to which it belongs* (authors' emphasis).
>
> (Mugerauer, 2008: 467)

Implicit in this idea of Gegnet as 'gathering in the abiding expanse' is a sense in which there is both the freedom and openness of mobility (being called into the novelty of open horizons) as well as the 'coming back home to itself' of dwelling (resting in the peacefulness of its own abiding). This togetherness of mobility and dwelling provides the possibility of well-being with both a 'rootedness' as well as a 'flow'. This rooted flow, this 'dwelling-mobility', is a space in which 'homecoming' can be found by embracing 'homelessness'. So in Gegnet there is always already the togetherness of dwelling and mobility. To sojourn in 'dwelling-mobility' is to. . .'endure in the abiding expanse' (Mugerauer, 2008: 469).

Summary of existential theory of well-being: dwelling-mobility

In this theory we approached the question of what it is about well-being that makes all kinds of well-being possible. Thus our phenomenon is about the structure of well-being before any particular categorisation of well-being, such as, for example, physical well-being, social well-being, emotional well-being, economic well-being. Our structure of well-being thus makes these categorical forms of well-being possible and provides the essence of well-being that coheres through all its variations.

Consistent with a phenomenological approach, well-being is both a way of being-in-the-world, as well as how this way of being-in-the-world is felt as an experience.

The deepest possibility of existential well-being lies in the unity of dwelling-mobility. Guided by Heidegger's notion of Gegnet, dwelling-mobility describes both the 'adventure' of being called into existential possibilities as well as the 'being at home with' what has been given. This deepest possibility carries with it a feeling of rootedness and flow, peace and possibility.

However, the variations of well-being lie in the dialectic of mobility and dwelling, as well as the relative emphasis that each dimension offers as a possible variation of well-being.

The essence of mobility lies in all the ways in which we are called into the existential possibilities of moving forward with time, space, others, mood and our bodies. The feeling of this 'moving forward' is one of energised flow.

The essence of dwelling lies in all the ways that we existentially 'come home' to what we have been given in time, space, others, mood and our bodies. The feeling of this 'coming home' is one of acceptance, 'rootedness' and peace.

Well-being, as we have articulated it, is a positive possibility that is independent of health and illness but is a resource for both. In other words, well-being can be found within illness and well-being is more than health. However, we wish to acknowledge that well-being, as an ontic everyday experience, is never complete, but something of the essence of well-being provides a possibility that always calls and can shine through. As such, our theory of well-being as 'dwelling-mobility' describes a capacity for movement and a capacity for settling.

Well-being possibilities: kinds and levels of well-being

Gegnet as an experiential possibility is inclusive of all the kinds and levels of well-being. It would appear to be an existential possibility that calls to us from deep within embodied being. In a sense, the body knows this unity of dwelling-mobility, even though one's life circumstances and conscious experience may not often present this deepest possibility of well-being. However the emphases that we have articulated as mobility and dwelling can also provide a conceptual foundation for considering various levels and kinds of well-being that stop short of the unity of dwelling-mobility. We would like to offer several kinds of well-being experiences in which dwelling and mobility occur with a number of different emphases. These emphases are informed by the following lifeworld constituents as articulated by Husserl and elaborated by Heidegger: spatiality, temporality, intersubjectivity, mood and embodiment. When dwelling is experienced in a spatial way one has a sense of being at home; when mobility is experienced in a spatial way one has a sense of adventure. When dwelling is experienced in a temporal way there is a sense of being grounded in the present moment; when mobility is experienced in a temporal way there is a sense of temporal 'flow' and forward movement. When dwelling is experienced in an intersubjective way there is a sense of kinship and belonging; when mobility is experienced in an intersubjective way there is a sense of mysterious interpersonal attraction. When dwelling is experienced as mood there is a sense of peace; when mobility is experienced as mood there is a sense of excitement or desire. When dwelling is experienced as a form of personal identity there is a sense of being at 'one with' the world; when mobility is experienced as a form of personal identity there is sense of 'I can'. When dwelling is experienced in an embodied way there is a sense of comfort; when mobility is experienced in an embodied way there is a sense of vitality.

All these experiential qualities, although overlapping, provide distinctive nuances or emphases. As such they can provide a conceptual framework for the range of distinctive resources that can be drawn upon or developed on in people's well-being journeys.

If one was trying to take this framework into a more applied direction one would be concerned with facilitating possibilities for 'movement' as well as possibilities for 'letting-be-ness' at both existential and literal levels.

We cannot pursue these applications in detail here, but this is the subject of Galvin and Todres, Chapter 30, Part 3, of this volume. The practical applications, however, proceed from a thoughtfulness about different kinds of mobility and dwelling at literal, metaphorical and existential levels, and how these different possible variations may be experienced within the context of fundamental lifeworld structures ('existentiale') such as temporality, intersubjectivity, embodiment, spatiality and mood. This sensitising (rather than prescriptive) way to consider the kind and level of well-being that may be possible in a concrete circumstance may offer some practical directions. So, for example, informed by the theory, one may think of one kind of possible well-being variation as 'spatial mobility', another as 'temporal mobility', and another as 'mooded dwelling', etc. In thinking about the question of what spatial mobility is possible for a person, one could, together with a person who has complex disabilities and can't go outside, consider what expansive spatial horizons may be possible within that context. An example of 'temporal mobility' may refer to the challenge of how to help a person access past memories (move into the past) when their short-term memory is failing. An example of 'mooded dwelling' may refer to the challenge of how to help a person feel more peaceful and 'at home' in a busy clinical care environment.

So, the theory itself may begin to provide a way of thinking about what the ontic possibilities and variations of well-being could be within the ontology of well-being as a human possibility.

Within this perspective of well-being, people find their own unique way towards well-being, and there is a play between all these nuances, one's personal history and the limitations that life presents. But in all these variations, the body knows something about well-being as 'dwelling-mobility', and such tacit knowing forms the experiential touchstone for guiding our quest towards homecoming within the homeless.

Acknowledgement

An earlier version of this Chapter was published in Galvin, K.T. and Todres, L. (2014) *Caring and Well-Being: A Lifeworld Approach.* Abingdon: Routledge.

References

Boss, M. (1979) *Existential Foundations of Medicine and Psychology.* Trans. S. Conway & A. Cleaves. New York: Jason Aronson.

Dahlberg, K., Todres, L. and Galvin, K.T. (2009) Lifeworld-Led Healthcare Is More Than Patient-Led Care: The Need for an Existential Theory of Well-Being. *Medicine, Healthcare and Philosophy*, 12: 265–271.

Gadamer, H.-G. (1996) *The Enigma of Health.* Trans. J. Gaiger & N. Walker. Cambridge: Polity Press.

Heidegger, M. (1962) *Being and Time.* Trans. J. Macquarrie & E. Robinson. New York: Harper & Row.

Heidegger, M. (1966) Conversations on a Country Path. In Trans. J.M. Anderson & E.H. Freund. *Discourse on Thinking*. New York: Harper & Row.

Heidegger, M. (1971) *Poetry Language and Thought.* Trans. Albert Hofstadter. New York: Harper & Row.

Heidegger, M. (1973) Art and Space. Trans. Charles H Seibert. *Man and World*, 6 (1): 3–5.

Heidegger, M. (1993a) Building Dwelling Thinking. In Krell, D. F. (Ed.). *Basic Writings: Martin Heidegger*. London: Routledge.

Heidegger, M. (1993b) Origin of the Work of Art. In Krell, D. F. (Ed.). *Basic Writings: Martin Heidegger.* London: Routledge.

Heidegger, M. (2001) *Zollikon Seminars.* M. Boss (Ed.). Trans. F. Mayr & R. Askay. Evanston, IL: Northwestern University Press.

Mugerauer, R. (2008) *Heidegger and Homecoming: The Leitmotif in the Later Writings.* Toronto: University of Toronto Press.

Svenaeus, F. (2000) *The Hermeneutics of Medicine and the Phenomenology of Health: Steps Towards a Philosophy of Medical Practice.* London: Kluwer Academic Publishers.

Toombs, K. (1993) *The Meaning of Illness – A Phenomenological Account of the Different Perspectives of Physician and Patient.* Philosophy and Medicine, 42. Boston: Kluwer Academic Publishers.

9
CAPABILITIES, WELL-BEING AND UNIVERSALISM

Gideon Calder

Introduction: the universal and the particular

'Well-being' risks becoming a hollow term, precisely because it matters so much. It seems by definition to be something we all seek and value – but at the same time, to be something we seek and value in different ways. This poses challenges at different levels: for theory, policy and practice. At the theoretical level, we struggle to identify necessary and sufficient conditions for well-being – and to distinguish contingent, temporary or culturally relative aspects of what contributes to human flourishing from elements which are somehow deeper, fixed or universal. Attempts to frame and promote well-being in policy or legislation may inevitably over-simplify what it means or the diversity of its components, or offer a reductive picture of how they relate to each other. There is a tendency to give primacy to one particular 'take' on well-being – perhaps medical, or psychological, or economic – and assume that the other dimensions of how we flourish can be gauged and fully accounted for through that lens. And in practice, knowing what our own or others' well-being consists in seems to demand a panoramic sense of the self and its social context. At each of these levels, the problem at stake might be expressed in a similar way. How can we generalize about what 'well-being' means, while also being suitably attentive to the very many nuances and circumstantial variations in how different people, in different social positions, with different beliefs and priorities, in different places, and different stages of their life, are 'well'? Amid such difference, is there anything universal about well-being at all?

Of course, versions of this question arise across this handbook, in a variety of ways. This chapter explores and assesses the insights on well-being emerging in what has come to be called the Capabilities Approach to social justice – with a particular focus on the work of Martha Nussbaum. Capabilities-based approaches to well-being are explicitly normative, concerning the principles by which we might understand well-being and evaluate how it is distributed in any given society. They sit in a distinct place in relation to two alternative ways of measuring how well we are doing in life. One is subjective. Viewed this way, my well-being depends on how well my preferences are satisfied, and so can be assessed on the basis of my feelings and experiences – my mental state. The other is objective. For accounts in this vein, certain things are good or bad for me *independently* (at least in part) of whether I desire them or whether they give rise to pleasurable experiences. For 'capabilitarians', by contrast, well-being is 'a matter of what people are able to do and to be, and thus the kind of life they are effectively able to lead' (Robeyns, 2016). The freedom to achieve well-being – an individual's real opportunity to do and be what they have reason to value – is morally paramount.

So the basic claim is that while different individuals may have reason to be and do different things – or to achieve different 'functionings', to use the term which covers both 'beings and doings' – the opportunity to achieve them is crucial for *anyone's* well-being. Your priority may lie in international travel, while mine is in meaningful relationships with a houseful of pets. But because we each have our own good reasons for seeking these different functionings, having real opportunities to achieve them is similarly crucial for us both. The range of such alternatives – what Amartya Sen calls our 'capability sets' (see especially 1992) – will differ between us. Whether in economics, politics or sociological analysis, a capabilities approach will assess the scale and distribution of such opportunities, or 'capabilities to function'. Thus if we want to compare how two different people are 'getting on', we should focus in on their respective capability sets. When evaluating a policy, we should gauge its impact on people's capabilities. If we want to compare quality of life across a range of countries, the capabilities of their inhabitants will give us a more precise and reliable guide than – for example – comparing those countries' levels of GDP. Or so the proponents of a capabilities approach will argue.

Discussing capabilities, we find ourselves in a complex debate about functionings, and about whether or not some ways we might be, or things we might do, are universal or definitive of the human condition. Famously, Nussbaum's work sits on the 'universalist' side of this line. So she has sought to identify the minimum conditions necessary for truly human functioning – with all the contentiousness that any such project will bring – and on that basis, to develop a specific list of the central human capabilities, from being able to live a life of normal length, to being able to laugh, to play and enjoy recreational activities. Of course, rather than settling the matter, this list – and the very idea that we might devise one – has been the prompt for extensive critique and debate, including among the strongest advocates of a capabilities-based approach.

After an initial setting-out of what is distinctive in the capabilities approach, as established by Sen and developed by Nussbaum, the following sections in this chapter explore two such areas of contention. One is the degree to which we can generalize about human capabilities across cultures and contexts. Another concerns the life course, and specifically whether children and adults should be seen as having mutually distinct capabilities, or a continuous, shared set. We will look at various examples along the way, in drawing out the significance of these themes – and assessing Nussbaum's fertile yet contentious 'take' on the capabilities approach.

A focus on 'actual living': what makes a capabilities approach distinctive

To capture what is distinctive about a capabilities approach, it helps to situate it against what it emerged as a response to. To a large extent, a stress on capabilities is an alternative to the dominant models of welfare economics up to the 1980s (within many quarters, their influence still, now, remaining quite robust). For Sen, as an economist-philosopher, the treatment of well-being in such models was starkly deficient. When faced with the question of how a society or an individual is doing, two kinds of answer tended to be reached for.

One was to gauge people's happiness – how satisfied they are with their life. So in these 'welfarist' or 'utilitarian' terms, well-being is promoted when more people's preferences are satisfied.[1] A 'better-off' person is one whose preferences are relatively well-satisfied. A 'better-off' country is one in which collective levels of happiness – or utility – are higher than in others. While they will argue between themselves about what kinds of distributions of happiness are fair or just, for all taking this approach the way to measure this is via levels of preference-satisfaction. The other kind of answer involved a focus on resources. Viewed this way, what matters for quality of life is people's access to certain goods or commodities. People are 'better' or 'worse' off according to the amount of resources at their disposal. Neither preferences nor resources, for Sen, is adequate as a gauge of how well an individual's life is going – or as a means by which we might compare 'quality of life' in different countries, or different groups.

Utilitarian approaches face problems in identifying what counts as a 'satisfied' preference or desire, and how to find a single common metric by which satisfaction might be weighed. One reason for this is that utility takes plural forms, within and between people's lives (Sen, 1981). So I may get satisfaction from a video game, or caring for a relative, or the paintings of Francis Bacon, or a spell of good weather – but there seems no obvious shared way of measuring the different pleasures at stake. The measurement problem is blown up to a larger scale by the fact that different people's lists of preferences will vary so widely – and that my neighbour's idea of a good painting, or whether painting matters at all, can reliably be expected to differ from mine. These objections to utilitarianism are well-trodden, and there are possible (if always contested) ways around them.

But Sen raises a deeper criticism, crucial for this chapter. It concerns 'adaptive preferences': the ways in which people's preferences are formed by the circumstances in which they live. To put it another way: in important respects, our preferences will be adapted according to social conditions. This comes into sharpest relief in the case of those whose circumstances are most deprived or constraining:

> A thoroughly deprived person, living a very reduced life, might not appear to be badly off in terms of the mental metric of desire and its fulfilment, if the hardship is accepted with non-grumbling resignation. In situations of long-standing deprivation, the victims do not go on grieving and lamenting all the time, and very often make great efforts to take pleasure in small mercies and to cut down personal desires to modest – 'realistic' – proportions. Indeed, in situations of adversity which the victims cannot individually change, prudential reasoning would suggest that the victims should concentrate their desires on those limited things that they can possibly achieve, rather than fruitlessly pining for what is unattainable.
>
> (Sen, 1992: 55)

We may pause here at some of the terminology – 'reduced life', 'victim' – which itself raises questions about the authority with which others can gauge the relative situations of different individuals. But the gist of the point stands apart from that. One way in which people adapt to adverse circumstances is to lower their expectations – like the fox in the fable of the sour grapes, who, having sought them, identifies them as 'sour' only after finding them to be out of reach (Elster, 1985). Learning not to want something unattainable is a sure way to increase one's satisfaction levels, and of bringing them under one's own control. For some, rather than their expectations being lowered, it may be more a matter of never having generating them. 'Knowing one's place' – knowing that people like me will never get access to goods like that – will seem a prudent approach for those whose position in society makes aspirations seem futile from the start. As we might also put it, 'it is unlikely that people who are badly off will be fully cognizant of what options could be made available to them' (Berges, 2007: 16). Thus a utilitarian metric will seem especially amiss in the cases of the 'underdogs in stratified societies': oppressed minorities, sweatshop labourers, women confined to a domestic role in severely sexist cultures (Sen, 1999: 62–63).

Any resource-based approach might seem more reliable with regards to just those people towards whom the utilitarian metric seems most unfair. If what matters is the amount of resources individuals have available to them, then clearly, the sweatshop labourer will rank badly in any interpersonal comparison, regardless of how accepting they are of their circumstances. The simplest indicator of access to resources is income. Hence the use of poverty trends and income inequality data in comparing standards of living across countries, or from one historical period to another. But as Sen observes, a focus on incomes or resources, or other 'means of good living' will also have its limitations. This is because in gauging well-being, we are interested not just in the means at people's disposal, but in 'the *actual living* that people manage to achieve' (Sen, 1999: 73). These two are related in complex ways – but are not the same thing. Those with more means are not always happier or more fulfilled. Those with less are not thereby simply condemned to a poor quality of life, in all respects. A steady rise in its GDP does not guarantee that a nation's population feels steadily better off. Meanwhile, the well-being derived from resources depends in large part on one's needs. An individual with a manageable chronic health condition is likely to need more resources to achieve the same standard of living as someone whose everyday living requires no specialist medication. £10 goes further for someone with modest tastes than for someone with expensive ones. A simple, equal distribution of identical resources to all would not, then, deliver equality of well-being, because people's needs are importantly different. And neither would it deliver equality of capability. It is not resources themselves which are valuable, we might say, but the functionings we are in a position to glean from them, or the capability sets of which they form a part.

So the capabilities approach is distinctive in assessing quality of life, and the distribution of advantage and disadvantage within and between societies, in terms not of how satisfied people are, or what people have, but of their 'freedoms to do' (Sen, 1984: 316). For Sen, it serves as a conceptual framework by which such assessments might be made. Rather than setting out a definitive list of capabilities or functionings, he leaves their identification to local democratic discussion and public analysis. So his case is, as it were, for a methodology rather than a method: an approach, rather than an itemized menu.

Nussbaum's list

Nussbaum differs here. Rather than leaving open to local decision-making or empirical data collection which capabilities matter for well-being, or which matter most, Nussbaum famously, and controversially, seeks to identify these upfront. This, in condensed form, is her list of central capabilities, a 'threshold level' of which is taken as necessary for 'a dignified and minimally flourishing life' (2011: 33):

1 *Life*. Being able to live to the end of a human life of normal length.
2 *Bodily Health*. Being able to have good health, nourishment and shelter.
3 *Bodily Integrity*. Being able to move freely about, being secure against violent assault, having opportunities for sexual satisfaction and reproductive choices.
4 *Senses, Imagination and Thought*. Being able to imagine, think and reason in a 'truly human' way, having access to the education required for this, and being able to use and express one's mind freely.
5 *Emotions*. Being able to have attachments to things and people outside ourselves; to experience love and grief and other basic emotional responses.
6 *Practical Reason*. Being able to form a conception of the good and to engage in critical reflection about the planning of one's life.
7 *Affiliation*. Being able to live with and toward others, to recognize and show concern for other human beings, to be treated as a dignified being whose worth is equal to that of others, and having the social bases of self-respect and nonhumiliation.
8 *Other Species*. Being able to live with concern for and in relation to animals, plants and the world of nature.
9 *Play*. Being able to laugh, to play, to enjoy recreational activities.
10 *Control over Environment*. Being able to participate effectively in political choices that govern one's life, and to have property rights and be able to seek employment on an equal basis with others and to work using one's practical reason; having freedom from unwarranted search and seizure.

(Paraphrased from Nussbaum, 2000: 78–80, 2011: 33–34)

Now any such list will point us back towards the critical challenges we identified earlier. Is this list comprehensive – does it indeed cover all the basic ingredients of a dignified and flourishing life? Does it apply to each of us, to the same extent? Does it apply across the lifespan? Are these *discrete* capabilities at all, or is each in practice always mutually entangled with the others? Can't we find examples of people flourishing more than minimally, while lacking one or more of these capabilities? Are they timeless – in which case, for most of human history, most human beings would have been living non-dignified, non-flourishing lives? If that's the case, and if such human beings nonetheless felt satisfied with their existence, does that suggest that there's more to life than dignity and flourishing? Or is it that such features of a life will be defined and lived out differently, according to one's historical context? For Nussbaum, the list, though abstract, offers a basic account of what every human being on earth should be morally entitled to. These are protected capabilities. Whether they matter is not itself something to be figured out context by context, via political deliberation. She is quite clear that these are universal standards reflecting what it is to 'function in a fully human way' (2000: 71). On the other hand, it remains open to local interpretation in terms of its implementation – and should be regarded as an open-ended proposal, up for contestation and revision (Nussbaum, 2000: 77, 2011: 36).

Thus Nussbaum's list is, in her wording, both 'thick' and 'vague'. It is 'thick' in the sense that it commits itself to a particular conception of human nature, or being. So whereas liberal accounts of social justice, for example, typically seek to avoid contentious claims about general features of a 'good life', Nussbaum is happy to affirm a series of definitively human ends, as an 'outline sketch' of what counts as human flourishing. But the list is vague in that it 'admits . . . of many concrete specifications' (Nussbaum, 1990: 217). Unsurprisingly, it has given rise to a wealth of critical discussion – the details of which are far beyond the scope of this chapter. (For helpful overviews, see for example Alexander, 2008; Robeyns, 2016; Sayer, 2011). Rather than trying to do justice to the whole range of debates to which Nussbaum's approach gives rise, the following sections pick out two areas in which we might unpack its strengths and limitations.

Example 1: capabilities and cultural contexts

There are long, influential traditions of understanding human life for which the most important aspects of it are culturally relative. Truth, moral values, ideas about human ends and purposes – all of these, on some accounts, are furnished by and limited to the specific cultural and historical context in which this or that set of people live. And put the other way around: any attempt to generalize about these things, across different cultures or different historical periods, will commit a certain kind of error which comes as soon as we think we can escape from the cultural parameters of our perspective, to view things in a more objective way. From this angle, as it is sometimes put: every universalism masks a particularism. Every supposedly general view or claim about human beings is a particular, localized one in disguise.

Such approaches are often born from a critical sense that in a diverse world of radically different beliefs and practices, we should be wary of extending our own ethnocentric assumptions about what counts as progress, or about appropriate ways of living. Instead, we should respect those of others, and allow them to persist on their own terms. So in the case of well-being, the full-on cultural relativist will insist that nothing about it is universal. This or that person's idea of their own flourishing will be relative to their culture, and should not be criticized in 'outsider' terms. To take a stark case, we might think about what counts as well-being in a remote hunter-gatherer community, with little or no direct contact with other cultures.

For the cultural relativist, we have to be careful even in raising this question. For even talking of 'what counts as well-being' might itself be seen a cultural imposition, given that 'well-being' is a contemporary, Western term whose resonance depends on its location in that setting. Even asking the question assumes that there is a transcultural 'thing' called well-being which might be understood or lived out differently, within different kinds of culture. But relativism bites at another level, too. For even if we do allow that every culture might have its own version of what well-being means and consists in, we cannot find a way either of reliably comparing or ranking those different versions of 'well-being', or considering whether an individual in *this* cultural setting is better or worse off than an individual in *that* one. To try to do so is arrogant (because it assumes that it's possible to take up a kind of superior position, from which to make such comparisons), morally wrong (because it inevitably involves a kind of violence, in imposing one culture's version on another) and futile, because such comparisons are in fact impossible.

Full-on cultural relativism is easy to pick holes in. For one thing, the idea that there is something mor-ally *wrong* in making judgements across cultures itself seems to require a kind of universal claim – i.e., that cultures should have the right not to be judged according to others. It looks as if relativists are claiming the same kind of superior moral vantage point which they started out by denying the grounds of. So the critic of relativism might just say 'ah, but the idea that you shouldn't impose your conceptions of well-being on people from radically different cultural backgrounds is itself a product of the society you live in'. Or they might point to the beliefs of a particular culture – which, say, sees itself as inherently superior to others, sees the existence of other ways of life, even elsewhere, as impeding the well-being of its own members, and for whom it seems morally imperative that all other cultures are exterminated. What objection could a full-on relativist have to that view, which wasn't itself the imposition of some 'outsider' perspective?

Or they might highlight an individual, within a particular culture, whose life doesn't seem to be going so well – denied opportunities or resources in ways which seem they are markedly worse off than others in the same culture, or elsewhere. Say they, in line with the dominant messages of the culture to which they belong, accept their position, believing it to be normal, natural, or anyway unchangeable. There seems to be no basis for the relativist to object to that individual's position, in that social set-up. To adapt the familiar phrase about Rome: the message might seem to be that when in drastically oppressive societies, we should simply do as drastically oppressive societies do. Or further: that no society can be judged as oppressive in the first place, as long as it successfully imposes its own dominant conventional views of what counts as flourishing, in ways accepted or internalized by those who seem, viewed from outside, to be oppressed. On these terms, if a dominant culture thinks female genital mutilation, or slavery, are good, then so it is (*for them*, which is the only way in which we can cash out the meaning of the term 'good').

This last criticism points us back towards adaptive preferences. Nussbaum, like Sen, mostly addresses the phenomenon through the lens of gender justice. Both cite examples of where women's current preferences seem to have been distorted by unjust background conditions – so for example where women report their health levels as higher than men, when evidence suggests that they are worse (Nussbaum, 2000: 136–142; cf. Chen, 1999). The reverse applies, as Nussbaum notes (139): 'privileged people get used to being pampered and cared for', and so may feel greater discontent at any given loss in services or resources than would their worse-off counterparts with lower expectations. This suggests that well-being is heavily relative to circum-stances. But to talk of adaptive preferences at all – to claim, for example, that a certain cohort of women are *really* worse off than they think they are, or that there is something *wrong* about a state of affairs where the 'adjustment to bad circumstances' which may help them cope with poor treatment – requires a rejection of full-on relativism. Nussbaum herself is firm on this point (2000: 48–49).

Even so, might her list of central capabilities be vulnerable to the criticism that they are falsely universal? Should it be seen as a projection of the values and intellectual habits of a certain time, place and milieu (roughly, contemporary liberal America) rather than a generalizable gauge of human flourishing? Does it suggest – in a way that just seems plain far-fetched when we take on board the sheer rich diversity of ways of human life – that there is only one good way of living? Any such list would be open to that charge. Yet for many sympathetic critics of Nussbaum, it is its 'thick, vague' quality that may help her list fend it off. One such commentator is the contemporary political economist and social theorist Andrew Sayer. Sayer defends an objectivist account of well-being, presented as compatible with pluralism, but not with relativ-ism. Pluralism is the notion that there are many kinds of well-being. Relativism is the notion that any way of life may constitute well-being. Splitting the two off allows us to weigh the significance of cultural dif-ferences to human flourishing, without fetishizing them, or inflating them to a level where they override all other factors:

> Different cultures provide different kinds and mixes of flourishing and suffering. Simply as human
> beings we don't need to pray or watch television in order to flourish, but because we necessarily
> always live within particular cultural forms, such as religions and modern media, our well-being

is affected by their nature and our place within them. To be denied access to the particular set of cultural practices to which we have become attached, through which we make sense of ourselves and construct our narratives, and without which we cannot earn the respect of our peers, is likely to cause suffering. . . . An objectivist view of well-being does not imply that there is only one kind of well-being, nor does it imply that western culture has any monopoly of them.

(Sayer, 2011: 135)

Nussbaum's list is objectivist in this sense: an attempt to set down conditions of human flourishing which might lend themselves to a wide variation of possible realisations – but which nonetheless set limits both on what is morally acceptable, and on what counts as adequate well-being. If we are to weigh up its convincingness, we should do so on those terms, rather than as if it were a heavy-handed, culturally blind blueprint for ideal human living.

Example 2: capabilities and the life course

First on Nussbaum's list is this:

1   *Life*. Being able to live to the end of a human life of normal length.

It comes first, presumably, because it is both fundamental in itself, and a precondition of any other condition of well-being. To have a good life, we first need to have a life to live. To experience the finer points of human flourishing, we might add, we need that life to endure.

But we need to be careful here. Just as it is risky to assume that flourishing means the same across cultures, it is not self-evident that it is tied up with the living of a life of a certain length. Within any human life, well-being will ebb and flow. The later stages of a long life are more likely to be characterized by loss and illness. Perhaps certain parts of a 'normal' human lifespan are more conducive to flourishing than others. It is not outrageous to suggest that new-born babies or 120-year-olds have, on average, less of a good time than people who are 50. Extending the lifespan is not, by definition, extending well-being. And there are also, of course, wide variations in life expectancy, both within countries and between them. Average life expectancy in the world is currently 71.2. In the EU countries, it is 80.4. Even within Europe, it varies between 83.1 (Iceland) and 70.8 (Kosovo). In sub-Saharan Africa, it is 56.9 (Ballas, Dorling & Henning, 2017: 36). Between local areas in the UK, it ranges between 68 and 83 (GCPH, 2015; ONS, 2015). So in terms of the lifespan, 50-year-olds sit in the middle of the population in some regions, and are very definitely 'older people' in others.

This suggests that Nussbaum's list may apply differently at different stages of the life course – and perhaps, that some items on the list may not apply to some life stages at all. To flourish as a young child, for example, will require (capability 2) shelter and nourishment – indeed more by way of protein nutrition, for example, than an adult (Nussbaum, 2011: 57). But it will not require the opportunities for choice in matters of reproduction mentioned under capability 3. (It will, on the other hand, require being free against violent assault, also included there.) Does that mean that the list is biased towards adulthood, or that it neglects the particularity of children's well-being? Is it based on the assumption that it's in the peak of mature and independent adulthood that capabilities really or mostly apply? Might that suggest that other stages of the lifespan are viewed as paler versions, inevitably constrained in terms of the opportunities for flourishing they offer?

Nussbaum herself suggests not. While she tends not to linger on childhood or later life in articulating its key elements, she clearly regards her approach as especially well equipped, compared to its normative alternatives, to take matters of the life course into serious account – and indeed to include groups of people neglected by other theories of social justice (Nussbaum, 2006). One relevant contention is that dignity applies from the word go – 'all human beings possess equal and inalienable human dignity', and 'children are no exception' (Nussbaum & Dixon, 2012: 557). Another reason is that the capabilities approach is inherently developmental. Becoming the kind of individual who is able to 'use the senses, to imagine, think and reason' (capability 4) is clearly not automatic: it requires that certain capabilities (e.g. life, bodily health and bodily integrity) are in place for long enough for the process of growing up to run its course. So it seems unsurprising to find reference to 'the centrality of early childhood to the realization of a range of human capabilities' (Nussbaum & Dixon, 2012: 553), and the claim that 'requiring certain kinds of functioning of [children] . . . is defensible as a necessary prelude to adult capability' (Nussbaum, 2011: 26; cf. 2000: 89–90).

This may, though, still point to a certain built-in assumption that being a fully fledged agent along the lines typically associated with adulthood is really, as it were, where flourishing is at. Childhood may be seen as a kind of conduit to adulthood, a period with no purpose of its own other than to deliver us to that destination, a stage valuable for what it leads to, rather than for its own sake. A life cut short at 14 would, at least on a simple interpretation of Nussbaum's list, appear to be an inferior version of a life. By the same token, children may be seen as inferior versions of adults. Such assumptions are familiar, even mainstream – but also deeply problematic. Adulthood is not indisputably more conducive to well-being than childhood. And the value of childhood is not obviously best seen simply in terms of its successful delivery of children into adulthood. Indeed, we can consider this by of Nussbaum's list itself. Take capabilities 5 and 9:

5   *Emotions.* Being able to have attachments to things and people outside ourselves; to experience love and grief and other basic emotional responses.
9   *Play.* Being able to laugh, to play, to enjoy recreational activities.

There are obvious senses in which these capabilities may come as readily to children as adults, or more so. Children learn to attach early, to appreciate those attachments, to build on them. When dealing with grief they can be differently skilled and literate, compared to adults. They are especially good at non-instrumental play: at recreation for its own sake, rather than as a means to an end (fitness, say, or the rewards of competitive success).

It may be that we see these features of childhood as *intrinsically* good, so that their value 'does not follow from their contribution to the goods of adult life' (Brennan, 2014). It may, alternatively, be that we see childhood as comparatively advantaged compared to adulthood, as a stage of life in which certain capabilities might be realized. So if there are goods of a human life, some may arrive sooner than others and fade, while others may emerge far further down the road. It may be that we see more starkly in childhood features of human existence which are key throughout, but which we later find it easier to play down – the need for friendship, for example, as a form of affiliation. And then again, it may also be that we tend to overgeneralize about 'childhood', which covers such a wide variety of states of being that there is arguably more diversity within the category of 'children' as there is within that of 'adults' (Skelton, 2018). From either direction, the point has a similar resonance. It seems that capabilities approaches, to avoid a complacent pro-adult bias, may need to look at childhood less as a period of incompleteness, and more as a distinct, and distinctly valuable, phase of human life.

We have taken childhood as an example here, to make a wider point about the life course. Childhood matters because the well-being of children is as much an issue of social justice as that of adults (see Calder, 2016). To avoid 'writing off' people early or late in life, we need to think carefully about the risks of installing a model of capabilities centred on one version of thriving mid-life, and using it as a yardstick by which other, ostensibly non-conforming stages seem automatically inferior. From another angle, we find strong arguments that the picture of the relatively independent, self-sufficient, vigorously individualized individual which many might take as emblematic of adulthood is itself a kind of ideological fiction. Dependency on others can be seen as a core feature of the human condition, rather than an aberration or blip – an inescapable feature of a full and flourishing life, rather than simply an impediment to it (Kittay, 1999; MacIntyre, 1999).

One way of thinking through this is to invoke a distinction, important for Sen, between well-being and agency. These are interdependent, but distinct. We have good reason to value both. Thus on the one hand, it matters whether we are well or ill. On the other hand, it matters whether we are in a position to act, or refuse to act, in one way or another (Sen, 1999: 189–192). As he puts it: because 'a person as an agent need not be guided only by her own well-being', her *achievement* of agency cannot only be measured in terms of how her actions contribute to her own well-being (Sen, 1992: 56). Agency is a vital thread running through Nussbaum's capability list (see Nussbaum, 2005). It is also something which we customarily associate with, or assume to operate most fully in, the 'prime' of adult life. This may lead us to assume that full agency in adulthood is the aim of the well-being of children. Yet as we have seen, this is a problematic assumption. To avoid bias against children, those with later-life conditions such as dementia, or people with diminished cognitive capacities, a capabilities approach needs to be careful to place agency in a duly complex interrelation with well-being (Wasserman, 2006).

Conclusion

This last issue shows both the promise of a capabilities approach, and the heavy demands that will be made of it. For Nussbaum herself, a strength of the capabilities approach is that it 'makes evident the complex forms of interdependence between human beings and their material, social, and political environments' (Nussbaum, 2004: 345). This is an exemplary articulation of a vital aim. A key question – for all the fertility of the approach as a way of thinking about the conditions and dimensions of well-being – is whether and how it can make good on that aim. For some commentators, one of the main deficiencies of the approach, particularly in Nussbaum's version, is that despite that wish to factor in complex relationships, in fact it focuses predominantly on individuals, rather than the multi-layered sources of their well-being (see e.g. Jordan, 2008; Dean, 2010; Sayer, 2011). It is not, by itself, social science. It does not provide a full explanation of the conditions under which people's lives go badly or well, or the influences of social structures on the shape of any individual life. These concerns are important. But rather than defeating the purpose of a capabilities approach in general, or Nussbaum's list in particular, they might be seen as highlighting the need for it to be complemented with robust, critical analysis of the social conditions of our lives.

For the promise of the capabilities approach lies in its pluralism about well-being. If it highlights complexities to which it then does not already provide all the answers, this does not mean that the complexities themselves are not the right ones to be thinking about. Nussbaum's list is brief to state, but long in the critical unpacking. Applying it across different versions of a human life highlights key areas for critical scrutiny. Yet it reminds us too of the immense promise – some might say, the moral necessity – of a duly sophisticated universalist approach to well-being.

Note

1 The relationship between the terms 'welfare', 'well-being' and 'happiness' are complex, in ways beyond the scope of this discussion – though for extended treatment see Jordan (2008) and Bruni, Comim and Pugno (2008). From here on, I will be using the term 'utilitarian' rather than 'welfarist', but not in a way which seeks to sideline those complexities.

References

Alexander, J. M. (2008) *Capabilities and Social Justice: The Political Philosophy of Amartya Sen and Martha Nussbaum*. Aldershot: Ashgate.

Ballas, D., Dorling, D. and Henning, B. (2017) *The Human Atlas of Europe*. Bristol: Policy Press.

Berges, S. (2007) 'Why the Capabilities Approach Is Justified', *Journal of Applied Philosophy*, 24 (1): 16–25.

Brennan, S. (2014) 'The Goods of Childhood and Children's Rights', in F. Baylis and C. McLeod (eds), *Family-Making*. Oxford: Oxford University Press.

Bruni, L., Comim, F. and Pugno, M. (eds) (2008) *Capabilities and Happiness*. Oxford: Oxford University Press.

Calder, G. (2016) *How Inequality Runs in Families: Unfair Advantage and the Limits of Social Mobility*. Bristol: Policy Press.

Chen, M. (1999) *Permanent Moving: Widowhood in Rural India*. New Delhi and Philadelphia: Oxford University Press and University of Pennsylvania Press.

Dean, H. (2010) *Understanding Human Need*. Bristol: Policy Press.

Elster, J. (1985) *Sour Grapes: Studies in the Subversion of Rationality*. Cambridge: Cambridge University Press.

GCPH [Glasgow Centre for Population Health]. (2015) 'Life Expectancy in Calton – No Longer 54'. Available at: www.gcph.co.uk/latest/blogs/555_life_expectancy_in_calton-no_longer_54 [Accessed 24 October 2016].

Jordan, B. (2008) *Welfare and Well-Being: Social Value in Public Policy*. Bristol: Policy Press.

Kittay, E. F. (1999) *Love's Labor: Essays on Women, Equality and Dependency*. New York: Routledge.

MacIntyre, A. (1999) *Dependent Rational Animals: Why Human Beings Need the Virtues*. Chicago: Open Court.

Nussbaum, M. C. (1990) 'Aristotelian Social Democracy', in R. B. Douglass, G. M. Mara and H. S. Richardson (eds), *Liberalism and the Good*. New York: Routledge.

Nussbaum, M. C. (2000) *Women and Human Development: The Capabilities Approach*. Cambridge: Cambridge University Press.

Nussbaum, M. C. (2004) *Hiding from Humanity: Disgust, Shame and the Law*. Princeton: Princeton University Press.

Nussbaum, M. C. (2005) 'Capabilities as Fundamental Entitlements: Sen and Social Justice', in B. Agarwal, J. Humphries and I. Robeyns (eds), *Amartya Sen's Work and Ideas: A Gender Perspective*. London: Routledge.

Nussbaum, M. C. (2006) *Frontiers of Justice*. Cambridge, MA: Belknap, Harvard University Press.

Nussbaum, M. C. (2011) *Creating Capabilities: The Human Development Approach*. Cambridge, MA: Belknap, Harvard University Press.

Nussbaum, M. C. and Dixon, R. (2012) 'Children's Rights and a Capabilities Approach: The Question of Special Priority'. University of Chicago Public Law & Legal Theory Working Paper No. 384: 549–593.

ONS [Office for National Statistics]. (2015) 'Life Expectancy at Birth and at Age 65 by Local Areas in England and Wales: 2012 to 2014'. Available at: www.ons.gov.uk/peoplepopulationandcommunity/birthsdeathsandmarriages/lifeexpectancies/bulletins/lifeexpectancyatbirthandatage65bylocalareasinenglandandwales/2015-11-04 [Accessed 24 October 2016].

Robeyns, I. (2016) 'The Capability Approach', revised entry, *Stanford Encyclopedia of Philosophy*. Available at: https://plato.stanford.edu/entries/capability-approach/ [Accessed 5 October 2016].

Sayer, A. (2011) *Why Things Matter to People: Social Science, Values and Ethical Life*. Cambridge: Cambridge University Press.

Sen, A. (1981) 'Plural Utility', *Proceedings of the Aristotelian Society*, 81: 193–215.

Sen, A. (1984) *Resources, Values and Development*. Oxford: Wiley-Blackwell.

Sen, A. (1992) *Inequality Reexamined*. Oxford: Oxford University Press.

Sen, A. (1999) *Development as Freedom*. Oxford: Oxford University Press.

Skelton, A. (2018) 'Children and Wellbeing', in G. Calder, A. Gheaus and J. De Wispelaere (eds), *The Routledge Handbook of the Philosophy of Childhood and Children*. London and New York: Routledge.

Wasserman, D. (2006) 'Disability, Capability, and Thresholds for Distributive Justice', in A. Kaufman (ed), *Capabilities Equality: Basic Issues and Problems*. New York: Routledge.

PART 2

How are understandings of well-being developing? Disciplinary and professional perspectives

10

WELL-BEING AND PHENOMENOLOGY

Lifeworld, natural attitude, homeworld and place

David Seamon

Introduction

Though 'well-being' is defined in a wide range of ways (Atkinson, Fuller and Painter 2012; Kearns and Andrews 2010; Pain and Smith 2010; Schwanen and Ziegler 2011; Ziegler and Schwanen 2011), the concept is most often associated with 'human flourishing' (Fleuret and Atkinson 2007: 109) and 'optimal psychological experience and functioning' (Deci and Ryan 2008: 1). In this chapter, I consider what a phenomenological perspective might contribute to research on well-being by examining two central phenomenological principles – first, *human-immersion-in-world*; and, second, *lived obliviousness*. Human-immersion-in-world refers to the phenomenological recognition that human beings are inescapably conjoined with and enmeshed in their world, which here relates to the person or group's sphere of action, understanding and experience, both firsthand and vicarious. That people are always already caught up in and enjoined with their world suggests that the well-being of an individual or group cannot be discussed apart from lived relationships with their worlds, including the places in which they find themselves. In other words, individual well-being and place well-being mutually presuppose and afford each other. In this sense, one might more accurately speak of the *well-being-of-person-or-group-in-place* (DeMiglio and Williams 2008; Eyles and Williams 2008; Malpas 1999; Relph 1976; Seamon 2014, 2018; Stefanovic 2008).

As a second relevant phenomenological principle, lived obliviousness refers to the recognition that well-being is not typically an explicitly experienced dimension of most peoples' everyday experiences; rather, life simply unfolds more or less automatically, and one may not be aware of or reflect upon any stressful, untoward or undermining elements of daily living that, to an outsider, might indicate a lack of well-being. For sure, human beings often experience self-conscious moments when, on one hand, they feel positive and hopeful about their lives or, on the other hand, feel negative and wish their life might be better. More typically, however, life simply happens. People 'just get on with things' and don't regularly give self-conscious attention to the lived fact that life might be otherwise (Moran 2014; Seamon 1979: 99–105).

In this chapter, I draw upon the phenomenological concepts of *lifeworld*, *natural attitude*, *homeworld* and *place* to clarify what human-immersion-in-world and lived obliviousness might mean for research in well-being. My real-world starting point is three narrative accounts of ordinary and out-of-the-ordinary place experiences: first, interior designer Jane Barry's first-person description of her ill father's last few months of life in the house he had inhabited most of his adulthood (Barry 2012); second, British-African writer Doris Lessing's novelistic account of the everyday world of Maudie Fowler, an impoverished old woman who is a central character in Lessing's *Diaries of Jane Somers* (Lessing 1984); and, third, sociologist Eric Klinenberg's empirical research on the significant role that urban place played in contributing to many of the several hundred deaths during a 1995 heat wave in Chicago (Klinenberg 2002).

Using these three examples as evidence, I contend that place is an integral, non-contingent aspect of human life and helps to explain why well-being can typically be out of sight and thus not recognized as a significant dimension of one's day-to-day experience. I conclude that, because of the always-already-present reciprocity between human-immersion-in-place and lived obliviousness, professional efforts to enhance individual and group well-being sometimes might be better accomplished indirectly by changing aspects of place, including creative neighborhood design and planning that facilitate place attachment and a strong sense of environmental belonging.

Lifeworld, natural attitude and homeworld

From a phenomenological perspective, there is no dualistic relationship between person and world or people and their environment (Casey 2009; Malpas 1999; Moran 2000; Seamon 2013a, 2018; Stefanovic 2008). Rather, there is only a people-world entwinement and commingling whereby what is conventionally understood as *two* – person/world, people/environment, subject/object – is existentially realized as *one* – people-immersed-in-world. As a means to specify this lived people-world connectedness, *lifeworld* is a valuable phenomenological concept because it spotlights a person or group's everyday world of taken-for-grantedness typically unnoticed and thus hidden as a phenomenon (Finlay 2011; Seamon 1979, 2013a; van Manen 2014). Unless it shifts in some noticeable way (for example, one's town is badly damaged by storm or flood), we are almost always, in our typical human lives, unaware of our lifeworld, which we assume is the only way our life could be. This unquestioned acceptance of everyday life is identified phenomenologically as the *natural attitude* via which we 'accept the world and its forms of givenness as simply *there*, "on hand" for us' (Moran 2005: 7). Because of the natural attitude, we habitually assume that the world as we know and experience it is the *real and only* world. Almost always, the lifeworld is transparent and pre-reflective in the sense that day-to-day life *just happens*, grounded in spatial-temporal actions and patterns more or less regular (Moran 2014; Seamon 1979).

A more localized, personalized dimension of one's lifeworld and natural attitude is the *homeworld*, which phenomenology founder Edmund Husserl identified as the tacit, taken-for-granted sphere of experiences, understandings and situations marking out the world into which each of us is born and matures as children and then adults (Donohoe 2011, 2014; Seamon 2013b; Steinbock 1995). The homeworld is the most intimate portion of one's lifeworld, marking out the experiences, actions, situations and meanings that are unself-consciously assumed to be appropriate, reasonable and accepted without question.

Because the homeworld is pre-given by the arbitrariness of birth and family, we have no choice in what our particular homeworld is. Some individuals are born into homeworlds that sustain kindness, freedom and beneficence, while other individuals experience homeworlds that are unkind, restrictive and bleak. In this sense, the homeworld is that lived portion of the lifeworld wherein one is most unwittingly and most primally who one is, largely because of the happenstance of time, place, birth factors, and familial and societal circumstances. The homeworld is 'a unity of sense that is manifest in a pre-givenness of the things of the world that constitute the norm by which we judge other worlds and by which the pre-givenness of other worlds becomes given' (Donohoe 2011: 30). Here, norms and normativity do not refer to some arbitrary ethical, ideological or metaphysical system of right and wrong or better and worse. Rather, they refer to 'a foundational standard to which other places are compared in terms of our embodied constitution of the world' (Donohoe 2011: 25). Steinbock (1995: 232) writes that the homeworld is

> indifferent to whether we like it or not, or to whether it makes us happy or miserable. The point is that the norms that guide the homeworld are our norms, our way of life, as that to which we have accrued.[1]

The phenomenological notions of lifeworld, natural attitude and homeworld are important for under-standing well-being because they demonstrate that, most of the time, we are unaware of and thus naively unconcerned with the degree to which our daily life accommodates 'human flourishing' (Fleuret and Atkinson 2007: 109) or 'optimal psychological experience and functioning' (Deci and Ryan 2008: 1). Rather, our particular way of life *is what it is and not typically envisioned or evaluated otherwise*. In this sense, our manner of living is pre-given, out of sight and unquestioned, even though, by an external evaluator, it might be judged as unsound, deleterious or life-threatening. This typical, unself-conscious unawareness of the lived quality of one's life does not mean that examining that life self-consciously is not possible or unimportant. Rather, it indicates the difficulty of motivating an individual or group to consider their life explicitly in terms of well-being and to make life changes whereby well-being might be improved.

Place and human-immersion-in-world

I next consider how a phenomenological understanding of place might be useful for well-being research. Phenomenologically, place can be defined as *any environmental locus that gathers together experiences, actions and meanings spatially and temporally* (Seamon 2013a: 150). By this definition, places range in spatial scale from a favorite chair or outdoor sitting place to a well-used room or building to an urban neighborhood, city as a whole or meaningful geographic region. In this sense, places are the typically pre-given, unreflected-upon environmental contexts that sustain particular lifeworlds and homeworlds – the locales, settings, resting points and pathways that provide the environmental, spatial and temporal grounding for one's everyday, taken-for-granted experiences, understandings and actions.

For research on well-being, the most important aspect of place phenomenologically is the recogni-tion that *human being is always human-being-in-place* (Casey 2009; Malpas 1999, 2001, 2009; Seamon 2013a; Stefanovic 2008). 'To be', wrote phenomenologist Edward Casey (2009: 14), 'is to be in place. There is no being without place'. To exist humanly, in other words, is always already to exist *somewhere*, spatially, envi-ronmentally and temporally: 'Place serves as the *condition* of all existing things. This means that, far from being merely locatory or situational, place belongs to the very concept of existence' (Casey 2009: 15). In this sense, being-in-place is a fundamental ontological structure of being human.

If this is the case, then human well-being is intrinsically emplaced, and any understanding of well-being must consider what this lived emplacement means for empowering quality of life, both individually and group-wise. In short, the quality of human life is intimately related to the quality of place in which that life unfolds, and vice versa. As phenomenologist Jeff Malpas (2001: 232) explained, the constitution and quality of one's life

> is directly tied to the way in which the lived relation to place comes to be articulated and expressed in that life. . . . To care for and attend to our own lives thus demands that we also care for and attend to place.

1. An elderly father's lifeworld

I next present three lived situations that illustrate the phenomenological interpretation offered here. My first example is Jane Barry's firsthand description of her father's intense attachment to the house he had lived in for 65 years (Barry 2012). In spite of failing health and declining well-being, he insisted that he die at home. For part of the last year of his life, Barry lived with him and attempted to improve his environ-mental well-being via physical changes like stair handrails, high-contrast step edging and relocating food items in more convenient locations. Because her father was completely inured to his place, however, he mostly ignored Barry's modifications and continued to conduct daily actions and tasks as he had before, even though these efforts were now often frustrating or unsuccessful. Barry offered a heartrending portrait of how his daily life 'was deeply rooted in his home. . . . The meaning of [this] place played a strong role in his behaviors and the choices he made, and in his resistance to making changes in his environment' (Barry 2012: 4).

I highlight Barry's account here because it demonstrates a lived situation of extreme lived obliviousness and embeddedness-in-place. Mr. Barry's house and home life had become a lifeworld so habitual and 'just so' that he was unable to accept physical changes that might return to that lifeworld a certain degree of comfortable taken-for-grantedness and, in that sense, an improvement in well-being. When, for example, Barry moved canned goods from the cellar to a kitchen cupboard upstairs, her father continued to trek downstairs to get similar canned goods still stored there, even though it would be physically easier for him to retrieve equivalent items from the new kitchen storage that Barry had provided. From her objective, professional perspective of interior designer, reconfiguring the home environment would improve her father's well-being. But because of his immersion-in-place and lived obliviousness – what Barry at first assumed to be 'stubbornness' – he was unable to understand or to accept these modifications: 'He refused to make changes. It seems that he couldn't (or wouldn't) imagine what helpful changes might be possible' (Barry 2012: 5). Barry's depiction demonstrates how the remarkable inertial power of immersion-in-place and lived obliviousness undermines a well-meaning effort to improve another's well-being.

2. An old woman's homeworld

A second narrative example relating to the phenomenological interpretation offered here is critically acclaimed novelist Doris Lessing's riveting portrayal of character Maudie Fowler, an indigent, 90-year-old Londoner who faces a life of limitations imposed by circumstances, happenstance and age (Lessing 1984; Seamon 1993). Lessing presents Maudie's situation through the eyes of character Janna Somers, a fashionable, middle-aged magazine editor who befriends Maudie after they meet accidentally waiting in line at a local apothecary. Placewise, Maudie's lifeworld is limited in that it includes only her apartment, the street where she lives and a corner grocery store run by an Indian man with whom she often quarrels because she feels he overcharges. The physical center of her lifeworld is the three-room apartment that Maudie has occupied for over 40 years, though her declining health has entirely interfered with efforts to keep the space clean and tidy: 'I have never', says Somers of her first impression, 'seen anything like it outside of condemned houses. . . . The whole place smelled, it smelled awful. . . . It was all so dirty and dingy and grim and awful' (Lessing 1984: 14).

Over time, however, Somers realizes that Maudie's squalid apartment is an integral part of her world. Somers's understanding is crucial to Maudie because it means that, if authorities demand that she move to housing they consider better, Somers will support Maudie's wish to stay in her own apartment. Early on in their friendship, Somers naturally assumes that Maudie would gladly accept new housing with modern conveniences. Once she becomes Maudie's closest friend, however, she understands that the apartment is the central anchor of Maudie's life. As she explains to Somers,

> "I've never not paid [the rent], not once. Though I've gone without food. No, I learned that early. With your own place you've got everything. Without it, you're a dog. You are nothing. Have you got your own place?" – and when I said yes, she said, nodding fiercely, angrily, "That's right, and you hold onto it, then nothing can touch you".
>
> (Lessing 1984: 18–19)

If Maudie's well-being were defined in terms of modern architectural and social criteria, then her moving to better housing would be the appropriate action for which to advocate. In terms of homeworld, lifeworld and place, however, Maudie, like Barry's father, is existentially bound to her dwelling; to propose that she move elsewhere would severely unsettle her sense of self. Somers comes to recognize that more comfortable material conditions are in the end irrelevant to Maudie, for whom physical difficulty and discomfort have long been taken for granted: 'By any current housing standard, [her apartment] should be condemned. By any human standard, she should stay where she is' (Lessing 1984: 103). Somers understands that Maudie is immersed in lifeworld and place; any improvement in Maudie's homeworld and well-being cannot be had by physical intervention alone:

> I've given up even thinking that she ought to agree to be 'rehoused'; I said it just once, and it took her three days to stop seeing me as an enemy.... I *am* housed, says she, cough, cough, cough from having to go out at the back all weathers into the freezing lavatory, from standing to wash in the unheated kitchen. But why do I say that? Women of ninety who live in luxury cough and are frail.
>
> (Lessing 1984: 86)

Maudie's situation is significant for well-being research because it demonstrates how her immersion-in-place via her apartment is an integral part of her homeworld – that she defines herself in terms of *this* place that, objectively, is largely unlivable and incompatible with well-being. Yet for Maudie, though not aware of this fact self-consciously because of lived obliviousness, the apartment is essential for her self-worth and personal identity. From an instrumentalist perspective, one would assume that the squalid apartment undermines Maudie's well-being. From an existential perspective, however, one understands that the apartment sustains her well-being because it is a taken-for-granted part of her homeworld that cannot and must not be questioned or changed. In her indelible portrait of Maudie's life, Lessing movingly depicts an old woman profoundly entrenched in homeworld and place.

3. Compromised lifeworlds and place

A third narrative example relating to the phenomenological interpretation offered here is Eric Klinenberg's *Heat Wave*, a book examining why some 700 Chicago residents, most of them elderly and poor, died in a five-day heat wave in 1995 (Klinenberg 2002). As one means to answer this question, Klinenberg studied two adjacent Chicago neighborhoods: first, North Lawndale, which was predominantly African-American; and, second, South Lawndale, which was colloquially known as Little Village and predominantly Latino. Klinenberg selected these two neighborhoods because, even though they were geographically adjacent and included similar proportions of seniors living in poverty and seniors living alone (the two groups the U.S. Center for Disease Control had earlier determined as most vulnerable in the heat wave), the neighborhoods had dramatically different heat-wave mortality rates. Klinenberg wondered whether this difference in deaths might at least partly be related to the two neighborhoods' contrasting environmental and place qualities.

As he became more familiar with North Lawndale and Little Village, Klinenberg realized that they were vastly different in terms of place structure and human sociability. These contrasting environmental and social differences included

> the ways in which residents use sidewalks and public spaces, the role of commercial outlets in stimulating social contact, the strategies through which residents protect themselves from local dangers, and the role of community organizations and institutions in providing social protection.
>
> (Klinenberg 2002: 86)

Klinenberg concluded that, during the heat wave, local place features inhibited vulnerable North Lawndale residents from finding the social contact that would help them survive. In contrast, Little Village's local place features assisted vulnerable residents in finding help mostly as it was already a part of their everyday lifeworld.

On a considerably broader environmental scale than the two examples above, Klinenberg's study demonstrates how human well-being and place well-being each afford the other. North Lawndale's well-being was weak in the sense that it was a neighborhood of derelict buildings, shuttered stores, second-tier fast-food eateries, abandoned lots, deteriorating housing stock, few employment opportunities and much crime, especially drug dealing. As North Lawndale's economy declined, residents able to do so departed the neighborhood, leaving behind unoccupied dwellings as well as neighbors who had not the resources or will to leave. These remaining residents often withdrew inwardly from North Lawndale, finding social support beyond the neighborhood or isolating themselves geographically and socially. Klinenberg determined that, during the heat wave, it was largely the place-alienated individuals who died because their personal well-being was at least partly dependent on the well-being of their place. These North Lawndale residents had neither the social contacts to assist them nor the courage to seek help in a threatening neighborhood offering few public or commercial establishments where they might escape the heat. There was little collective life or environmental well-being to protect them, most of whom were older persons living alone 'with limited social contacts and weak support networks during normal times' (Klinenberg 2002: 41).

In contrast, Little Village's much more vibrant well-being played a major role in the well-being of its residents, particularly during the heat wave. Even though Little Village had similar proportions of poor elderly and elderly living alone, the neighborhood incorporated lively retail, bustling sidewalks and many more intact dwellings, all of which were occupied. Whereas North Lawndale as a place undermined neighborhood activity, Little Village facilitated 'public life and informal social support for residents' (Klinenberg 2002: 109). This exuberant place activity was particularly important for older residents living alone because it drew them out of their dwellings into the streets and public places where they made the social contact that isolated individuals in North Lawndale were much less able to establish. During the heat wave, the activity of nearby streets provided shops, eateries and other places where these individuals might find respite from the heat. Most vulnerable during the heat wave were older white residents remaining in the neighborhood after it had become mostly Latino. For the most part, however, they too were protected. Klinenberg (2002: 110) concluded that 'the robust public life of the region draws all but the most infirm residents out of their homes, promoting social interaction, network ties, and healthy behavior'.

Immersion-in-place, lived obliviousness and well-being

Via the phenomenological principles of lived obliviousness and human-immersion-in-world, I have attempted to describe an entrenched, lived dimension of human experience and understanding that is pre-given, taken-for-granted and thus often out of sight in professional discourse attempting to understand and to improve human well-being. In the current research literature, well-being is typically defined in two contrasting ways (Ziegler and Schwanen 2011: 763): either *objectively*, as a situation related to an individual or group's observable, measurable living conditions (e.g., income level or housing quality); or, *subjectively*, as an individual or group defines well-being for themselves experientially (e.g., in terms of happiness or life satisfaction).

A phenomenological criticism of these objective and subjective definitions is that both assume well-being to be an accessible phenomenon explicitly identifiable and describable – the objective version, using publically definable features often evaluated quantitatively; the subjective version, using first-person reports of what the individual or group appreciates or questions in regard to their relative happiness or dissatisfaction with life. Here, in contrast, I have emphasized a dimension of human experience and awareness that is transparent, taken-for granted and thus regularly unnoticed, both for the researcher and for the individuals whose well-being is the focus of concern. I have illustrated how this hidden, unspoken dimension of human life can be given direct presence via a phenomenological vantage point.

Because of lived obliviousness and immersion-in-place, an individual or group may not realize how changes in everyday actions or environmental modifications might improve their lifeworlds, homeworlds and well-being. For individuals or groups thoroughly inured to their place, motivating them to recognize how shifting everyday behaviors or reshaping existing environments might enrich their well-being becomes difficult and often impossible as demonstrated by the entrenched situations of Barry's father and Lessing's Maudie Fowler. Mr. Barry paid little heed to the thoughtful household improvements made by his daughter, and Maudie resolutely refused to consider moving to better housing even though, objectively, the material quality of her life would no doubt improve.

Place making and well-being

For both Mr. Barry and Maudie Fowler, lived obliviousness and unchangeable entrenchment in place brooked no possibility for the improvement of their well-being directly. In the same way, the isolated elderly who died in the Chicago heat wave took their social and environmental isolation for granted and had little will or active means to shift their situation in time of crisis. If, therefore, the inertia of lifeworld is an integral feature of many human lives, then positive change in human and place well-being might be more effectively advanced by making supportive changes in the worlds of individuals and groups rather than in their understandings, attitudes and actions. If human beings are always already embedded in place, then one important effort is to recognize how environmental and spatial reconfigurations might contribute to robust neighborhood place making. Can we, in other words, draw on design, planning and policy to recreate, self-consciously, dynamic urban neighborhoods like Klinenberg's Little Village that in the past developed organically without deliberate plans or actions?

In relation to this question, Klinenberg's research is instructive because it offers support for this claim that a benign manipulation and rehabilitation of neighborhood places might reconfigure lifeworlds and thereby strengthen environmental and human well-being. On the one hand, it was very much North Lawndale's fragmented, collapsing neighborhood that limited vulnerable elderly in finding help during the heat wave. On the other hand, it was very much Little Village's intact, animated neighborhood that allowed the same vulnerable elderly to survive. The key point phenomenologically is that *this support just happened or did not happen largely because of contrasting place qualities.* Klinenberg (2002: 230–235) emphasized that, during the heat wave, officially sponsored institutional structures and agencies did little formally to guarantee this support, which was much more usefully provided (or not) by informal environmental and social features grounded in the everyday lifeworld dynamics of neighborhood place.

There is a flourishing research literature on how creative place making might facilitate individual and group well-being.[2] These studies lay out practical ways to regenerate a better quality of life via place-supportive policy, planning and design. One example is the work of urban theorist Jane Jacobs (1961), who demonstrated how place diversity and exuberance, at least in urban neighborhoods, are sustained by short blocks, a range in building types, a sufficient concentration of people and a mixture of primary uses – i.e., anchor functions like home and work to which users must necessarily go. Another example is urban designer Vikas Mehta's observational studies of urban pedestrian behavior (Mehta 2013). He demonstrates how sidewalk sociability can be enhanced or weakened by designable and policy-regulated features such as seating, sidewalk width, variety of goods and services, permeable storefronts and so forth. A third example is urban designer Ian Bentley and colleagues' efforts to create *responsive environments* – urban neighborhoods that 'respond' to users in the sense that their everyday needs and activities – work, shopping, services, recreation, sociability and so forth – are conveniently accessible walking-wise from home (Bentley et al. 1985). The underlying aim in all of this work is provision of lively, mixed-use neighborhoods that, within their immediate surroundings, offer a wide range of people, functions, activities and events. The aim is a sense of place and environmental well-being *readily at hand* for residents and other place users. The potential result is neighborhoods with many of the place qualities that Klinenberg identified in Chicago's Little Village.

In short, one potential way to circumvent lived obliviousness and immersion-in-world is to reconfigure places that facilitate lifeworlds in which people feel a part rather than apart. This approach for strengthening well-being is indirect in that helpful change arises, not straightforwardly via individual and group assistance and services, but roundabout via physical intervention that makes an individual or group's place better materially, spatially and environmentally. Residents and others associated with that place feel a sense of attachment and belonging. The hopeful result is spirited, vigorous environments that sustain and strengthen the well-being of individuals and groups as they simply carry out their everyday lives in place.

Notes

1 Husserl emphasized that the homeworld is always in some mode of lived mutuality with an *alienworld*, which is the world of difference and otherness but is only provided awareness because of the always already givenness of one's homeworld; see Donohoe (2014: 12–20; Steinbock 1995: 178–185).
2 Overviews include Alexander 2012; Atkinson, Fuller and Painter 2012; Carmona et al. 2010; Cooper and Burton 2014; Frumkin, Frank and Jackson 2004; Kopec 2017; Mehta 2013; Seamon 2014, 2018; Steinfeld and White 2010.

References

Alexander, C. (2012) *Battle for the Life and Beauty of the Earth*, New York: Oxford University Press.
Atkinson, S., Fuller, S. and Painter, J. (2012) 'Well-being and place', in S. Atkinson, S. Fuller and J. Painter (eds.), *Well-Being and Place*, Farnham, UK: Ashgate.
Barry, J. (2012) 'My dad's house', *Environmental and Architectural Phenomenology*, 23 (2): 4–10.
Bentley, I., Alcock, A., Murrain, P., McGlynn, S. and Smith, G. (1985) *Responsive Environments*, London: Architectural Press.
Carmona, M., Tiesdell, S., Heath, T. and Oc, T. (2010) *Public Places, Urban Spaces*, London: Architectural Press.
Casey, E. S. (2009) *Getting Back into Place*, 2nd edn, Bloomington, IN: Indiana University Press.
Cooper, R. and Burton, E. (eds.) (2014) *Well-Being and the Environment*, New York: Wiley-Blackwell.
Deci, E. L. and Ryan, R. M. (2008) 'Hedonia, eudaimonia, and well-being', *Journal of Happiness Studies*, 9: 1–11.
DeMiglio, L. and Williams, A. (2008) 'A sense of place, a sense of well-being', in J. Eyles and A. Williams (eds.), *Sense of Place, Health and Quality of Life*, Farnham, UK: Ashgate.
Donohoe, J. (2011) 'The place of home', *Environmental Philosophy*, 8 (1): 25–40.
Donohoe, J. (2014) *Remembering Places*, New York: Lexington Books.
Eyles, J. and Williams, A. (eds.) (2008) *Sense of Place, Health and Quality of Life*, Franham, UK: Ashgate.
Finlay, L. (2011) *Phenomenology for Therapists*, Oxford: Wiley-Blackwell.
Fleuret, S. and Atkinson, S. (2007) 'Well-being, health and geography', *New Zealand Geographer*, 63: 106–118.
Frumkin, H., Frank, L. and Jackson, R. J. (2004) *Urban Sprawl and Public Health: Designing, Planning, and Building for Healthy Communities*, Washington, DC: Island Press.
Jacobs, J. (1961) *Death and Life of Great American Cities*, New York: Vintage.
Kearns, R. and Andrews, G. (2010) 'Geographies of well-being', in S. J. Smith, R. Pain, S. A. Marston and J. P. Jones (eds.), *The SAGE Handbook of Social Geographies*, pp. 309–328, London: Sage.
Klinenberg, E. (2002) *Heat Wave*, Chicago: University of Chicago Press.
Kopec, D. (2017) *Environmental Psychology for Design*, 3rd edn, New York: Fairchild.
Lessing, D. (1984) *The Diaries of Jane Somers*, New York: Vintage.
Malpas, J. (1999) *Place and Experience*, Cambridge: Cambridge University Press.
Malpas, J. (2001) 'Comparing topologies', *Philosophy and Geography*, 4: 231–238.
Malpas, J. (2009) 'Place and human being', *Environmental and Architectural Phenomenology*, 20 (3): 19–23.
Mehta, V. (2013) *The Street*, New York: Routledge.
Moran, D. (2000) *Introduction to Phenomenology*, London: Routledge.
Moran, D. (2005) *Edmund Husserl*, Cambridge: Polity Press.
Moran, D. (2014) 'Edmund Husserl's phenomenology of the habitual self', *Phenomenology and Mind*, 6: 26–47.
Pain, R. and Smith, S. J. (2010) 'Introduction geographies of well-being', in S. J. Smith, R. Pain, S. A. Marston and J. P. Jones (eds.), *The SAGE Handbook of Social Geographies*, London: Sage.
Relph, E. (1976) *Place and Placelessness*, London: Pion.
Schwanen, T. and Ziegler, F. (2011) 'Well-being, independence and mobility', *Ageing & Society*, 31: 719–733.
Seamon, D. (1979) *A Geography of the Lifeworld*, New York: St. Martin's.

Seamon, D. (1993) 'Different worlds coming together: A phenomenology of relationship as portrayed in Doris Lessing's *Diaries of Jane Somers*', in D. Seamon (ed.), *Dwelling, Seeing, and Designing*, Albany, NY: State University of New York Press.

Seamon, D. (2013a) 'Lived bodies, place, and phenomenology', *Journal of Human Rights and the Environment*, 4 (2): 143–166.

Seamon, D. (2013b) 'Phenomenology and uncanny homecomings', in D. Boscaljon (ed.), *Resisting the Place of Belonging*, Farnham, UK: Ashgate.

Seamon, D. (2014) 'Physical and virtual environments: Meaning of place and space', in B. Schell and M. Scaffa (eds.), *Willard & Spackman's Occupational Therapy*, 12th edn, Philadelphia: Wippincott, Williams & Wilkens.

Seamon, D. (2018) *Life Takes Place: Phenomenology, Lifeworlds, and Place Making*, New York: Routledge.

Stefanovic, I. L. (2008) 'Holistic paradigms of health and place', in J. Eyles and A. Williams (eds.), *Sense of Place, Health and Quality of Life*, Franham, UK: Ashgate.

Steinbock, A. (1995) *Home and Beyond*, Evanston, IL: Northwestern University Press.

Steinfeld, E. and White, J. (2010) *Inclusive Housing*, New York: Norton.

van Manen, M. (2014) *Phenomenology of Practice*, Walnut Creek, CA: West Coast Press.

Ziegler, F. and Schwanen, T. (2011) 'An exploratory analysis of mobility and well-being in later life', *Ageing & Society*, 31: 758–781.

11

HERITAGE AND WELL-BEING

Therapeutic places, past and present

Timothy Darvill, Vanessa Heaslip, and Kerry Barrass

Introduction

Physical and mental well-being are universal concerns amongst human societies. Many ancient sites, from prehistoric stone circles to great medieval churches, hosted ceremonies to maintain or restore the health of peoples' bodies and souls. The World Heritage Site of Stonehenge on Salisbury Plain, UK, is believed to have been a place of healing based on the presence of powerful stones brought to the site from the Preseli Hills of west Wales (Darvill 2016; Darvill & Wainwright 2014). Healing ceremonies have been held at the cathedral in Santiago de Compostela in Galicia, northwest Spain, also a World Heritage Site, for more than a thousand years because of the presence of powerful human remains believed to be those of St James the Apostle (Roux 2004). And in eastern Turkey, ancient Anatolian rock monuments closely connected with healing traditions are still used therapeutically by local communities who see them not as relics of the archaeological past but as part of the lived present (Harmanşahe 2015: 150). So can heritage play a role in promoting health, well-being, and quality of life in modern Western societies?

Recent surveys suggest that many people certainly think so (Fujiwara et al. 2014a). The "Taking Part" survey aimed at providing a measurement of how engaging with sport and culture might increase people's happiness found that those who "visited a heritage site in the last 12 months are significantly happier than those who had not" (DCMS 2014: 4, 2016a). A study by the Heritage Lottery Fund found that 81 per cent of residents questioned said that local heritage was important to them personally, of whom 50 per cent estimated that it had an impact on their personal quality of life which they rated at 7 out of 10 or higher (HLF 2015: 5). In addition, the economic value of visiting heritage sites in terms of improved well-being has been calculated at £1646 per person per year, based on the amount of money that would have to be taken away from a person to restore them to their level of well-being had they not visited a heritage site (Fujiwara et al. 2014b: 26).

Against such a background it is not surprising that the contribution of heritage to well-being is deeply enshrined in legislation and public policy at many levels. The Council of Europe's 2005 *Framework Convention on the Value of Cultural Heritage for Society* (also known as the Faro Convention) emphasized that: "the conservation of cultural heritage and its sustainable use have human development and quality of life as their goal" (CoE 2005: Art. 1). In Britain at the same time Tessa Jowell, then Culture Secretary, issued a personal essay entitled *Better Places to Live* which discussed the role of the historic environment in building and maintaining identity, noting that historic places form part of peoples' lives and that "we should do more to make this connection between people and places" (Jowell 2005: 13–14). A decade later the

Government's *Culture White Paper 2016* contained an undertaking to "develop and promote the contribution of the cultural sectors to improving health and well-being" (DCMS 2016b: 9), acknowledging that "we are beginning to understand better the profound relationship between culture, health and well-being" (DCMS 2016b: 13). Throughout the paper there was strong emphasis on the role that culture plays in the well-being both of society as a whole and of individuals, including contributions to improving mental health (DCMS 2016b: 15).

In this chapter we contextualize these public perceptions and aspirational public policies by reviewing the development of interest in therapeutic places, and summarizing the achievements of heritage-based projects that promote physical and mental well-being through engagements with landscapes, encounters with museum collections, and participation in archaeological fieldwork. We conclude with a brief account of the Human Henge project based in the Stonehenge landscape. This programme aims to provide qualitative and semi-quantitative assessments of the impact of using cultural heritage to enhance mental well-being, and allows consideration of some of the implications for developing further initiatives in this field.

From pilgrimage roads to designed gardens

Stonehenge and Santiago de Compostela were, like many sacred sites closely associated with healing across the ancient world, places of pilgrimage, and it is in this simple activity that we find the roots of the connection between heritage and well-being. Pilgrimage itself concerns spiritual renewal, emotional enrichment, renunciation of the past, guidance about the future, performing rites of passage, or searching for physical and spiritual healing (Armstrong 2012: 21). But as Slavin points out, the pilgrim's journey is not merely a means to an end; it is a process of personal development, an opportunity to be reflective, and a healing experience (2003: 17). Monuments and structures along the route, as well as those at the journey's end, are significant and form enduring locations in changing landscapes (2003: 6). Powell discusses the performative aspects of medieval pilgrimage, specifically that related to St Æbbe, in which pilgrims had to follow a prescribed series of movements through difficult terrain to reach the healing location (Powell 2014: 84). This itinerary defining how places are encountered gives a commonality of experience and also allows the pilgrims a sensation of preparing themselves to be healed, heightening their anticipation that, when they correctly complete the set requirements, they will increase the likelihood of a cure or miracle. Doughty (2013) also explores the pilgrimage to Santiago de Compostela as a way of experiencing a landscape in a bodily sense, as well as being an opportunity to socialize with others and accumulate the physical benefits of the activity itself. Tim Ingold comments further on the social potential of moving around the landscape with others; interacting and constantly adjusting to their presence (Ingold 2000: 196). Pilgrimage as a tool for self-healing is suggested by Rountree (2006), while Edensor (2000) explores walking as a way of distancing oneself from the everyday (2000: 84 and 103) and as a restorative activity (2000: 86).

Pilgrimage involves an active engagement with landscape – conventionally defined as the natural or imagined scenery – and it was perhaps this link that triggered an interest in landscape as a therapeutic entity in Britain during the early nineteenth century. In the context of institutionalizing those diagnosed with mental health conditions (Rutherford 2004: 28), asylum landscapes were designed to act as aids to recovery that facilitated the return of patients to a functional role in society. Indeed, the creation of such landscapes became a recognized specialization within landscape gardening (Rutherford 2005: 62). Examples include the grounds of Brislington House in Bristol, opened as a private asylum in 1806 (Hickman 2005: 47), where landscape features designed by Edward Long Fox included pathways, walks, leisure facilities, and a grotto, created in the hope of improving the emotional state of patients (Hickman 2005: 59).

As new clinically based approaches to mental healthcare gained popularity in the mid-twentieth century so the earlier focus on environment and landscape as therapeutic tools declined (Collins et al. 2016). But the tide has turned again, and over the last 30 years there has been renewed interest in the role of therapeutic landscapes built upon new research (Collins et al. 2016: 675).

A trigger for a re-evaluation of the environment as an element of recovery in a clinical setting came in 1984 with a paper by Robert Ulrich in *Science*. Here he outlined a study in which hospital patients with a view over a natural landscape recovered from surgery significantly faster, and with lower intake of painkillers, than those with a view of a plain brick wall (Ulrich 1984). In 1991, Ulrich and colleagues published a second study that examined the effect on stress recovery of watching videotapes; those watching films of natural environments recovered faster than those whose viewing was confined to urban environments (Ulrich et al. 1991). Significantly, these differences between rural and urban landscapes also appear in a later study by Hartig and colleagues who used clinical measurements to show that exposure to rural environments had a calming and restorative effect, whereas the urban environment exacerbated negative factors such as feelings of anger and aggression (Hartig et al. 2003: 121–122; Hartig & Cooper Marcus 2006).

The work that Ulrich and others started was extrapolated to underpin the concept of a "therapeutic landscape" by Wil Gesler in 1992. He described how landscapes might be experienced as "therapeutic" and how they become more than a passive physical entity in order to exert a restorative or healing influence (Gesler 1992). Gesler proposed a fusion approach, involving not only the medical community but also a range of other social sciences (Gesler 1992: 744). Expanding on this, Gesler then proposed that a medical geographic response was an appropriate way of addressing the perceived crisis in modern healthcare which he characterized as being based on a largely biomedical approach to well-being (Gesler 1993). Using the ancient healing centre of the Asclepian Sanctuary near Epidauros, Greece, as an example, Gesler explored how its natural landscape setting, buildings, history, mythology, reputation, and appeal to experts rendered it an accepted "therapeutic landscape" (1993: 178–184). He suggested that these factors could be applied more successfully to healing locations in the modern world, improving their effect on well-being by widening their remit to include physical, mental, and spiritual dimensions (1993: 186).

Therapeutic landscapes in theory

Shifting from a biomedical approach to a socioecological one as Gesler (2006) suggested, means stepping beyond conventional understandings of the landscape as a physical entity to allow it agency and power. As Tim Ingold discussed, landscape in a cultural sense is "the world as it is known to those who dwell therein, who inhabit its places and journey along the paths connecting them" (Ingold 2000: 193). This approach expanded a landscape's therapeutic potential beyond that which is physically experienced, known, or understood, to encompass what might in addition be felt or sensed through emotional and intellectual responses (Darvill 2015). This was an idea echoed by Edmunds Bunkše's description of how a landscape is "a way of being in the world" (2007) and that reconciling an internal landscape with the external environment can be significant for shaping an individual's place in the world (Bunkše 2007: 219). See also Mugerauer, Chapter 3; Seamon, Chapter 10; and Rapport, Chapter 2, this volume, in illuminating the complex relation between place and well-being. Taking a psychoanalytic approach, Emma Rose (2012) suggests that a participant's mind is an active component of a therapeutic landscape, as the perceived landscape is transformed by the participant just as it transforms them (2012: 1382–1383). However, Rose also cautions that we need to distinguish between real and imagined landscapes, with negatives contained within the imagined landscape where they can be controlled and modified, and familiar real landscapes playing a role in psychoanalysis (2012: 1385–1386).

Two other important dimensions of the ongoing relationship between landscapes and well-being emerged for discussion in the early twenty-first century. First was the matter of what was being achieved. Terry Hartig and Clare Cooper Marcus (2006: S36) sounded a timely alarm that "healing" is an unfortunate term when used in a medical sense, as it implies "cure" or complete recovery from a condition. They noted that more appropriate terms might be "therapeutic" or "restorative". No engagement with an environment or landscape can promise a cure, but participants can be given the opportunity to experience some level of improvement in their conditions. This perspective sits well with work by Les Todres and Kathleen T. Galvin

(2010, Chapters 8, this volume) exploring the nature of well-being in existential terms, emphasizing its individuality and the potential for wide-ranging differences of experience (Galvin & Todres, Chapter 30, this volume).

Second was a recognition that the issue was multi-disciplinary. Whilst Ulrich's original ideas regarding the nature of indoor medical or medicalized settings remain under discussion (e.g. Gesler & Curtis 2007), the concept had been expanded to include anthropological considerations, population-specific landscapes, and some locations which might be considered both therapeutic and harmful. Kaplan had earlier been concerned that a greater connection between disciplines and a synthesis of approach was still needed when considering the therapeutic landscape, also arguing that both physical and non-physical engagement with a landscape could have a therapeutic effect (Kaplan 1995: 179–180). These concerns were echoed by Andrews (2004). Williams's edited volume *Therapeutic Landscapes* (2007) presented papers which expand the concept to include interior and cognitive, as well as exterior environments and a range of interpretations of what might be considered "therapeutic".

Why therapeutic landscapes have the effects that are claimed, and what exactly they represent, remains far from clear (Cleary et al. 2017: 122). Different population groups are probably affected in different ways (Ward Thompson 2011: 194), and the perception of and interaction with such landscapes differs between individuals; there is no "one-size-fits-all" intervention (Ward Thompson 2011: 126). Reviewing a range of sources on landscape and well-being, Abraham and colleagues concluded that the highlighted benefits derived from opportunities for physical activity, relaxation, and social support led to improved concentration and emotional stability (Abraham et al. 2010: 66), all traits that can be seen in recent case studies.

Therapeutic landscapes in action

Through the first two decades of the twenty-first century many residential institutions have embraced the idea of landscaped gardens as a therapeutic element, although Moon and colleagues have argued that in many cases these were as much a marketing ploy as a therapeutic strategy (Moon et al. 2006: 145). At the same time, the move towards non-institutionalized care (Gleason & Kearns 2001: 61) has increased opportunities for project-based initiatives that build on the theme of therapeutic landscapes, as the following case studies show.

Livability Holton Lee in Dorset is described on its website as "a well-being discovery centre" (Livability Holton Lee 2016) which offers engagement with nature and outdoor activities in a natural landscape, as a way of coping with mental health issues and other disabilities. Conradson's (2005: 342–345) discussion of the impact of the centre is based on direct feedback from users, but does not attempt to use formal assessment methods. Three key benefits of the centre's approach are emphasized: distancing from the attendees' usual environment; interaction with the natural environment; and the creation of new social contacts (Conradson 2005: 346).

Engaging with walkers on the coastal footpath around the southwest of England resulted in a study by Bell and colleagues (2015a) which emphasized that the coastal landscape has value as a therapeutic environment, with well-being in this study measured using a methodology based on GPS and geo-narratives (Bell et al. 2015b). It is a project that may link across into the recreational and respite opportunities offered by seaside resorts (Darvill 2009: 371), suggesting that this is a particular kind of therapeutic landscape in its own right.

"Thrive" is the name of a small-scale social and therapeutic horticulture project in Reading. Its promotional material lists a series of benefits linked to the type of outdoor exercise and activity encouraged by gardening, including improved mental health through a sense of purpose and achievement, the opportunity to connect with others thereby reducing feelings of isolation or exclusion, and "Just feeling better for being outside, in touch with nature and in the 'great outdoors'" (Thrive 2016). At a slightly different scale, the NHS Forest initiative is currently planting areas of woodland on NHS-owned land to provide a potential therapeutic resource (NHS 2016). No evaluation of the impact of these projects appears to be taking place, although this field of research is still developing. They show how gardens of various kinds remain important in the range of therapeutic landscapes utilized, although Parr cautions that the nature of outdoor engagement is not inherently inclusive. Some of the target participants may lack the physical ability to engage in planned activities, which may also be limited – or reduced in therapeutic effect – by uncontrollable factors such as poor weather (Parr 2007: 558).

Museum collections

Weather is not such a problem when treating museums and their collections as a kind of indoor therapeutic landscape. The Arts Council-funded "Happy Museum Project" launched in 2011 was set up to investigate ways in which museums could "develop a holistic approach to well-being and sustainability" (HMP 2016). The project sought to re-imagine museums so that they could support institutional and community well-being and resilience (HMP 2016). Work was undertaken at more than a dozen institutions, with formal statistical analysis – the Wellbeing Valuation approach (Fujiwara & Campbell 2011) – used to examine effects on well-being. This work showed that visiting museums has "a positive impact on happiness and self-reported health" (Fujiwara 2013: 35). Similarly, a study of the benefits of health interventions in museums and galleries outside the usual medical settings concluded that physical and institutional distance from traditional locations is a benefit of this approach (Camic & Chatterjee 2013: 69).

Taking artefacts to hospitals and care homes provides an experience that has been well trialled with UCL's 2008 pilot "Heritage in Hospitals" project (Chatterjee et al. 2009). The work has given rise to a number of publications and further studies, as well as the development of the "Museum Wellbeing Measures Toolkit" (Thomson & Chatterjee 2013). Chatterjee and Noble (2009) documented a training exercise for medical students where it was found that physically interacting with archaeological artefacts provided a useful improvement in the quality of patients' lives whilst in hospital, measuring well-being with visual analogue scales (Chatterjee & Noble 2009: 45). Ander and colleagues discussed the difficulties inherent with measuring well-being outcomes in this type of project and proposed the use of a standardized "Well-being Outcomes Framework" (Ander et al. 2011). They went on to use grounded theory method data collection and analysis (Ander et al. 2013: 233) supported by the New Economics Foundation's well-being indicators (Ander et al. 2013: 231) in a qualitative study of museum artefact handling in hospitals. This demonstrated that engagement with museum artefacts in a hospital setting provided a range of benefits to patients with both mental and physical health issues, and that this approach was accessible and versatile (Ander et al. 2013: 240). Working in an unspecified NHS psychiatric hospital in the UK, Solway and colleagues (2015) confirmed short-term benefits to older psychiatric in-patients when they undertook museum artefact handling.

A Bournemouth University initiative explored the therapeutic effects of engagement with maritime archaeology for people with dementia (Cutler et al. 2016). This tied in with the "Prime Minister's Challenge on Dementia 2020" (DoH 2015), the aim of which was that people with dementia should be helped to "remain active and engaged, with regular opportunities for social interaction and activities focused on the individual" (DoH 2015: 33). It also addressed the integrative societal aspect of dementia caring raised in Green and Lakey (2013). Data collection took the form of ethnographic field notes, end of session discussions, and evaluation forms, with a data coding system and a thematic psychological analysis method (Cutler et al. 2016: 2). However, the published paper does not include the detailed results of this dataset, limiting itself to a summary of perceived benefits that included access to information, access to activities, access to education and learning, and access to support (Cutler et al. 2016: 3).

"Doing" as well as "looking" can be important, as shown by an all-male occupational therapy group run as a pilot at Beamish Museum (Kindleysides & Biglands 2015). This explored the opportunities afforded by the open-air heritage environment to improve health issues and social isolation. Participants engaged in a range of "Do It Yourself" building and toy-making activities using traditional tools from the museum collections (Kindleysides & Biglands 2015: 273–274). Whilst observation and monitoring revealed definite benefits for the participants (Kindleysides & Biglands 2015: 276), it concluded that the Well-Being Measures Toolkit (Thomson & Chatterjee 2013, 2015) was not particularly effective at evaluating this type of therapeutic activity (Kindleysides & Biglands 2015: 274) and that alternatives were needed.

Slightly different again was the "GalGael" project in Glasgow, a community-based charitable initiative that seeks to "offer hospitality to the margins" (GalGael Trust 2016a) through involvement with traditional boatbuilding and associated heritage skills and crafts. Whilst it has no aspirations to academic engagement or the formal measurement of participants' well-being, the case studies provided on their website illustrate the positive benefits to some participants (GalGael Trust 2016b). As with other aspects of the therapeutic landscapes movement, participation is emphasized.

Archaeological fieldwork

The most visible way in which heritage and well-being are connected is through archaeological fieldwork of various kinds, mainly under the wide-ranging banner of community archaeology that developed strongly in Britain from the 1980s (Marshall 2002). Many community archaeology projects include an intention to promote well-being in various ways, although few provide measured assessments of their impact.

Faye Sayer conducted research across six archaeological excavations, to explore whether participation in such fieldwork had an inherent capacity to improve the happiness of those taking part (Sayer 2015). The 170 participants were a mix of students undertaking the work as part of their educational courses, and volunteers involved with community projects. Formal measurement techniques included the Positive and Negative Effects Schedule (PANAS) and Modified Visual Analogue Scale (MVAS) (Sayer 2015: 251–252). Sayer concluded that archaeological work alone did not necessarily improve well-being because other external factors were significant. For example, volunteers in community projects scored more highly under the MVAS measurements than students undertaking mandatory fieldwork, suggesting that choice in participation may be a critical factor (Sayer 2015: 257). Similarly, the PANAS results indicated more negative outcomes for the students when compared with the community volunteers. External influences on negative outcomes might include factors such as the weather, which was poor during the pilot project, and tensions within the participant group (Sayer 2015: 258). A factor which significantly increased satisfaction was making archaeological discoveries, but this is a random occurrence and could not be planned or anticipated (Sayer 2015: 258). Key positive findings highlighted the benefits of the physical activity involved in archaeological work, together with the interactions with other participants and levels of job satisfaction. Sayer concludes that it is possible to design archaeological fieldwork projects that factor in many of the attributes identified as providing positive improvements to the participants' well-being (2015: 258).

Inclusivity is a major theme running through most community archaeology projects. One such project in Bristol sought to involve the homeless community in an archaeological investigation of their own city landscape, as they experience it. The project, undertaken in 2009, was designed to involve a minority community in an activity not usually open to them and they excavated a contemporary location used by the homeless community at "Turbo Island" in Stokes Croft, Bristol (Kiddey 2014). The impact on some participants was significant, apparently giving them the motivation to move beyond their situation at the beginning of the project (Kiddey & Schofield 2011: 20).

The Workers' Educational Association Heritage Lottery Funded project "Digability" aimed to involve disadvantaged people in a range of structured archaeological activities including surveys, small-scale excavations, artefact handling sessions, finds processing, creative workshops, and field trips across Yorkshire and Humberside from 2011 to 2014. Target participants included those with mental health issues (WEA 2016a) although therapeutic benefits to participants were initially seen as something of a side issue. Later, the project aims were updated on its website to "demonstrate how archaeology can develop a wide range of skills, both specific and transferable, build confidence and self-esteem and promote a sense of well-being and help community cohesion" (WEA 2016b: aim 3). An online forum related to the project encouraged discussion of the question "How can we measure and evidence the health and well-being benefits of participation in heritage activities?" amongst others, although it was noted that there was limited engagement with this (Beauchamp et al. 2014: 36). Anecdotal structured feedback from participants was very positive (Beauchamp et al. 2014: 39–42), with outcomes described as "significant and in some cases life-changing" (Beauchamp et al. 2014: 74).

"Past in Mind" was a Heritage Lottery Funded project run by Herefordshire Mind, to explore the potential for mental health recovery offered by engagement with archaeological activities (McMillan 2013; Lack 2014). The work suggested that archaeology was an analogy to uncovering and discovering elements of mental health in a way that promoted self-awareness and might prompt the recovery of participants (Lack 2014). Participants were involved in documentary research, surveys, and excavations at the lost medieval village of Studmarsh on the National Trust's Brockhampton Estate. Whilst the reported results were positive, no formal methods were used to measure the well-being of participants at the start, during the work, or at the conclusion of the project. Reported outcomes cover the ways in which participants developed and pursued interests in history and archaeology, and how the community became engaged with the project (McMillan 2013: 199).

Elmet Archaeological Services Ltd ran a 24-week therapeutic archaeological initiative, "The Mental Wellbeing Project", in partnership with the NHS Rotherham Commissioning Group (EASL 2016). The aim of this initiative was to deliver mental health therapies and services within the framework of archaeological activities by reducing social isolation, providing access to physical activity, and a variety of psychological health interventions including mindfulness, relaxation, and positive visualization. No assessment of its impact appears to have been published to date.

Operation Nightingale is a Ministry of Defence initiative founded in 2012 by the Defence Archaeology Group working in partnership with a range of archaeological units and universities, to provide rehabilitation for military personnel recently returned from operations in Afghanistan through participation in archaeological excavations (DAG 2017; MOD 2012; University of Glasgow 2015; University of Leicester 2014; Wessex Archaeology 2016). Excavations have been undertaken at Barrow Clump and Chisenbury Midden, Wiltshire, Caerwent, Glamorgan, and on the route of the A1 near Catterick, North Yorkshire. Whilst the project has an internet presence across various partner websites, little has been published concerning formal evaluation of its benefits. However, Alan Finnegan (2016) reviewed two Operation Nightingale excavations that took place in 2015 based on semi-structured interviews with participants and also a short survey to provide demographic background information. This revealed biological, psychological, emotional, and social benefits, with a suggestion that monitoring long-term benefits would be useful (Finnegan 2016: 21). It was also noted that the archaeological work was part of a broader set of activities that participants felt had been of use to them (Finnegan 2016: 21). It highlighted the benefits of working in a non-medical setting and accepting that the enjoyment of doing archaeology was as much a valued output as the academic knowledge that the research produced. Interestingly, Operation Nightingale has also been adopted as a military rehabilitation initiative in the United States (ONUSA 2016).

Big Heritage's 2015 "Dig Blacon" project near Chester, Cheshire, was a community archaeological dig partly funded by the local Public Health Team as a health and social inclusivity initiative (BH 2016). The work focused on the area around St Theresa's Catholic Primary School, Blacon, and involved surveys, test-pitting, excavations, and finds processing. The project issued a Health Evaluation report which stated that this was the first UK project where archaeological work had been commissioned by a Public Health Team specifically in order to improve health and well-being (BH 2015: 3). Formal evaluation of the planned benefits formed part of the project design and measurement was carried out using a variety of techniques. Two volunteers wore Fitbit technology to monitor their physical activity as they participated in the excavation of archaeological test-pits (BH 2015: 6–10). Qualitative results were gathered through feedback from participants and participating group organizers (BH 2015: 12–18) and a structured survey (BH 2015: 19–24), although the survey did not follow a previously established methodology. Approximately 92 per cent of respondents felt that the social aspect of the project had improved their health and/or well-being (BH 2015: 22). The project concluded that monitoring over a more sustained period of time would be beneficial.

Human Henge

Drawing on the results of many of these projects, Human Henge was undertaken in 2016–2017 in the Stonehenge landscape to combine archaeology and creativity as a way of improving mental health and reaching out to marginalized communities. Run by the Restoration Trust in partnership with Bournemouth University, the Richmond Fellowship, English Heritage, and The National Trust, participants take journeys of discovery to explore relationships between people and place in the past and the present (Human Henge 2016). The aim was to open up new ways of looking at the landscape and thereby break down some of the emotional barriers that underpin many mental health issues. By spending time at a selection of the sites, singing, dancing, making music, and looking both inwards and outwards it became possible for participants to connect with the landscape, the skyscape, the monuments, and, most importantly, with themselves and with other participants.

Each programme involved ten half-day sessions held in different parts of the landscape, including Durrington Walls and Woodhenge, the Cuckoo Stone, the King Barrow Ridge Barrow cemetery, and the reconstructed houses and displays at the Stonehenge visitor centre. A night-time walk along the Cursus provided a chance to experience the largest monument in the landscape under a star-lit sky. Each programme culminated in an early-morning ceremony inside Stonehenge, designed and executed by the participants themselves. Linking back to Rose's point (2012: 1395), the Stonehenge landscape becomes a familiar landscape, and one that allowed participants to move away from compartmentalized thinking in clinical settings and permitted a range of non-standard, creative, cross-disciplinary ways of thinking to influence care and therapeutic decisions, putting people back into the centre of care processes (Galvin & Todres 2007; Todres et al. 2009).

Unlike some of the previous projects mentioned in this chapter a key aspect of Human Henge was the formal evaluation that ran alongside the project. This research set out to review the impact of Human Henge on the mental well-being of its 25 participants through a mixture of qualitative and semi-quantitative surveys. At the start participants completed a baseline questionnaire capturing their thoughts and feelings about the project; the Short Warwick Edinburgh Mental Wellbeing Scale (Tennant et al. 2007) was used, supplemented by questions regarding their interests in history, heritage, and archaeology. The same questionnaire was repeated in the middle and at the end of the ten-week programme, and will be run again in 2018 a year after the sessions finished. Additionally, participants, volunteer helpers, and staff were involved in a series of focus groups to assist with evaluating the project and its impact using thematic analysis.

Conclusions

Heritage and well-being have deep-rooted and ancient connections extending back to the early days of pilgrimage. In modern times there have been many projects forging links between dimensions of heritage and well-being, and running through these are a number of common themes, three of which may be highlighted here. Especially important is the idea of journeying, a concept that can be applied at many scales; it is not only the physical act of moving through space, but also the emotional and intellectual progress towards improved well-being as part of the metaphysical journey of life. Second is the principle of structured engagement with people and places. And third is the range of opportunities offered for human interaction and making sense of empirical experiences. Much of the work undertaken to date highlights the value of inter-disciplinary approaches, the urgent need for more fully evaluated studies, and the opportunities to theorize the relationship in such a way that it generates productive approaches to managing heritage sites in sensitive, imaginative, and meaningfully engaging ways.

Acknowledgements

This chapter is based on research carried out as part of the Human Henge project funded by the Heritage Lottery Fund, Amesbury Area Board, Restoration Trust, Bournemouth University, Richmond Fellowship, and English Heritage, with assistance from the National Trust (http://humanhenge.org/). In preparing the text we would like to thank Laura Drysdale, Sara Lunt, Yvette Staelens, Daniel O'Donoghue, Toby Sutcliffe, Colin Caldow, Martin Allfrey, Katherine Snell, Briony Clifton, and all the participants in the Human Henge project for their enthusiasm and valuable insights into the evolving relationship between heritage and well-being.

References

Abraham, A., Sommerhalder, K. & Abel, T., 2010. Landscape and well-being: a scoping study on the health promoting impact of outdoor environments. *International Journal of Public Health*, 55, 59–69.

Ander, E., Thomson, L., Noble, G., Lanceley, A., Menon, U. & Chatterjee, H., 2011. Generic well-being outcomes: towards a conceptual framework for well-being outcomes in museums. *Museum Management and Curatorship*, 26 (3), 237–259.

Ander, E., Thomson, L., Noble, G., Lanceley, A., Menon, U. & Chatterjee, H., 2013. Heritage, health and well-being: assessing the impact of a heritage focused intervention on health and well-being. *International Journal of Heritage Studies*, 19 (3), 229–242.

Andrews, G., 2004. (Re)thinking the dynamics between healthcare and place: therapeutic geographies in treatment and care practices. *Area*, 36 (3), 307–318.

Armstrong, K., 2012. Pilgrimage: why do they do it? In: V. Porter (ed), *Hajj: journey to the heart of Islam*. London: The British Museum Press. 8–25.

Beauchamp, V., Hindle, R. & Thorpe, N., 2014. *"Digability": Inclusive archaeology education project. Evaluation report*. [Available online at: https://digability.files. wordpress.com/2015/01/archie-report-master1.pdf. Accessed 10 May 2017].

Bell, S., Phoenix, C., Lovell, R. & Wheeler, B., 2015a. Seeking everyday wellbeing: the coast as a therapeutic landscape. *Social Science & Medicine*, 142, 56–67.

Bell, S., Phoenix, C., Lovell, R. & Wheeler, B., 2015b. Using GPS and geo-narratives: a methodological approach for understanding and situating everyday green space encounters. *Area*, 47, 88–96.

BH [Big Heritage], 2015. *Dig Blacon: health evaluation*. Chester: Big Heritage. [Available online at: http://bigheritage. co.uk/files/2015/07/Dig-Blacon-Health-Evaluation-2016-1.pdf. Accessed 10 May 2017].

BH [Big Heritage], 2016. *Dig Blacon: project overview*. Chester: Big Heritage. [Available online at: http://bigheritage. co.uk/digblacon/. Accessed 10 May 2017].

Bunkše, E., 2007. Feeling is believing, or landscape as a way of being in the world. *Geografiska Annaler* (Series B, human geography), 89 (3), 219–231.

Camic, P. & Chatterjee, H., 2013. Museums and art galleries as partners for public health interventions. *Perspectives in Public Health*, 133 (66), 66–71.

Chatterjee, H. & Noble, G., 2009. Object therapy: A student-selected component exploring the potential of museum object handling as an enrichment activity for patients in hospital. *Global Journal of Health Science*, 1 (2), 42–49.

Chatterjee, H., Vreeland, S. & Noble, G., 2009. Museopathy: Exploring the healing potential of handling museum objects. *Museum and Society*, 7 (3), 164–177.

Cleary, A., Fielding, K., Bell, S., Murray, Z. & Roiko, A., 2017. Exploring potential mechanisms involved in the relationship between eudaimonic wellbeing and nature connection. *Landscape and Urban Planning*, 158, 119–128.

CoE [Council of Europe], 2005. *Council of Europe Framework convention on the value of cultural heritage for society: council of Europe treaty series – No. 199*. Strasbourg: Council of Europe. [Available online at: www.coe.int/en/web/conventions/full-list/-/conventions/rms/0900001680083746. Accessed 10 May 2017].

Collins, J., Avey, S. & Lekkas, P., 2016. Lost landscapes of healing: the decline of therapeutic mental health landscapes. *Landscape Research*, 41 (4), 664–677.

Conradson, D., 2005. Landscape, care and the relational self: therapeutic encounters in rural England. *Health & Place*, 11, 337–348.

Cutler, C., Palma, P. & Innes, A., 2016. Tales of the sea: Connecting people with dementia to the UK heritage through maritime archaeology (innovative practice). *Dementia: The International Journal of Social Research and Practice*, 1–5. [doi:10.1177/1471301216666171]

DAG [Defence Archaeology Group], 2017. *Defence archaeology group*. London: Defence Archaeology Group. [Available online at: www.dag.org.uk/. Accessed 10 May 2017].

Darvill, T., 2009. Review of 'Therapeutic landscapes' Edited by Allison Williams. *Time and Mind*, 2 (3), 271–274. [doi:1 0.2752/17516909X12464529903533]

Darvill, T., 2015. Making futures from the remains of the distant past: archaeological heritage, connective knowledge, and the promotion of well-being. In: M. van den Dries, S. van der Linde & A. Strecker (eds), *Fernweh: crossing borders and connecting people in archaeological heritage management. Essays in honour of Prof. Willem J.H. Willems*. Leiden: Sidestone Press. 42–46.

Darvill, T., 2016. Roads to Stonehenge: a prehistoric healing centre and pilgrimage site in southern Britain. In: A. Ranft & W. Schenkluhn (eds), *Kulturstraßen als konzept: 20 jahre straße der Romanik*. Regensburg: Schnell und Steiner GmbH. 155–166.

Darvill, T. & Wainwright, G., 2014. Beyond Stonehenge: Carn Menyn Quarry and the origin and date of bluestone extraction in the Preseli Hills of south-west Wales. *Antiquity*, 88, 1099–1114.

DCMS [Department for Culture, Media and Sport], 2014. *Culture, sport and wellbeing: an analysis of the Taking Part survey*. London: Department for Culture, Media and Sport. [Available online at: www.gov.uk/government/uploads/sys tem/uploads/attachment_data/file/476322/Culture_Sport_and_Wellbeing-An_analysis_of_the_Taking_Part_Sur vey.pdf. Accessed 10 May 2017].

DCMS [Department for Culture, Media and Sport], 2016a. *Taking part survey*. London: Department for Culture, Media and Sport. [Available online at: www.gov.uk/guidance/taking-part-survey. Accessed 10 May 2017].

DCMS [Department for Culture, Media and Sport], 2016b. *The culture white paper*. London: Department for Culture, Media and Sport. [Available online at: www.gov.uk/government/ uploads/system/uploads/attachment_data/ file/510798/DCMS_The_Culture_White_Paper_3_.pdf. Accessed 10 May 2017].

DoH [Department of Health], 2015. *Prime Minister's challenge on dementia 2020*. London: Department of Health. [Available online at: www.gov.uk/government/uploads/ system/uploads/attachment_data/file/215101/dh_133176.pdf. Accessed 10 May 2017].

Doughty, K., 2013. Walking together: the embodied and mobile production of a therapeutic landscape. *Health and Place*, 24, 140–146.

EASL [Elmet Archaeological Services Ltd], 2016. *The mental wellbeing project*. Rotherham: Elmet Archaeological Services Ltd. [Available online at: www.elmetarchaeology.co.uk/ mentalwellbeing.html. Accessed 10 May 2017].

Edensor, T., 2000. Walking in the British countryside: reflexivity, embodied practices and ways to escape. *Body and Society*, 6 (3–4), 81–106.

Finnegan, A., 2016. The biopsychosocial benefits and shortfalls for armed forces veterans engaged in archaeological activities. *Nurse Education Today*, 47, 15–22.

Fujiwara, D., 2013. *Museums and happiness: the value of participating in museums and the arts*. Stowmarket: Museum of East Anglian Life. [Available online at: http://happymuseumproject.org/happy-museums-are-good-for-you-report-publication/museums-and-happiness/. Accessed 10 May 2017].

Fujiwara, D. & Campbell, R., 2011. *Valuation techniques for social cost-benefit analysis: stated preference, revealed preference and subjective well-being approaches*. London: Department for Work and Pensions and HM Treasury. [Available online at: www.gov.uk/government/uploads/system/uploads/attachment_data/file/209107/greenbook_valuationtech niques.pdf. Accessed 10 May 2017].

Fujiwara, D., Cornwall, T. & Dolan, P., 2014a. *Heritage and wellbeing*. London: English Heritage. [Available online at: https://content.historicengland.org.uk/content/heritage-counts/pub/2190644/heritage-and-wellbeing.pdf. Accessed 10 May 2017].

Fujiwara, D., Kudrna, L. & Dolan, P., 2014b. *Quantifying and valuing the wellbeing impacts of culture and sport*. London: Department for Culture, Media & Sport. [Available online at: www.gov.uk/government/uploads/system/uploads/ attachment_data/file/304899/Quantifying_and_valuing_the_wellbeing_impacts_of_sport_and_culture.pdf. Accessed 10 May 2017].

GalGael Trust, 2016a. *GalGael: roots*. Glasgow: The GalGael Trust. [Available online at: www.galgael.org/about-us/roots. Accessed 10 May 2017].

GalGael Trust, 2016b. *GalGael: case studies*. Glasgow: The GalGael Trust. [Available online at: www.galgael.org/folk/ case-studies. Accessed 10 May 2017].

Galvin, K. & Todres, L., 2007. The creativity of 'unspecialization:' a contemplative direction for integrative scholarly practice. *Phenomenology and Practice*, 1 (1), 31–46.

Gesler, W., 1992. Therapeutic landscapes: medical issues in light of the new cultural geography. *Social Science and Medicine*, 34 (7), 735–746.

Gesler, W., 1993. Therapeutic landscapes: theory and a case study of Epidauros, Greece. *Environment and Planning D: Society and Space*, 11, 171–189.

Gesler, W., 2006. Geography of health and healthcare. In: B. Warf (ed), *Encyclopedia of human geography*. Thousand Oaks: Sage Publications, Inc. 205–206.

Gesler, W. & Curtis, S., 2007. Application of concepts of therapeutic landscapes to the design of hospitals in the UK: the example of a mental health facility in London. In: A. Williams (ed), *Therapeutic landscapes*. Aldershot: Ashgate. 149–164.

Gleason, B. & Kearns, R., 2001. Remoralising landscapes of care. *Environment and Planning D: Society and Space*, 19, 61–80.

Green, G. & Lakey, L., 2013. *Building dementia-friendly communities: a priority for everyone*. London: Alzheimer's Society. [Available online at: www.alzheimers.org.uk/downloads/file/1916/ building_dementia_friendly_communities_a_priority_for_everyone. Accessed 10 May 2017].

Harmanşahe, Ö., 2015. *Place, memory and healing: an archaeology of Anatolian rock monuments*. Abingdon: Routledge.

Hartig, T. & Cooper Marcus, C., 2006. Essay: healing gardens – places for nature in healthcare. *The Lancet*, 368 (Supplement 1), S36–S37.

Hartig, T., Evans, G.W., Jamner, L.D., Davis, D.S. & Gärling, T., 2003. Tracking restoration in natural and urban field settings. *Journal of Environmental Psychology*, 23 (2), 109–123.

Hickman, C., 2005. The picturesque at Brislington House, Bristol: the role of landscape in relation to the treatment of mental illness in the early nineteenth-century asylum. *Garden History*, 33, 47–60.

HLF [Heritage Lottery Fund], 2015. *20 years in 12 places: improving heritage, improving places, improving lives*. London: Heritage Lottery Fund. [Available online at: www.hlf.org.uk/about-us/research-evaluation/20-years-heritage. Accessed 10 May 2017].

HMP [The Happy Museum Project], 2016. *The happy museum: about*. London: The Happy Museum Project. [Available online at: http://happymuseumproject.org/about/. Accessed 10 May 2017].

Human Henge, 2016. *Human Henge: about*. London: The Restoration Trust. [Available online at: http://humanhenge. org/about/. Accessed 10 May 2017].

Ingold, T., 2000. *The perception of the environment*. Abingdon: Routledge.

Jowell, T., 2005. *Better places to live: government identity and the value of the historic and built environment*. London: Department for Culture, Media and Sport.

Kaplan, S., 1995. The restorative benefits of nature: toward an integrative framework. *Journal of Environmental Psychology*, 15 (3), 169–182.

Kiddey, R., 2014. Turbo Island, Bristol: excavating a contemporary homeless place. *Post-Medieval Archaeology*, 48, 133–150.

Kiddey, R. & Schofield, J., 2011. Embrace the margins: adventures in archaeology and homelessness. *Public Archaeology*, 10 (1), 4–22.

Kindleysides, M. & Biglands, E., 2015. 'Thinking outside the box, and making it too': piloting an occupational therapy group at an open-air museum. *Arts and Health*, 7 (3), 271–278.

Lack, K., 2014. *Past in mind: a heritage project and mental health recovery*. Hereford: Privately Published.

Livability Holton Lee, 2016. *Livability Holton Lee: a place to discover wellbeing*. Poole: Livability Holton Lee. [Available online at: www.holtonlee.org/. Accessed 10 May 2017].

Marshall, Y., 2002. What is community archaeology? *World Archaeology*, 34 (2), 211–219.

McMillan, I., 2013. Making a mark on history with the past in mind. *Mental Health and Social Inclusion*, 17 (4), 195–201.

MoD [Ministry of Defence], 2012. *Op Nightingale*. London: Ministry of Defence. [Available online at: www.army.mod. uk/royalengineers/units/32526.aspx. Accessed 10 May 2017].

Moon, G., Kearns, R. & Joseph, A., 2006. Therapeutic landscapes and the (re)valorization of confinement in the era of community care. *Transactions of the Institute of British Geographers* (New Series), 31 (2), 131–149.

NHS, 2016. *NHS forest: Growing forests for health*. London: NHS Forest. [Available online at: http://nhsforest.org/. Accessed 10 May 2017].

ONUSA [Operation Nightingale USA], 2016. *Operation Nightingale USA*. Michigan: Operation Nightingale USA. [Available online at: www.opnightingaleusa.com/. Accessed 10 May 2017].

Parr, H., 2007. Mental health, nature work, and social inclusion. *Environment and Planning D: Society and Space*, 25 (3), 537–561.

Powell, H., 2014. Pilgrimage, performance and miracle cures in the twelfth century *miracula* of St Æbbe. In: E. Gemi-Iordanou, S. Gordon, R. Matthew, E. McInnes & R. Pettitt (eds), *Medicine, healing and performance*. Oxford: Oxbow Books. 71–85.

Rose, E., 2012. Encountering place: a psychoanalytic approach for understanding how therapeutic landscapes benefit health and wellbeing. *Health & Place*, 18 (6), 1381–1387.

Rountree, K., 2006. Performing the divine: neo-pagan pilgrimages and embodiment at sacred sites. *Body and Society*, 12 (4), 95–115.

Roux, J., 2004. *The roads to Santiago de Compostela.* Vic-en-Bigorre: MSM.

Rutherford, S., 2004. Victorian and Edwardian institutional landscapes in England. *Landscapes*, 5 (2), 25–41.

Rutherford, S., 2005. Landscapers for the mind: English asylum designers, 1845–1914. *Garden History*, 33 (1), 61–86.

Sayer, F., 2015. Can digging make you happy? Archaeological excavations, happiness and heritage. *Arts & Health*, 7, 247–260.

Slavin, S., 2003. Walking as spiritual practice: the pilgrimage to Santiago de Compostela. *Body and Society*, 9 (3), 1–18.

Solway, R., Thomson, L., Camic, P. & Chatterjee, H., 2015. Museum object handling groups in older adult mental health inpatient care. *International Journal of Mental Health Promotion*, 17 (4), 201–214.

Tennant, R., Hiller, L., Fishwick, R., Platt, P., Joseph, S., Weich, S., Parkinson, J., Secker, J. & Stewart-Brown, S., 2007. The Warwick-Edinburgh Mental Well-being Scale (WEMWBS): Development and UK validation. *Health and Quality of Life Outcome*, 5, 63. [doi:101186/1477-7252-5-63]

Thompson, C.W., 2011. Linking landscape and health: the recurring theme. *Landscape and Urban Planning*, 99 (3–4), 187–195.

Thomson, L. & Chatterjee, H., 2013. *UCL museum wellbeing measures toolkit.* London: University College London. [Available online at: www.ucl.ac.uk/culture/resources?nid=673. Accessed 10 May 2017].

Thomson, L. & Chatterjee, H., 2015. Measuring the impact of museum activities on well-being: developing the Museum Well-Being Measures Toolkit. *Museum Management and Curatorship*, 30 (1), 44–62.

Thrive, 2016. *Thrive: what is social and therapeutic horticulture?* Reading: Thrive. [Available online at: www.thrive.org.uk/what-is-and-social-and-therapeutic-horticulture.aspx. Accessed 10 May 2017].

Todres, L. & Galvin, K., 2010. "Dwelling-mobility": an existential theory of well-being. *International Journal of Qualitative Studies on Health and Well-Being*, 5 (3), 1–6.

Todres, L., Galvin, K. & Holloway, I., 2009. The humanization of healthcare: a value framework for qualitative research. *International Journal of Qualitative Studies on Health and Well-Being*, 4 (2), 1–10.

Ulrich, R., 1984. View through a window may influence recovery from surgery. *Science*, 224 (4647), 420–421.

Ulrich, R., Simons, R., Losito, B., Fiorito, E., Miles, M. & Zelson, M., 1991. Stress recovery during exposure to natural and urban environments. *Journal of Environmental Psychology*, 11 (3), 201–230.

University of Glasgow, 2015. *Archaeologists and veterans to explore what lies beneath Waterloo Battlefield, 200 years on.* Glasgow: University of Glasgow. [Available online at: www.gla.ac.uk/news/headline_392886_en.html. Accessed 10 May 2017].

University of Leicester, 2014. *Military operations on the archaeological front.* Leicester: University of Leicester. [Available online at: www2.le.ac.uk/offices/press/press-releases/2014/may/military-operations-on-the-archaeological-front. Accessed 10 May 2017].

WEA [Workers' Educational Association], 2016a. *Digability: about the project.* Leeds: Workers' Educational Association Yorkshire and Humber Regional Office. [Available online at: https://digability.wordpress.com/about/about-the-project/ Accessed 10 May 2017].

WEA [Workers' Educational Association], 2016b. *Digability: stated aims of the project.* Leeds: Workers' Educational Association Yorkshire and Humber Regional Office. [Available online at: https://digability.wordpress.com/about/stated-aims-of-the-project/ Accessed 10 May 2017].

Wessex Archaeology, 2016. *Operation Nightingale.* Salisbury: Wessex Archaeology Ltd. [Available online at: www.wessexarch.co.uk/OperationNightingale. Accessed 10 May 2017].

Williams, A. (ed), 2007. *Therapeutic landscapes.* Aldershot: Ashgate Publishing.

12

DISABILITY AND AMBIGUITIES

Technological support in a disaster context

Minae Inahara

Introduction

The 2011 Tōhoku earthquake and tsunami and the Fukushima Daiichi nuclear disaster has provided additional difficulties and challenges to daily life for all human beings in Japan, perhaps especially those with disabilities or chronic illnesses (including the elderly). In particular, people with disabilities and chronic illnesses required specific accessible forms of evacuation and shelter, for example, location and accessibility of shelters, accommodation and facilities available at shelters.

When the 9.0-magnitude earthquake hit off the east coast of Japan on 11th March 2011, I was in Tokushima (Shikoku island – mid-Western part of Japan). I did not feel any quake at all. In fact, a seminar talk was planned for me on 13th March at the University of Tokyo, so I was packing my bag and getting ready. I turned on the TV and watched some afternoon gossip shows with my grandmother. At 2.45 pm, the TV screen suddenly changed into the emergency information for the earthquake and tsunami warnings. I was so shocked; however, I did not know how big the earthquake was at that moment. Gradually, I came to realise that the quake was one of the largest in recorded history, and triggered a 23-foot tsunami that battered Japan's coast, killing more than 15,000 people (at least 2500 people are still missing) and sweeping away massive numbers of cars, homes, buildings, and boats.

Then, the whole nation was in complete panic and has been since the 3.11 disasters. It has been dreadful for most of victims, but in particular for those with disabilities and chronic illness. The natural and manmade disasters have disrupted their social contacts and support network, and resulted in incredible human suffering and countless humanitarian catastrophes. The 3.11 disasters have underscored the importance of two of human securities: 'freedom from terror and anxiety', where the natural and manmade disasters disrupted people's day-to-day lives, and 'freedom from need', where the disasters led to mass disruptions, a failure of the public health system, and lack of the basic requirements of life. Thus, the 3.11 disasters have raised serious human security questions for the international community and made me rethink how to voice silent people who have been vulnerable under these special circumstances. In this chapter, I want to argue for the phenomenological observation of the world from an embodied perspective, that is, a view of the embodied subject who experiences a complex, constructing, transforming, and living body, as opposed to the fixed assumption of the human body and the world.

I consider that an understanding of perception reveals that the world (all knowledge) cannot be detached from an embodied subject and that, as Donna Haraway (1991) considers, all knowledge is situated. The 3.11 disasters have made me realise that the world, like the human body, is living and transforming and that all knowledge has to be revised and altered regarding the lived world. Like Haraway (1991) who argues for her deconstructive thoughts of the masculinised and fixed metaphors and narratives that lead the science of primatology, I want to discuss that we need to question the able-bodied and normative metaphors and narratives that lead the technology for the able-bodied world. This is my "Cyborg Manifesto", wherein I use Haraway's theory of the cyborg to undermine traditional demarcations, dichotomies, conceptual divisions, and social constructions regarding human abilities and vulnerabilities, and to suggest a cyborg phenomenology to challenge the normative assumption of the world where we have been forced to believe that the human culture can control nature. Moreover, in this chapter, my desire is to find a way to voice the silent — those with disabilities or illnesses who have become even more vulnerable in the 3.11 disasters.

Silencing the lived voice

Both in normal times and during disasters, the burden of health problems, disease, and death lies heaviest on vulnerable groups who are least able to afford medical treatment and preventive measures, and whose Japanese government has the least capacity to meet these urgent needs. Simultaneously, the human cost of the natural and manmade disasters has been increasing in Japan. In order to conserve electricity and prevent unexpected power cuts, Tokyo Electric Power Company (TEPCO) enforced the government-scheduled blackouts across the region. Japan has been in the midst of a major, nationwide energy crisis. Three-fourths of Japan's nuclear power plants were offline for safety checks after the disaster that began unfolding at Fukushima following the earthquake and tsunami. We have reduced energy consumption, and consequently we have had to change our life-style in order to use less electricity. However, the change of our life-style has been problematic, in particular, for those with disabilities and illness.

The problems arising from the change of our life-style (our living space) have been very serious, for example, for those who use an electric wheelchair and those with amblyopia. Those in an electric wheelchair cannot leave their house if they do not have special equipment such as an extra 'condenser'. Those with amblyopia cannot walk around the home, because they cannot see anything in the dark. Moreover, in the case of a patient using an artificial respirator, he or she needs a constant electricity supply. In normal times, people with disabilities have the voice and access to the world where they can protect themselves from death and danger; however, in disasters, they become silent — no voice. Most able-bodied people after the earthquakes and tsunami have become *ecologically* disabled, and then those with disabilities have become more vulnerable than before, and in the end, have become completely silent.

As a researcher of health and welfare studies, Kaori Iwasaki (2011) has reported the situation of people with disabilities in the affected areas. She states:

> [A]t evacuation shelters which they reached after escaping the disaster, disabled persons were forced to face many inconveniences due to difficulties moving in wheelchairs and lack of medical equipment, medications, and nursing care products, as well as difficulties communicating with others.
>
> (Iwasaki, 2011)

Thus, Iwasaki has mentioned the real problems about people with disabilities because their needs are diverse, and has suggested that environmental changes can deteriorate their disabilities and medical conditions. More importantly, she has revealed the ecological circle of those with disabilities. When each ecosystem is broken down due to the disasters, those with disabilities become more vulnerable. Here, I give an example.

I read the online newspaper story about a 53-year-old Sendai man, Masashi Tsuchiya, who has ALS (amyotrophic lateral sclerosis) and he depends upon an artificial respirator to breathe (*The Mainichi Daily News* on 23rd March 2011). When the power went out in Sendai on 11th March 2011, his wife, Kayoko, and other family members kept him alive through the dark night. They did the job instead, manually pumping air into his lungs with a special rubber bag. When the city lost power, so did the artificial respirator, thus, if there was no power, he would have stopped breathing. More detailed narratives from the *Mainichi Daily News* are as follows:

> Pumping the bag by hand was simple but tiring, and Masashi's family took turns; Kayoko for an hour, and their two sons for two hours each. . . . [T]hose not at the pump managed to hook the external battery up to a car battery, giving the respirator power again for a while.
>
> (*The Mainichi Daily News* on 23rd March 2011)

In the context of the 3.11 disasters, the disabled cyborg (i.e. Mr Tsuchiya as mentioned above) has blurred the distinctions between the natural and artificial, mind and body, self-developing and externally (de/re) constructed, and many other distinctions that used to apply to humans and machines. Machines that exist in nature are disturbingly lively, and humans are passive. Here, I want to draw attention to the disabled cyborg and his hybrid status. The narrative about Mr Tsuchiya has provided one such complex example, including his embodied experience of being connected to a respirator when the power went off and the many difficulties experienced to get the power back into it. The readers of the narrative have come to realise that the love from his family members and many friends saved his life. They all tried to find a way to get his respirator working under the special circumstances, and it succeeded for him. Thus, the narrative about Mr Masashi Tsuchiya, his family, friends, and doctors around him has raised two questions: 1) Can we simply see Mr Tsuchiya as a cyborg, and consider his embodied experience in Haraway's theory? 2) Understanding the ecology of Mr Tsuchiya (his embodied relationship with respirator and the lived world), can we simply apply Haraway's theory to Mr Tsuchiya's condition? (the disabled cyborg in the affected area).

Embodying cyborg and situated knowledge

In the "Cyborg Manifesto", Donna Haraway (1991) deploys the metaphor of a cyborg to challenge feminists to engage in a politics beyond naturalism (the nature, body, feminine) and essentialism (technologies and masculine). She also uses the cyborg metaphor to offer a political strategy for her interests in socialism and feminism. Haraway (1991: 150) states, "We are all chimeras, theorized and fabricated hybrids of machine and organism; in short, we are cyborgs". She defines a cyborg as:

1   a cybernetic organism,
2   a hybrid of machine and organism,
3   a creature of both fiction and lived social reality.

(Haraway, 1991: 149)

Thus, Haraway argues against essentialism, which claims to recognise a universal foundation or constitution of gender identity or patriarchy. Such masculine and essentialist theories, she argues, either exclude women who do not follow the theory and segregate them from real women or characterise them as inferior. Here, Haraway (1991) argues that masculine essentialism excludes the nature and its fluid transformation. Masculine essentialism reduces the experience of a group category (i.e. gender, class, ability, race, sexuality) to the experience of one sub-group (i.e. white American men), and stabilises the boundaries between men and women and between culture and nature. In short, most of us have assumed that we (humans) can control nature and that the well-ordered world can be maintained for good. Control of all things (including the natural world) is considered as both human obsession and of human nature. Furthermore, the idea of control that most people embrace is also a myth. We control to keep the world, objects, our minds, and our bodies fixed; however, at the same time we are aware of the impossibility of fixity. We seek power we do not and cannot have, because in fact, there is no such thing. We have been seeking power over others to control their perceptions and their behaviours, and power over nature. However, when the disasters hit the land so badly, the essentialist assumption about the world radically collapsed.

Haraway has been considering the relationship between scientific human nature and machinery. She proposes an interpretation of these relationships in terms of "situated knowledge". By blurring the boundary between subject and object, Haraway's idea about cyborg discourse becomes inhabited with hybrid subjects/objects. She offers an account of the feminist involvement in the masculinised customs of scientific discourse and the multiple and complex theories of objectivity and points to situated knowledge. The concept of situated knowledge refers to "location, partial embodiment, and partial perspective" (Haraway, 1991: 191). A situated knowledge reveals the "particular and specific embodiment" of the subject that reflects her subjective position in social relations (Haraway, 1991: 190). The embodied position is a position for the various and complex social practices that form all knowledge claims, whether techno-scientific or feminist and whether objective or subjective. However, Haraway also recognises the partiality of scientific knowledge and she can be reflexive because she recognises the partiality and, thus, limits any possible account of technology that can be offered. Haraway (1991: 191) argues "for situated and embodied knowledges and against various forms of unlocatable, and so irresponsible, knowledge claims". Here, I want to ask: How does Haraway conceive of its reconstructive elements, which would allow us to construct new accounts of technology?

Haraway (1991) addresses the birth of the cyborg, which is the human being in his/her technological becoming – as some creature that may undermine gender boundaries and that should be fully supported by feminists. Haraway's (1991: 181) famous statement, "I would rather be a cyborg than a goddess" can be read as her optimism that the new technologies can liberate women from the burden of the patriarchal system. That new technologies can liberate many people from putting their bodies under the service of maintaining the essential norms under the patriarchal and the able-bodied system remains contested. However, the cyborg unchained from the essential norms challenges our ways of thinking about the relationships between men and women, between able-bodied and the disabled, and about our own identities.

Here, I consider that Haraway (1991) diffracts philosophical studies of technologies. Her work aims to establish an alternative model of techno-scientific studies for feminism. In this context, the cyborg should be understood as a political intervention in technology studies that intend to create a different depiction of how we see technologies. Rosi Braidotti (1999) reconsiders Haraway's alternative models of technologies from her reading of Gilles Deleuze:

> Deleuze works primarily on the formulation of alternative conceptual forms of representation for these subjects-in-becoming. The aim here is to provide a materially based practice of representation of the fast-shifting social landscape of post-industrial societies. Furthermore, poststructuralists attempt to connect these changes to fundamental shifts in the conceptual fabric of philosophy. In his classical text *What is Philosophy?*, Deleuze, with Guattari, makes it quite explicit that what he is after is a new form of conceptual creativity which would allow us to think and represent change and transformation.
>
> (Braidotti, 1999: 91)

Thus, Braidotti argues that Haraway's work is to understand reflexivity as a feminist practice. Like Deleuze with Guattari, as Braidotti sees, Haraway acknowledges that embodied and political practices construct technologies, and she reconfigures reflexive feminist science studies in terms of its constitution by our embodied and political subjectivities. Haraway questions feminist studies of science to recognise the formation of its accounts of science in terms of these practices.

Haraway (1991: 164–165) considers technologies (in particular, communication technologies and biotechnologies) as "the crucial tools recrafting our bodies", in relation to the formation of "natural technical objects of knowledge in which the difference between machine and organism is thoroughly blurred; mind, body, and tool are on very intimate terms". Expanding Haraway's theory of the cyborg, I recognise the undermining of the dualistic boundaries that have controlled to establish and maintain the normative and the able-bodied self. Challenging to the common distinctions between organism (human) and machine, between nature and culture, the cyborg offers the possibility for a new politics. The fixed assumption through which disabled bodies have habitually been demarcated in terms of vulnerability, passivity, silence, and absence is questioned by the idea of the cyborg. Within this idea, our relation to technologies (machine) is not one of subject to object – rather it is one in which such a distinction is disturbed. Haraway (1991) states:

> The machine is not an it to be animated, worshipped, and dominated. The machine is us, our processes, an aspect of our embodiment. We can be responsible for machines; they do not dominate or threaten us. We are responsible for boundaries; we are they.
>
> (Haraway, 1991: 180)

Thus, Haraway's cyborg is both phenomenological and discursive, not only an imaginary creature of myth and science fictions, but also our embodiment. Our day-to-day engagement with technologies involves us in our lived world and alters our sense of our own embodiment, our positioning as an embodied subject within time and space. In particular, for those with disabilities and illness, as these technologies become more indispensable, so the disabled cyborg becomes capable and engages with things which she could not do before. However, I consider, the disabled cyborg, in the affected Japanese area, demonstrates that not only the distinctions between humans and machines, but also the distinctions between nature and culture, have become leaky.

The cyborg embodiment – a phenomenological reading of the "Cyborg Manifesto"

The ecological changes the 3.11 disasters bring to bear on the way we experience embodiment of technologies has been the main focus in this chapter. The unstable relationship between nature and culture (between humans and technologies) with which we engage when we faced the huge disasters (both natural and manmade disasters) involves us in modes of subject formation and socio-cultural relations which are very different from those which we experience in the day-to-day world. Here, I begin to understand the issue of disabled embodiment in normal times and expand my understanding to the specific case of the 3.11 disasters. In this section, I shall explore Merleau-Ponty's (2002 [1945]) understanding of perception and his description of how the embodied subject experiences the world in relation to a particular embodiment of technologies.[1]

Like Haraway (1991), Merleau-Ponty undermines the fixed assumptions of the world where we live in. Merleau-Ponty (2002 [1945]) explains the relationship between the body and the world – the embodied knowledge:

> A movement is learned when the body has understood it, that is, when it has incorporated it into its 'world', and to move one's body is to aim at things through it; it is to allow oneself to respond to their call. . . . In order that we may be able to move our body towards an object, the object must first exist for it, our body must not belong to the realm of the 'in-itself'.
>
> (Merleau-Ponty, 2002 [1945]: 160–161)

Merleau-Ponty's observation of the body points to its adaptability as expressed in more complex movements and deeds extending over time and space. Such a deed is routine – a set of incorporated actions that accomplish a certain task, for example, typing keyboards, driving a wheelchair. For example, the wheelchair, as an embodied subject that experiences the world through the sensation of the wheelchair and the kinesthetic understanding of the wheelchair-in-the-world, becomes another way that the subject makes sense of human spatiality and movement. The subject comes to understand the wheelchair, an everyday experience, as an embodied orientation that she then uses to comprehend and judge things like speed, distance, road surface. This field of perception changes from one moment to another, but her attuning to this changing world includes a set of perception that organises and locates our sense of self. Merleau-Ponty writes:

> We do not merely behold as spectators the relations between the parts of our body, and the correlations between the visual and tactile body: we are ourselves the unifier of these arms and legs, the person who both sees and touches them.
>
> (Merleau-Ponty, 2002 [1945]: 173)

Thus, considering this person with disability, and her relationship with a wheelchair, she perceives the lived world from a position that she feels the surface of the road through her touch to the seat and that she feels the vibration as the wheelchair moves. In short, her perception creates a particular mode of being in the world.

The disabled cyborg overlooks the subjective lived experiences with technologies, where patriarchal and normative values continue to be practiced through and on disabled bodies. The phenomenological engagement with the cyborg is concerned with Merleau-Ponty's (2002 [1945]) thought of embodiment as a lived experience of "being-in-the-word" (Heidegger, 2005 [1962]), and with the relationship between embodiment, technology, and disability. Through such understandings, the reality of lived experience and embodiment and the embedded specificity of disability, emphasise that while the cyborg can undermine the dualistic assumption of the world, the disabled cyborg should not be simply considered a post-disability paradise.

The lived experience of the disabled body and its intentionality is seen in the hybrid embodiment with the wheelchair, where the wheelchair can be ambivalently a part of her body in a multi-dimensional ontology of the subject (humans)/the object (machines)/the abject (nature). Consequently, I argue that our understandings of the disabled body should not only be perceived as transcending the flesh, but also dependent upon our lived experiences of the disabled body in a certain world and at a certain time. An example of this disabled cyborg experience is not simply the dominant transition of the vulnerable human body to an enhanced body, but the kinesthetic transition and extension of the particular body to the body with the embodied objects (i.e. wheelchair, respirator, etc.). This reassertion of bodily transformations occurs through techno-scientific knowledge.

To return to the narratives about the disabled cyborg in the 3.11 disasters, as I have discussed above, the disabled cyborg in the affected geographical area has become more vulnerable than able-bodied people. Moreover, the landscape of the affected areas dramatically changed into 'the abyss', and the lived world has been extremely disrupted for them. Under the dreadful circumstances, most people have come to realise that our knowledge of the relationship between nature and technologies was not right; in particular, our knowledge of the relationship between earthquakes (including tsunami) and nuclear energy was wrong. The disabled cyborg reconsiders our ecological relationship between humans, technologies, and nature, and blurs the distinction between the three in order to find a new way of being-in-the world. Furthermore, the lived experience of the disabled body in the 3.11 disasters continues to reassert the need to be aware of human vulnerabilities within the relationship between technologies and nature and to connect ourselves to nature through technologies. In turn, the interrelation between technologies and nature is important in the reconstruction of Japan. Thus, unlike Haraway who acknowledges the social influences on cyborgs, I focus on the lived experience of the disabled cyborg; it is important to reconsider what the 3.11 disasters actually mean for the lived experiences of disabled cyborg bodies.

Shin-do-fu-ji (身土不二): "the body and the earth are not two"

Katsuhiko Ishibashi, a professor in the Research Center for Urban Safety and Security in the Graduate School of Science at Kobe University and a seismologist, points out (2007) that the study of earthquakes is not a fully established science even now and we should not underestimate the possibility of disasters.[2] However, paying no attention to his warnings, the Japanese government insisted that all nuclear power plants in Japan were safe, as they were in compliance with the earthquake resistance guideline for nuclear facilities. According to Ishibashi, there are two major problems. The first problem derives from defects in the guideline itself, in consideration of modern seismologic theory, and the second problem involves safety concerns over nuclear power plant construction, based on the opinion of a nuclear power plant construction supervisor with more than 20 years of experience. Since the earthquake tsunami and nuclear meltdown at Fukushima Daiichi, the Japanese government and TEPCO's opportunistic estimations have been criticised by many specialists.

The 3.11 disasters have recalled to mind an old Japanese (Buddhist) phrase *shindo-fuji*, which literally means, "the body and the earth (land) are not two". As I understand it, it means that the body and the earth are inseparably connected as one.[3] This phrase reflects the awareness of ecology in the world after the 3.11 disasters.[4] Further, biomedical sciences have diagnosed injury of the human body, tried to prevent it, and to cure it, and in the same way, technologies have tried to predict and to find a way to control any natural condition. Here, I emphasise the limitation of both technological and biomedical sciences, and therefore, the need to accept any vulnerability of human body and the earth without depending on technological and biomedical knowledge.

Although Descartes believed that the body was a machine and the mind was what runs the machine, Merleau-Ponty reconsiders that the body is not a machine, but a living organism. We are our bodies, and consciousness is not just locked up inside the head. In his later thought, Merleau-Ponty considers the body as 'flesh', made of the same flesh of the world, and it is because the flesh of the body is of the flesh of the world that we can know the world. Thus, Merleau-Ponty's thought of the flesh, to me, is very similar to *shindo-fuji*, which reveals that the lived body and the lived world are inseparably connected as one.

Following Merleau-Ponty, I begin my phenomenology by giving primacy to lived experiences, and I want to return to "the world which precedes (scientific description), (the world) of which science always speaks, and in relation to which every scientific characterization is an abstract and derivative sign language as is geography in relation to the country-side" (Merleau-Ponty, 2002 [1945]: x). I see that both wheelchair and respirator, for example, do not simply impose themselves on consciousness as atomistic sense impressions, nor do the users form both objects in their minds. Rather, both, as the users experience them are discovered through a subject-object dialogue. In order to grasp how Merleau-Ponty sees this subject-object dialogue, and in order to expand the subject-object dialogue to the dialogue between humans and technologies, I need to understand the ecological idea of the lived body.

Concluding remarks: the ecology of cyborgs and the disabled "Cyborg Manifesto"

As a helpless spectator of the 3.11 disasters who could not do anything at all, I felt numb when I watched the TV news (even now, I feel numb). My feeling went beyond sadness. When I read the online news article about Mr Tsuchiya, I imagined myself in his situation. I felt extremely helpless and vulnerable. As I mentioned above, Mr Tsuchiya needs a respirator to maintain his life. In the 3.11 disasters, the power cut at the TEPCO nuclear power plant meant his respirator stopped working; this means he would have lost his life if no one was there to look after him. For Mr Tsuchiya, the machine cannot be seen as separate parts but must be understood as a whole, as it is lived. His respirator is as much part of his body and his lived being as his heart or lungs; in the essence, the respirator is his lungs. Accordingly, the respirator is not 'just' an aid or 'mere' piece of technology; rather the respirator is essential to Mr Tsuchiya's very existence and crucial to his continued well-being.

Crucial to any sense of well-being is a sense of 'home'. It is when we are 'at home' that we feel safe; at home we are free from any danger that the outside world might pose. The idea of 'home' as a 'safe place' is common to many cultures, and is certainly not unique to Japan, but perhaps Japan has a specific way of viewing the 'home'; there could be a reason why Japanese people always take off their shoes and wash their hands on entering their home, as if they are removing the debris they acquired in the apparently dangerous outside world.

Illness and disablement, or more specifically, the problems associated with such phenomena threaten our sense of home. Illness and disablement remind us that we are vulnerable. And if we are unable to feel safe, the place where we live is no longer a home; it becomes something threatening and unfamiliar, as Les Todres and Kathleen T. Galvin explain:

> Heidegger uses the term 'uncanniness' (unheimleich) to indicate this kind of existential homelessness that is faced when one is able to embrace the 'resolute' responsibility of moving away from the 'taken for granted' securities of the familiar 'at-homeness'. Within this perspective, ill health can be one of the ways in which human vulnerability reminds us of an existential homelessness that cannot be denied.
>
> (Todres & Galvin, 2010; Chapter 8, this volume)

When the power cut occurred and Mr Tsuchiya's respirator stopped working, it wasn't just that Mr Tsuchiya had a medical or a technological problem to deal with, his 'homeliness' and 'well-being' were disrupted. Heidegger, as Todres and Galvin explain in the context of well-being, sees homeliness as a kind of attunement, a willingness to 'dwell', and necessary if one is to have any kind of harmony with one's body and environment:

> To dwell is to come home to one's situation, to hear what is there, to abide, to linger and to be gathered there with what belongs there. When such dwelling is able to be fully supported, there may be a mood of peacefulness. But peacefulness is only one possible attunement within dwelling. The essence of dwelling is simply the willingness to be there, whatever this 'being there' is like. One can come to dwelling in many ways such as sadness, suffering, concern, attentiveness, acceptance, relaxation or patience. Dwelling is intentional in its attunement in that it allows the world, the body, things, others and the flow of time to be what it is.
>
> (Todres & Galvin, 2010; Chapter 8, this volume)

Mr Tsuchiya was meant to be safe in his house, on his respirator, but the power cut all but destroyed his homeliness. If he had an independent power source that could keep his respirator working, his sense of home could have been preserved. Of course, some may object that illness and disability make any idea of well-being impossible, but that is simply not the case. It is possible to be ill or disabled and have well-being:

> Well-being, as we have articulated it, is a positive possibility that is independent of health and illness but is a resource for both. In other words, well-being can be found within illness and well-being is more than health.
>
> (Todres & Galvin, 2010; Chapter 8, this volume)

As a disabled cyborg, I declare my own cyborg manifesto in order to voice the silent. My life always exists in the world. My life is bound to a certain space and in an embodied relationship to others or objects. My life can be regarded as being-in-the-world. I part company with Heidegger, who laments the modern age. For Heidegger (1977), technology can only inhibit human ability. I want to develop a new way of understanding embodied subjectivities in relation to their worlds. The world and the body are not two and we need to find an ecological way of being in the body and in the embodied world. The ecological way, to me, is not a way of developing power structures, and deciding whom/what-controls-who/what, but a way of co-existing with the world (nature), the body, and technologies. Thus, the disabled cyborg manifesto is not simply to proclaim a process of blurring the boundaries of two, but rather to suggest the phenomenological reduction towards the holistic nature (gestalts) of the world without eliminating technologies.

The disabled cyborg manifesto requires that I reject all conceptualisations, generalisations, and all assumption of what are 'natural' or 'artificial'. Technologies are for me objects, devices, and processes that enable me to experience the world and increase my well-being. We cannot stop earthquakes or a tsunami, but we can rethink how we live with them. We can stop using nuclear energy with its risk of dreadful accidents (i.e. Fukushima Daiichi). We can certainly find a way to provide every patient who uses a respirator with a generator so they can get through long stretches without power. In order to do so, we need to voice the silent and to listen to their voice. In the disabled cyborg manifesto, we need to remove the fixed conceptions and knowledge that mask the phenomenon and experience, and which prevent us from seeing the phenomenon and experience in a phenomenological manner. The best way to support technologies is not to simply ignore them, but rather examine them for any phenomenological insights or understandings hidden and silenced in them. It is also helpful to examine how technologies improve or worsen our lived experience and the lived world where such technologies are used. Technologies can be used to control phenomena that are not really understood in a lived or concrete sense. Thus, the disabled cyborg must voice ourselves and ask: how is this phenomenon really experienced? How can we situate ourselves in a particular world? My own inquiry is repeatedly turned back to the beginning place in order to experience as a lived subject.

Notes

1 Most people probably assume that phenomenology cannot theorise cyborg. I think it is because Heidegger (1977: 5). considers the technological quantification of everything as a "will to mastery" which "becomes all the more urgent the more technology threatens to slip from human control". Control and fixed knowledge structures: all are strands in the technological world. For Heidegger, technology appears to be about human power over anything that disrupts human activities, and technology is instrumental.
2 Seismotectonics is the study of the relationship between the earthquakes, active tectonics, and individual faults of a region. It understands which faults are responsible for seismic activity in an affected area by analysing a combination of regional tectonics, recent instrumentally recorded events, accounts of historical earthquakes, and geomorphological evidence.
3 This phrase is consisted of four characters 身 (body), 土 (earth), 不 (not), and 二 (two).
4 Ecology is "the scientific study of the interrelationships among organisms and between organisms, and between all aspects, living and non-living, of the environment" (Allaby, 1998: 136).

References

Allaby, Michael. 1998. *The Oxford Dictionary of Ecology*. New York: Oxford University Press.
Braidotti, Rosi. 1999. "Response to Dick Pels". *Theory, Culture and Society* 16 (1): 87–93.
Haraway, Donna. 1991. *Simian, Cyborgs and Women: The Reinvention of Nature*. London: Routledge.
Heidegger, Martin. 1977. *The Question Concerning Technology*. (trans. W. Lovitt). New York: Harper and Row.
Heidegger, Martin. 2005 [1962]. *Being and Time* (trans. J. Macquarie and E. Robinson). Oxford: Blackwell Publications.
Ishibashi, Katsuhiko. 2007. "Why worry? Japan's nuclear plants at grave risk from quake damage". *International Herald Tribune and The Asia-Pacific Journal: Japan Focus* (August 11, 2007).
Iwasaki, Kaori. 2011. "The Great East Japan Earthquake and the disabled". *Daily Yomiuri Online* (The Daily Yomiuri), Waseda Online, 24 October, 2011. www.yomiuri.co.jp/adv/wol/dy/opinion/earthquake_111024.htm
Mainichi Daily News, The. 2011. "Family bands together to keep Sendai man on respirator alive through long blackout". *The Mainichi Daily News*, 23 March, 2011.
Merleau-Ponty, Maurice. 2002 [1945]. *Phenomenology of Perception* (trans C. Smith). London: Routledge.
Todres, Les & Galvin, Kathleen T. 2010. "Dwelling-mobility: An existential theory of well-being". *International Journal of Qualitative Studies on Health & Well-Being* 5 (3): 1–6. doi:10.3402/qhw.v5i3.5444

13

THE EXISTENTIAL SITUATION OF THE PATIENT

Well-being and absence

Stephen Burwood

Good health, like peace, is an absence of something more deleterious. Also like peace, a fully adequate understanding of good health requires an acknowledgement of its enabling conditions and its obtaining requires their sustenance, particularly when understood as part of overall well-being and when this is construed as flourishing. Good health and well-being do not exist in a vacuum. However, at its heart good health is still an absence. It is, of course, an absence of suffering and, again like peace, an absence of conflict and, in this latter respect, it is also to a large degree an experiential absence of one's body. When accounting for the absence of illness as a major theme in literature, Virginia Woolf points to the literary erasure of the body in favour of the mind. The body, she says, "is a sheet of plain glass through which the mind looks straight and clear, and, save for one or two passions such as desire and greed, is null, and negligible and non-existent" (2002: 4). This is a description of the body in good health, and the healthy body's experiential absence, or what we might term its transparency, has been a major theme in work on the phenomenology of lived experience, as has the body's experiential resurfacing in adverse circumstances.

What we mean by good health or a healthy body is mostly relative, of course, and even for the relatively healthy it is a dynamic reality, as is its transparency. Equally, ill health and those bodily conditions taken as contrasts to the healthy body are themselves heterogeneous categories, so that making glib generalisations is an ever-present danger in this context. Nonetheless, the healthy body is the homely and familiar body. This is the body that is mostly compliant with one's wishes and desires and is the means by which we achieve our projects in the world and with others. "The body", notes J. H. van den Berg in his seminal little book, *The Psychology of the Sickbed*, "is the healthy person's faithful ally" (Berg 1966: 66). The compliant body's familiarity, normality, and routine contribute to its invisibility, and so this very familiarity may breed forgetfulness. We become lost in our projects, whatever they are and whatever their value or desirability. Hence van den Berg's paradoxical, and somewhat melancholic, assessment of our prospects for well-being: "Probably there is no better guarantee of a really unhealthy life than perfect health" (ibid.: 74). Paradoxical and melancholic the assessment may be, but it is not entirely disconsolate. It embodies a profound truth about the experience of illness and health that reveals illness, apart from its obvious physiological or psychological characteristics, to consist in a number of existential 'conflicts' – with oneself, one's body, one's surroundings, and with others – which could be said to constitute the existential situation of the patient. What was once familiar or routine becomes agonistic and takes on a distant and uncanny aspect. One's experience of good health, on the other hand, consists largely, though not entirely, in the absence of these conflicts. In good health, one might say, one is at home with oneself, one's body, one's environment, and with others.

And yet, perhaps to be in *really* good health, such conflicts must not be completely absent from our lives. Without underplaying the suffering illness visits on the sick, the consolation van den Berg suggests illness may bring is that it is the "giver of little things" (ibid.: 68). After all, it is the little things that often form the wellspring of our sense of well-being. Thus, amidst the travail and anguish we can find a positive reminder of important things familiarity and routine made us forget. There is, therefore, what van den Berg calls a 'light side' in addition to the 'dark side' of the sickbed. "The patient who does not stubbornly cling to the memory of his healthy days", he explains, "discovers a new life of surprising intensity. He becomes sensitive to little things" (ibid.). This is precisely the experience so exquisitely recounted by Laurie Lee in *Cider with Rosie*, when he describes a bout of childhood fever and delirium that brought home to him for the first time the realisation that he might die.

> What gross human wastes, dull jellies, slack salts I had been purged of I could not say; but my senses were now tuned to such an excruciating awareness that they vibrated to every move of the world, to every shift and subsidence both outdoors and in, as though I were renewing my entire geography.
>
> (1959: 199–200)

Alongside what he calls the terror, the accustomed fires of the fever, and the corroding darkness, Lee recalls his finely tuned and acute senses, noticing his environment in a way unavailable to the busy and hurried well: for example, hearing the faintest sounds of nature – "streams running, trees stirring, birds folding their wings" – and the comforting familiarity of the human soundscape – the cosy murmurs from the kitchen, footsteps on the road, a voice saying Goodnight – and describes being "moved to stupidity by these precious sounds" (ibid.: 194).

That illness has a light side, as van den Berg puts it, has been noted before – as well as Laurie Lee's account, similar thoughts were a feature of Virginia Woolf's own reflections on the phenomenology of being ill – and it is something that has again received attention (e.g. Carel 2007, 2013, 2016), with the suggestion that well-being and illness are not merely compatible, but that illness may provide a condition for and stimulus to well-being. Certainly, its gifts are reflection and re-evaluation and the re-ordering of priorities and attitudes – arguably necessary for a fulfilling, healthy life, as van den Berg suggests. And yet, these are possible only where circumstances and some degree of absence allow. In the midst of an illness of sufficient moment to generate life audits, there is usually no space in which such reflective evaluation or contemplation can take place.

What illness reveals particularly starkly is two aspects to the body-as-lived: on the one hand, the subject-body as a set of capacities and one's mode of being-to-the-world, including others, and on the other hand the object-body as a biological materiality in the world. To speak, as Woolf does, of the body as null and negligible recalls Husserl's (curiously contemporaneous) description of the body of the perceiver as "a null-point of orientation, or a null-thing" (1977: 121). In other words, the sensorimotor body in its subjective mode of perceiving and acting is never objectively capturable as a thematised entity within perception (i.e. one that is the object of perceptual experiences). Rather, it is a focal point from which the world as perceived and acted upon radiates outwards, but which itself, qua subject, remains a phenomenological nothing at the heart of this world.[1] Of course, our bodies can also be objects for ourselves. The body is therefore what Merleau-Ponty calls the enigma that is a sensing-sensible: that which "simultaneously sees and is seen. That which looks at all things can also look at itself and recognize, in what it sees, the 'other side' of its power of looking. It sees itself seeing; it touches itself touching; it is visible and sensitive for itself" (1964: 162). And yet, as was also famously noted by both Merleau-Ponty and Sartre, although the seeing eye can also be seen and the touching hand can also be touched, one cannot "see the seeing" or "touch the touching" themselves.

The sensorimotor body is thus the vehicle of the subject's being-to-the-world and it is in the nature of this subject-body that it recedes or disappears in this manner from the world it is disclosing. Indeed, the intentional transparency of the body that Woolf describes is necessary for us to achieve our motile goals with fluidity: the dancer who thinks about her feet is unable to execute the move with grace, the speaker stumbles over her words because she is aware of the movement of her lips and tongue, the athlete suffers the yips as a result of self-focused performance anxiety and over-thinking the play, and so on. As W. Timothy Gallwey (1974) laments in *The Inner Game of Tennis*, the statement "I can never do anything I try to!" comes close to expressing an important truth. Fluid motility is, if you like, a 'technique of the body', when performance has become second nature, so that the intrusion of reflective awareness, in which my body appears to me as a thematised object of attention, renders the body opaque and disrupts the harmony of the body engaged in the act. My body experienced from the first-person perspective – that is, my body as lived and engaged in my intentional tasks – is not normally experienced by me as a physiological organism but as that, as Sartre puts it, which is continually 'forgotten' or 'surpassed' as I pursue my projects in the world. As he says,

> My body as it is *for me* does not appear to me in the midst of the world. Of course during a radioscopy I was able to see the picture of my vertebrae on a screen, but I was outside in the midst of the world. I was apprehending a wholly constituted object as a *this* among *thises*, and it was only by a reasoning process that I referred it back to being *mine*: it was much more my *property* than my being.
>
> (1956: 402)

This elemental divergence between the experiencing, phenomenological body – as it is for me – and the experienced, objective body never quite allows a complete merger of the two. I can attend to the eye or hand as thematised objects but cannot at that same moment experience them in their subjective modes of operation. As soon as I do that, they 'disappear' as fully thematised objects from my awareness and the null-point phenomenon reoccurs. Nonetheless, the transparency of the sensorimotor body is a dynamic phenomenon: in the usual course of things, there is a continuing interplay of the body qua sensory-motor subject and body qua object of attention, in which different elements surface, disappear, and resurface in awareness depending on their role in achieving the tasks at hand.

In his detailed treatment of what I have termed the intentional transparency of the sensorimotor body, Drew Leder identifies two primary, and complementary, ways in which the body tends to what he calls 'self-concealment'. The first he terms 'focal disappearance', which refers to the way in which the perceiving body is unable to become its own object of perception precisely because it is itself the focal origin of that perception. We have already discussed this aspect of embodiment to some degree above. The second Leder calls 'background disappearance' (Leder 1990: 25–27). This is something that arises directly out of the dynamic nature of the sensorimotor body and the fact that this manifests itself as a 'synergic system' – what Richard Zaner (1981) termed a 'contexture': a system in which the employment of any one part at a given moment must be viewed in the context of the engagement of the whole body forming a 'background attitude'. As such, the body is actually a complex harmony of bodily regions; this harmony requiring certain bodily regions to play a supporting role in sensorimotor activity and for others to switch between playing active and supporting roles or for them to be simply 'out of play' in a form of a complex corporeal Gestält.

For example, whilst sitting and reading this text your eyes obviously play a primary role and are thus clearly characterised by focal disappearance; yet we see not just with the eyes alone, but with the eyes-in-the-head-on-the-body-resting-on-the-ground, to adopt a phrase (Gibson 1979). Much of the body therefore continues to perform a secondary but nevertheless necessary supporting role – the trunk maintains an upright posture, the neck muscles adjust the head's position, the hand and forearm buttress the chin. Given the specific requirements of the task at hand, obviously other elements may not be put to use at all: in a sitting position this would probably be true of your lower legs and feet. Both sets of constituent elements are thus characterised by background disappearance, but each in its own way. Unless circumstances are such that a certain posture is or becomes uncomfortable (e.g. that after a long period of sitting and reading, one's neck muscles become stiff and painful), one is likely to be unaware of and untroubled by one's body. "The healthy person", van den Berg notes, "is so much his body that he usually forgets about it. He passes on to it the duties it has to perform. It is those duties that tell him he has a body. . . . Everywhere it is proved to him that his body is an instrument, a condition. This evidence is sought in vain by the patient. . . . It is not an instrument but an object, a prey to disease. It's a thing that is ausculated, tested and palpated by the physician (1966: 67–68)."

Of course, the forgetfulness of the healthy is what Woolf suggests accounts for the literary absence of the body, as well as illness. A similar idea has been proposed by Leder, who argued that the phenomenology of subjective embodiment can, to some degree, account for our cultural and philosophical neglect of the body – so that the body is not only surpassed in experience but also in thought – encouraging psycho-physical dualism and a tendency to identify the self with an homuncular and incorporeal mind (1990: 103).[2] What van den Berg makes plain is that, on a personal level, corporeal forgetfulness is a luxury of good health, and is not something easily available to the ill. Rather, it is the background against which a number of interrelated conflicts play out.

The key conflict is that with one's body. In illness the body resurfaces in awareness in a particularly insistent way, so that it is no longer straightforwardly experienced by us as our mode of being-to-the-world and as a set of capacities or an 'instrument', as van den Berg puts it, but as something objectified,[3] obeying a call that is not ours, to be examined and treated by another. In other words, my body-as-lived also includes my experience of my own body as a materiality. Thus, standing back to back with experiences of embodiment characterised by intentional transparency and modes of bodily disappearance are other experiences in which, as Merleau-Ponty says, the intentional arc 'goes limp' (1962: 136) and the body resurfaces and imposes itself on us in all its contingency and materiality. These moments of resurfacing of the body are what Leder terms modes of 'dys-appearance' – a term he employs to deliberately emphasise their often insalubrious and alienating nature (1990: 69–99). "The healthy person", van den Berg explains, "is allowed to *be* his body and he makes use of this right eagerly: he *is* his body. Illness disturbs this assimilation. Man's body becomes foreign to him" (1966: 66). Deleterious conditions such as illness, pain, and bodily impairment are thus commonly accompanied by a sense of dissociation, in which one's body takes on an uncanny aspect: at one and the same time it presents as close and familiar and as an external reality or, as Zaner says, as both "intimately alien, strangely mine" (1981: 54), hence his conclusion that a fundamental truth of human embodiment is captured in the phrase "I *am* my body: but I am as well *not* my body" (1973: 119; cf. 1981: 50). This sense of the uncanny is carried over into aspects of our former lives that now belong to a different world. In the new circumstances even my clothes, van den Berg notes, though familiar and imbued with personality, simultaneously lie outside the horizon of my present existence (1966: 31–35). The overwhelming feeling is that "I no longer belong to the life which none the less is still mine" (ibid.: 35).

The conflict with one's body is thus the central aspect of a broader conflict with oneself, throwing into question one's relationship with others and one's environment, even one's identity and sense of self. As van den Berg relates, a transition occurs, where one acquires a new identity and status: one becomes a patient. "Normal life is at an end. Another life takes its place, a life of a completely unknown nature" (1966: 38). It is a life, he says, that seems to the patient to be one "which cannot be really lived; it has to be passively endured" (ibid.). It is marked by uncertainty about things most taken for granted: faith in the future and in the integrity of the body, and the indispensability of what he calls "the personal function in the existence of others" (ibid.). Since Michael Bury's influential paper, these sorts of conflicts have been termed 'biographical disruption', where illness, and he argues especially chronic, and not just episodic, illness "is precisely that kind of experience where the structures of everyday life and the forms of knowledge which underpin them are disrupted" (1982: 169). As well as "attention to bodily states not usually brought into consciousness and decisions about seeking help", the substantial readjustments required by the on-set of a serious condition challenge taken-for-granted assumptions and behaviours, disrupt normally reciprocal and mutually supportive relationships, and require a "fundamental re-thinking of the person's biography and self-concept" (ibid.).[4]

One key element of such disruption is, of course, the loss of independence and autonomy, primarily as a result of the collapse of the intentional arc. For van den Berg, being a patient means being a 'non-participant' in the life that preceded the illness and which is still the reality for others, a reality the ill are forced to relinquish. He describes how the normal routines of daily life also appear uncanny: at once homely and yet increasingly remote. "The day outside the house, in which 'outside' has acquired a new special meaning for me, a meaning emphasizing my exclusion" (1966: 26). Spaces previously accessible without a second thought inside the house also become unreachable *terra incognita*. "The horizon is narrowed to the edge of the bed and even this bed is not completely my domain" (ibid.: 27). Corresponding to this conflict with one's surroundings – including, not least, with the sickbed itself, in which the bed acquires a wholly different character and meaning to the bed of the healthy – one's temporal horizons also shrink and plans become meaningless, so that one lives in the 'confined present'. "All that awaits me becomes tasteless, or even distasteful. The past seems saturated with trivialities" (ibid.: 27). Thus, my lived world, and the "horizon of my existence", becomes spatially and temporally constricted to the here and now, so that the possibilities it once offered me no longer seem ready-to-hand.

And as the world recedes in face of the body's exigencies, so do other people. Increasingly, van den Berg notes, the healthy appear remote to the patient (and vice versa), who now inhabits a different world barely graspable by others who themselves represent a life of which the patient is no longer a part. This is particularly and inescapably true, he suggests, for healthy visitors. While the patient's former world and the "life outside his small existence has become strangely foreign, his visitors transform this strangeness into a hostile distance" (ibid. 43–44). They do this by well-meaning but ill-chosen behaviour and ways of speaking, particularly an 'unjustifiable levity' in matters of real moment for the patient; but also merely by being representatives of that former, lost world.

Although more often occurring in disagreeable circumstances, not all cases of bodily resurfacing occur as a result of disagreeable somatic sensations such as nausea and pain, or physiological morbidity or dysfunction. Nor do they always result in existential conflict. There are many circumstances in which I notice my body as a material existence that may be unpleasant but are non-biological in origin, and there are others, whatever their origins, which are either neutral, pleasurable, or at least have a positive aspect and could be viewed as life enhancing. Examples of the neutral and the pleasurable could include: checking myself in the mirror, deliberately regulating my breathing, feeling for my pulse, revelling in the caress of a partner's hand, or the feel of a cool breeze on the skin on a hot day, feeling the physical glow of my body after vigorous exercise, the arousal of sex and its culmination, and so on.

Nonetheless, in many of the neutral circumstances where the body resurfaces there is a degree of licence about whether or not we adopt the relevant stance towards our bodies. This is partially true of pleasurable circumstances as well, although it is often the case that these take us beyond ourselves and the confines of our bodies into the company of others: in the case of the pleasurable, the experiences are what F. J. J. Buytendijk describes as being the release of "an inner expansive movement, in which the personality reaches outside itself, oblivious of self" (1961: 25, cf. Leder 1990: 75). Only the narcissistic or those excessively prone to navel gazing are likely to pay any attention to their bodies in such circumstances. On the other hand, as Buytendijk also notes, "suffering in all its forms is conducive to recollection. It isolates a man from the rest of the world and from all that is without some connexion with suffering" (ibid.). It is the power of these more deleterious circumstances to isolate and concentrate one's attention, to gather one's life into the area of the body, congealed in space and time, which singles them out.

Good health, I have suggested, is at its core an absence of these sorts of existential conflict, and primarily the conflict with one's body. Nonetheless, to be in *really* good health, van den Berg argues, such existential conflicts must not be completely absent from our lives, for these may also be, as paradoxical as this may initially seem, life enhancing, by being a significant part of the enabling conditions for living a properly healthy life. If the foregoing conflicts constitute what van den Berg calls the dark side of the sickbed, there is, he suggests, also a light side conducive to well-being (1966: 68). As the giver of little things – including "articles so much devoted to utility that they used to disappear behind the goal they served" (ibid.: 29) – such conflicts change our perspective on the all too easily overlooked features of everyday life and prompt a necessary re-evaluation of their significance.

> Who misses more of life, the healthy person, when he throws himself into the avalanche of ever more respect, with an ever more wonderful house, an ever more expensive car and ever further reaching holiday trips, and consequently a frantic drive for money; when he throws himself into this avalanche which bears the dazzling name of 'career'? Or the sick person who makes his room, his window sill, his window and his view a world full of significant and breathtaking events? Who – now in a completely different sense – is more ill? The illness of the body can be the condition for a soundness of mind which the healthy person misses easily.
>
> (ibid.: 73)

The healthy can also be distanced from the world, which may be just as remote for them, though in a different way, as it is for the ill. Indeed, in some ways the dimensions of "our useful, busy, noisy, healthy existence (which are often insignificant)" appear to be at a greater remove than in the constricted dimensions of the sickbed (ibid.: 74). At the discovery of a serious illness, life and the world becomes clearer and dearer than ever to the sufferer, little daily matters more desirable, and their importance more plainly resolved. "The certainty of a chronic illness," he remarks, "stresses the blessings of health. The astonishment felt by the patient at this discovery never really disappears as long as his illness lasts" (ibid.: 40). The lesson van den Berg draws is "that health and an existence without conflict are not synonymous" (ibid.). As well as acquiring an appreciation of the little things, their value and significance, those whose lives contain the conflicts visited on the ill also acquire an awareness of the vulnerability of the body. "This", he concludes, "results in a certain responsibility and this responsibility is never a matter of course" (ibid.).

That illness can have a role in the service of well-being, and that a truly healthy life is not necessarily one lived in the absence of conflict, has been a theme that has been taken up more recently by Havi Carel. Central to Carel's approach is the idea that illness, in requiring the adjustment of the sufferer across a number of interrelating registers (physical, psychological, social, and temporal) to changes within one's body, illness encourages 'adaptability' and 'creativity' in response to the new circumstances (2007). For example, in compensating for lost capacities, new ways are found to tackle old tasks, new activities are found to participate in with others; or in response to biographical disruption, "a new meaning must be found for the new narrative; the ill person seeks an explanation for her suffering and limitations; a new approach to one's future must be created" (ibid.: 106). Carel's point is that 'health within illness' is possible and that illness demands a diverse set of responses from the sufferer that are characteristic of what it is to live the good life. This is not to minimise the dark side of the sickbed, with its conflicts or constraints. "Rather", she argues, "cultivating well-being within illness and learning to live well with physical and mental constraints requires conscious effort and is an *achievement* that should be recognized as such" (2016: 149).

The suggestion of van den Berg goes beyond this: his argument is that the conflicts and constraints of illness are actually necessary for truly leading the good life, and are not merely compatible with it. Without the reminder of our vulnerability or mortality provided by the sickbed, we lack the stimulus to live a life elevated above insignificance. This argument assumes that illness has a singular cognitive value: that it reveals the constituent elements of our lives in their true perspective. Illness, even one that is particularly serious or life-threatening, may not be alone in this – one can see how similar claims could be made for other intense and challenging experiences – but it is likely that for most of us, it is an illness that provides the spur to therapeutic reflection, or what would nowadays be termed mindfulness, an attitude and frame of mind that clears the numbing fog of habituation and discloses the real values of life. The last of these claims is not entirely convincing. From the viewpoint of the sickbed, the concerns of a healthy existence may indeed appear insignificant, absurd even; but this does not mean that they are insignificant or absurd. Some may be, but many will not be. As well as giving us back little things that we value, illness can also have an unrealistically distorting effect on our view of the big things that we value. Therefore, we should not be too quick in assuming that the view of these that illness bestows is always an accurate one. The foregoing description van den Berg offers of our everyday concerns, for example, is a somewhat tendentious one: the drive for money is frantic, one's career is a dazzling avalanche. Yet, an income is a necessity that may also enable valuable and life-enriching projects as well the accumulation of possessions – many of which, in any case, will have a deeper significance for us than merely being an indication of status. And, given that work is a substantial part of life, a happy and fulfilling career may be a part of – and a significant part of – a happy and fulfilling life, as well as providing one with an income and so indirectly enabling other things. While illness offers a palliative against letting an imbalance develop, so that we are consumed with the concerns of a healthy life to an unhealthy degree, it does not reveal that these concerns have no significance, or are simply trivial.

It is also worth noting that it is not incidental that the light side of the sickbed is a liminal aspect of illness, rather than one at its core. Laurie Lee's autobiographical morning reverie, "damp with weakness" but lying in "a trance of thanks", was of course the start of his recovery and rehabilitation when the dimensions of one's horizons may again begin to expand so one can renew one's geography. In van den Berg's imaginary scenarios of the sick father, the person who learns of a serious illness, and Robert Louis Stevenson's fictional Keawe[5] who contracts leprosy, all of the protagonists are in the early stages of illness or have just discovered that they have a serious condition, before the illness takes grip. The possibility of reflection and re-evaluation or the re-ordering of priorities and attitudes exists at the margins of illness, or during interludes, or in response to the shock of discovery, or when the ebb and flow of the insistent demands of the debilitated body permits.

Although an episodic illness that is little more than a simple inconvenience may result in a biographical disruption of some degree, it is unlikely that it would lead to a significant change in perspective and to what I earlier called a life audit. To produce such a fundamental re-evaluation, the condition would have to be of sufficient moment in the life of sufferer. However, in many instances, such as the pneumonia Lee describes, when we are in the throes of the illness, the demands of the body are so complete that the body occupies one's whole existence: we are our bodies and nothing but our bodies. This does not defeat van den Berg's insistence on the necessity of existential conflicts for general well-being. Arguably, if we want to avoid the fate of a banal life – such as that lived, for example, by H. G. Wells's easy living Eloi[6] – we need such reminders of our vulnerability. But if the achievement of well-being is possible in the context of illness, it is only in the absence of such conflicts and the body's experiential absence, or when they and its presence sufficiently retreats. In other words, the light side of the sickbed is possible in the liminal space where absence allows and before absence dominates once more, with its attendant forgetfulness.

Laurie Lee and Virginia Woolf were able to compile their accounts because they were lucky enough to live through a serious illness and recover enough to write. In contrast, a poignant literary testament to the power of illness to completely disrupt is Alphonse Daudet's unfinished work, *In the Land of Pain*. Suffering from *tabes dorsalis*, Daudet could only work during periods of remission from the extreme pain that he says blots out the horizon and fills everything. And yet, when the pain ebbs it is difficult to place oneself back in the midst of the suffering. "Words only come when everything is over, when things have calmed down. They refer only to memory, and are either powerless or untruthful" (2016: 15).

Notes

1 It is not a complete phenomenological nothing, for it is implicitly present in experience in the way the world we perceive is imbued with values and information that reflects back to us the nature of our embodiment, its possibilities for action, and the constraints on this: e.g. whether something is large or small, hard or soft, upright or upside-down, manipulable or unwieldy, safe or requires caution, etc. (cf. Gibson 1979; Leder 1990). With different bodily architecture and different capacities, the world would look significantly different.

2 Leder suggests that the phenomenology of embodiment more generally, including experiences in which the body resurfaces as an alien presence (as discussed hereafter), provides grounds for dualism. "Philosophical doctrines arise out of the life-world", he argues, "and attain popularity and credibility only to the extent that they harmonize with lived experience". I have previously cautioned against a view in which phenomenology is said to ground theory, for there is a danger that we ignore the influence of culture and theory on the shaping of lived experience itself. The apparent harmonisation may thus be a product of our doctrinal commitments (Burwood 2008).

3 The degree to which the unhealthy body presents as an object – a pure "this amongst thises" – is circumscribed, despite it widely being described as such in the literature. If it were experienced literally as an object, this would render the experiences unintelligible.

4 The exact nature and degree of disruption appears to be dependent on the condition and its cause and can also vary according to factors such as the age, affluence, cultural context, and clinical history of those affected. This was illustrated, for example, in a recent study of the experience and significance of tooth loss (Rousseau et al. 2013), though another study suggests that disruption can be equally relevant for groups where it has been argued to be less of an issue, e.g. those in later in life and those with early on-set chronic conditions (Taghizadeh Larsson & Grassman 2012).

5 Robert Louis Stevenson's short story 'The Bottle Imp', in *Island Nights' Entertainments*. London, Paris & Melbourne: Cassell & Company Ltd, 1893.

6 H. G. Wells, *The Time Machine*. London: William Heinemann, 1895.

References

Berg, J. H. van den, 1966. *The Psychology of the Sickbed*. Pittsburgh, PA: Duquesne University Press.

Burwood, S., 2008. 'The apparent truth of dualism and the uncanny body', *Phenomenology and the Cognitive Sciences*, 7 (2): 263–278.

Bury, M., 1982. 'Chronic illness as biographical disruption', *Sociology of Health and Illness*, 4 (2): 167–182.

Buytendijk, F. J. J., 1961. *Pain: Its Modes and Functions*, E. O'Shiel (trans.). London: Hutchinson.

Carel, H., 2007. 'Can I be ill and happy?' *Philosophia*, 35: 95–110.

Carel, H., 2013. 'Ill, but well: a phenomenology of wellbeing in chronic illness', in Bickenbach, J., Felder, F. & Schmitz, B. (eds.), *Disability and the Good Human Life*. Cambridge: Cambridge University Press.

Carel, H., 2016. *Phenomenology of Illness*. Oxford: Oxford University Press.

Daudet, A., 2016. *In the Land of Pain*, J. Barnes (ed. & trans. 2002). New York: Vintage Classics.

Gallwey, W. T., 1974. *The Inner Game of Tennis*. New York: Random House.

Gibson, J. J., 1979. *The Ecological Approach to Visual Perception*. Boston, MA: Houghton Mifflin.

Husserl, E., 1977. *Phenomenological Psychology: Lectures, Summer Semester 1925*, J. Scanlon (trans.). The Hague: Martinus Nijhoff.

Leder, D. 1990. *The Absent Body*. Chicago, IL: University of Chicago Press.

Lee, L., 1959. *Cider with Rosie*. London: The Hogarth Press.

Merleau-Ponty, M., 1962. *Phenomenology of Perception*, C. Smith (trans.). London: Routledge & Kegan Paul.

Merleau-Ponty, M., 1964. *The Primacy of Perception and Other Essays on Phenomenological Psychology, the Philosophy of Art, History and Politics*, J. M. Edie (ed.). Chicago, IL: Northwestern University Press.

Rousseau, N., Steele, J., May, C. & Exley, C., 2013. '"Your whole life is lived through your teeth"; biographical disruption and experiences of tooth loss and replacement', *Sociology of Health and Illness*, 36 (3): 1–15.

Sartre, J.-P., 1956. *Being and Nothingness*, H. E. Barnes (trans.). New York: Washington Square Press.

Taghizadeh Larsson, A. & Jeppsson Grassman, E. 2012. 'Bodily changes among people living with physical impairments and chronic illnesses: biographical disruption or normal illness?' *Sociology of Health and Illness*, 34 (8): 1156–1169.

Woolf, V., 2002 (1930). *On Being Ill*. Ashfield, MA: Paris Press.

Zaner, R. M. 1973. 'The subjectivity of the human body', *Main Currents in American Thought* 29: 117–120.

Zaner, R. M., 1981. *Context of Self*. Athens, OH: Ohio University Press.

14

ECOLOGICAL HEALTH AND CARING[1]

Helena Dahlberg and Albertine Ranheim[2]

Suppose that everything is linked together, that the world is a web of relationships in which every being is included, and which consequently affects and is affected by every individual's actions. Suppose that every single decision we make in life, e.g. within health contexts, is part of a larger continuum. If we, throughout life, are part of structures, systems and processes that are substantial to how we manage to form our lives, it must be of great interest to see what these relationships do to health and our experience of well-being.

We argue for an expanded awareness in order to find satisfactory answers to some essential questions within the area of "health and care". Our aim in this chapter is to illuminate possible answers to the following questions:

How can we understand the concept of ecology within health and care? What can ecological caring be?
How can we deepen our understanding of caring and its focus on health based on the knowledge of our lived contexts?
What is caring's and e.g. nursing's focus on health in relation to nature, vegetation, the life of animals, nutrition and environment?
How can we understand the professional caring relationship, e.g. between nurses and patients, if we consider it an ecological relationship?

To declare a background for answering these questions we begin with some statements about health and caring, as well as our recognition of ecology. An important element of our analysis is the findings from an empirical study of caring practice, which are included in our assumption of what ecological health and caring can be. We present this study and the meanings of ecological care that we see there. Finally, we deepen the idea of ecological health and caring by drawing all threads together with the support of Merleau-Ponty's philosophy.

The notion of health and caring

We understand health and caring from a phenomenological approach, i.e. from a lifeworld theory position, and consequently we talk about lived health, i.e. health as it is experienced in everyday life, and lived caring, i.e. how caring is experienced by patients and/or carers. Such an approach also unites the natural and human science perspectives on health and caring, i.e. we include biological health in our approach as well as a perspective where health is understood in terms of existential vitality. In this understanding, health means well-being as well as the capacity of being able to realize one's minor and major life projects. In such an approach caring should support patients' health processes and help them participate in caring processes, with the goal of existential vitality (Todres et al., 2007; Dahlberg et al., 2009; Dahlberg & Segesten, 2010; Ranheim & Dahlberg, 2012; Todres et al., 2014). Consequently, the focus upon health is superior to the focus upon illness, i.e. all caring of illness must be directed towards health and the experience of well-being as well as the capacity of running one's life projects.

The notion of ecology

Ecology, in our understanding, means an existential web of relationships. It is the science of living creatures' relation to and interaction with the environment, i.e. the milieu and contexts that we are living and sharing. In ecological studies, the intention is to understand life processes and the development of ecological systems, as well as relations between different organisms and their environment.

The term "ecosophy", as described by Arne Naess (1976), means ecology in practice. According to Naess, "sofia", i.e. wisdom, is manifested in practical complex situations: "you cannot be an ecosophist purely theoretically or academically" (p. 84). This is an essential understanding of what ecology can mean to health care: lived wisdom of how health is related to the living context.

Naess asks for a scientific approach that includes the web of life. We argue that phenomenology is such an approach, being a philosophy that connects with an ecological ontology. With the aim to deepen the understanding of what an ecological caring could mean, we use Merleau-Ponty's philosophy and especially his understanding of corporeal being and flesh (Merleau-Ponty, 1995; Dahlberg, 2013). This philosophy shows us how there is a deep connection, and at the same time an irreducible difference, between human being and nature, between humans, and – not least – between the person and his or her body. With this philosophy, we can understand how we as humans take part in and form a part of the world.

An empirical study of caring practice

As a foundation for our analysis of ecological care, and in order not to dwell only within the realm of theory and philosophy, we chose empirical data from an investigation at an anthroposophic clinic in Sweden. The caring practices at this clinic should be understood as an example of ecological caring, and not as a definition. We use the empirical data from this clinic as an opportunity to explore what ecological health and care is and can be.

Anthroposophic care integrates theories and practices of modern medicine with alternative, nature-based treatments and a spiritual scientific view of the human being (Arman et al., 2008). Anthroposophic medicine and care is offered to patients in many countries. It is a complementary initiative that integrates an anthroposophic health care convention with conventional medicine to an integrative synthesis. Health care personnel in this field have a specialized medical education, and today there are more than 25 hospitals within Europe that are specialized in this form of medicine and care (Arman et al., 2011).

Developing from the idea of Rudolf Steiner, anthroposophic medicine rests on three pillars: nursing care, therapeutic treatment and medical treatment (Therkleson, 2005; Arman et al., 2008). Anthroposophic therapy treatment is always individually prescribed by a physician, and might include conventional medication accompanied by any of the following complementary therapies: natural remedies (herbs, plant extracts, essential oils, natural substances), therapeutic baths, external compresses and rhythmical body oiling, artistic therapies (clay modeling, painting, music therapy and therapeutic song), therapeutic eurhythmy (movement therapy), rhythmical massage (a form of light-touch massage), psychological and biographical counseling and anthroposophic nursing care.

The participants were 16 patients diagnosed with various kinds of cancer and the patients had gone through a rehabilitative caring process (mainly during 14 days). The patient interviews that compose our data were part of a larger study with health care staff and patients at the clinic, inquiring into the meaning of existential care (Arman et al., 2011).

Interview data were analyzed from a reflective lifeworld research (RLR) approach presented by Dahlberg et al. (2008). RLR means an interest in phenomena, i.e. how aspects of human existence present themselves to and are experienced by humans. In this study, focus is upon the phenomenon of health and caring, and the aim of our analysis was to describe the phenomenon's meaning structure, i.e. the essential and more general meanings as well as contextual nuances and more individual meanings, as they appear in the analysis of the interviews.

Lived experience of health and caring in an ecological context

Articulating the essential meaning of the phenomenon of ecological health and caring, we wanted to avoid the concept holistic, which is ambiguous and imprecise. However, the patients are very explicit about the importance of care that addresses them as whole beings. The anthroposophic care is experienced as "a life-line", i.e. care that relates to the patients as persons who have a vivid life context. Also explicit is the objection against care that is fragmented and that addresses only piece by piece of them. The investigated anthroposophic care means the experience of being cared for as someone who is body, soul and spirit all together.

The experience of this complete form of caring is built up by the therapies and the attitude of the carers, together with a caring milieu: the architecture, choice of genuine materials in the buildings as well as in linen and cloth, and including choice of colors and forms, as well as organic healthy food and contact with nature. The caring warmth together with the caring milieu is meant to nurture the patients and their existence, and be understood as health supporting.

The anthroposophic care can be described as giving possibilities for patients to be both passively receiving care and actively acting for their own health processes to be strengthened. On the one hand, they are received and accepted as patients, that is, as persons with caring needs, wanting to be taken care of. As a consequence they are given enveloping, nursing care that meets their vulnerability.

On the other hand, they are seen as persons with resources and as experts on their own life. They are supported with "tools" for self-reflection and personal growth through carefully chosen treatments and other creative activities that address their health processes.

The care is characterized by a high degree of responsiveness and sensitivity in order to bridge the individual patients' process between passively receiving care and becoming active and creative in one's own healing processes. The patients must be invited to participate in both health and caring processes. Such support from carers is strengthening their experience of life power and life meaning, and it has a centering and balancing meaning to the patients, who experience a movement towards well-being and a new capacity to realize their life projects, the minor as well as the major ones.

The phenomenon is further described by its constituents, which make the essential meanings more explicit. The constituents open up for more contextual meanings and individual descriptions from the interviewees. The constituents are:

- Caring concern, peacefulness and letting be
- Realization of one's intentions as the other side of letting be
- Cultural input
- The meaning of the environment
- Green and white caring

Caring concern, peacefulness and letting be

Existential vulnerability increases when one is being diagnosed with severe illness or other conditions, which threatens well-being and the capacity to realize one's life projects. In such situation, care that expresses concern and attention is immensely important. The patients in this study express how they felt welcome to a big warmth and experience that they were taken care of and that they were being protected from all the threats that can come with illness.

Some excerpts from data:

"I experience carers who really care, they care about me."

"I was touched by how they tucked me up in the bed in the evening, and I was given gentle massage with oils, was strengthened by this and my life-spark came back."

"The first thing I felt was that I could leave all troubles outside, let go of all that, and just receive attention."

Close to the experience of receiving care that expresses concern and attention is the experience of peacefulness. The anthroposophic clinic is offering a milieu that is silent and without disturbing impressions, such as traffic, intensive discussions or TV and computers. Instead the patients are offered e.g. experiences from the surrounding countryside landscape, storytelling, conversations on peaceful subjects, or such activities as making handcrafts or jigsaw puzzles. The patients appreciate that "even the carers speak carefully (with small letters)". They express that "everything here is careful". The interviews display more such expressions:

"To be offered rest and daring to rest. Previously I was tired, the whole time, because I never found rest."

"I have looked at myself here – I thought I had to do things all the time, now I have been offered tools to make rest possible."

"The health care staff submits quietness. The feeling of others' hands on you is more important than tranquilizing pills. Both tears and laughter; the staff catches both."

To be in such peaceful milieu helps one's own peacefulness to grow. There are expressions in the interviews that such care gives room for new insights that give room for an experience of letting be.

"One feels comfortable and calm here; almost like a little child // The environment – the colors, treatments, massage, embrocation and the herbs are all calming. The health care staff as well. It is tranquilizing – and then the body initiates self-healing."

Descriptions like the feeling of not being in a hospital but rather some kind of resting or rehabilitative home came forth. The interviewees refer to the importance given to reaching into deeper conditions of rest, "there is no background noise here, as there is on other hospitals, nor any luminous tubes or noisy air vents here or doors that slammers; it becomes clear that someone has done some thinking about this".

Expressions of the opposite are also present, giving the insight that even the experience of peacefulness is individual. Some descriptions express restlessness and frustration from the silenced mood that is a permeated atmosphere at the hospital:

"[S]ometimes I just wanted to spin off – or wish for someone to get stressed, so that I could feel that the usual life conditions were present here as well."

"I came upon myself of thinking of taking some provocative dance steps of salsa or such to tear the harmony apart."

The anthroposophic clinic makes up a kind of "caring cocoon". The perhaps brutal reality is for some time kept at a distance by the care that wraps the patients in caring attention; they are enveloped by health-oriented caring intentions. The interviewees express appreciation of the nursing care, which made them feel understood, that they had time to express their experiences, that they felt safe.

The carers in particular but also the whole caring context including other patients invite health-promoting stillness.

"I am allowed both to laugh and to cry, and the carers are attentive to both."

"One really experiences oneself as important, the carers care about you, here is no stress, no pressure, no rush, instead here are foot baths, enveloping treatments and such, and they take their time with you."

"I feel the ground beneath me now."

Peacefulness and letting be seems to be closely connected with being grounded, in a manifest way as well as existential. When illness is there, the sense of being grounded is important for the ability to grow the experience of well-being.

Realization of one's intentions as the other side of peacefulness

The experiences of peace, stillness, rest and letting be are not necessarily the opposite of being active. Being able to let go of everyday demands and the distress that illness causes, one's apt for well-being and a capacity of realizing one's intentions for life can be strengthened. The anthroposophic care seems to infuse the patients with energy and growth.

"If I was asked to use figurative language I would describe the care as a movement, a light green upward movement, as a spiral, or a plant, something that is growing within me and make change possible."

The care that is in focus in the interviews is experienced as providing the patients with desirable pauses from a sometimes hectic everyday situation. The importance of rhythm in the daily routines is appreciated by the patients. They have time for reflection and become able to establish a new and healthier life rhythm, which includes both movement and stillness: "In between treatments and other activities there are pauses, and that is very important".

The interviewees expressed how the attentive care was experienced as confirming and strengthening. Such care gives room for accepting and affirming oneself, to see oneself in new light. And then the possibility to change something in one's situation increases. The patients are given an opportunity to build up the strength that illness demands from them.

"The importance of finding one's own voice."

"Came in contact with creative processes – and something happens in my body."

Inpatient care always runs the risk of forgetting that patients are persons with a majority of their lives outside of the hospital. It is therefore of interest to note how the interviewees in this study express how they experienced support for their further existence, in particular when they should leave the clinic. The care that addresses the patients as whole beings enables them to find themselves and what and how they want to do in the future. For example, they learn strategies for how to feel what is right and what is wrong for them, they learn how to protect themselves, they find ways to say "no" to too much work or other engagements, they learn how to care for others by caring for themselves. Maybe most important is the insight of how much they themselves can have impact on their lives. The participation in both health and caring processes during the time in care awakes one's power to take responsibility for one's health even further on. Some examples of such support:

"I have learned how to live in a way that means balance."

"I have power to change things and achieved new routines."

"I have been out in deep water, 'treading water', but there was help on the other side – friends, family and the clinic."

The anthroposophic care, and the opportunity to realize one's own intentions, is but the other side of peacefulness. It can provide a way forward, to better understand, carry out and maybe reorganize one's health-oriented everyday life.

Cultural input

There exists a variety of tools within anthroposophic medicine and care. Nurses, physicians and various therapists work together in teams addressing the individual patient. Dwelling on the anthroposophic view that the human being needs the threefold of truth, good and beauty to develop and to heal, the care offers a variation of cultural inputs and activities to stimulate the individual patient. There is a library with scientific literature, as well as essays and poetry. There are concerts held and live music played as well as performative arts and theater on a local basis. Architecture is intentionally constructed to make a healing environment in terms of forms and color.

Contributing cultural inputs or happenings such as storytelling evenings was expressed as both a kind of entertainment and a source for deeper reflection. The stories have the possibility of explaining life situations or essentialities of life in allegoric meanings: "Stories or fairy-tales have the ability to explain the larger questions in life".

The storytelling evenings, which took place in the common living room where the patients and staff gathered there to listen, were appreciated: "I haven't heard stories told since I read them for my children". One's own reflection on the stories could be shared with the others, or just be restrained and privately contemplated.

Other forms of optional cultural inputs in the evenings are the possibilities of sharing thoughts concerning paintings together with professional art-interpreters. Contemplating on paintings together, the patients are taking part of its idiom, colors and meanings. This may open up to possibilities of getting wider perspectives of the expressions of art. The patients may achieve new insights of themselves through the works and activities done with painting. Important was the room for being creative without being judged or validated, letting the process itself be what mattered: "No judgments were made in the creative processes, and getting inspiration to become creative was a central experience"; "I can be creative without anyone judging my abilities". Another interviewee described: "I begin to relate to art in a new way now. Something wants to come out that has not dared to be let out earlier". And another said: "I baked my anger into the clay in modeling". The art therapy is an example of how a therapy could give rise for reflections and how the patients could express themselves in a new way. To get involved in the creative or artistic expressions was described as relieving and challenging at the same time. Not least was it a challenge and meant resistance to try to express something through a medium or material that was previously relatively unknown.

A special kind of cultural input is eurythmy, which in addition to physiotherapy is an often used movement therapy. The principle of such therapy is that certain movements stimulate life processes. Therapeutic eurythmy attempts enlivening and supporting flux in processes.

"When I came I had a lot of fatigue in my body, then in the eurythmy sessions things happened, it affects me a lot and I become thirsty and tired. Working with movements in relation to the central points in self, my experience was that I was building up stamina within myself on which I can hold on to."

The interviewees display how eurythmy therapy movements had been a way of getting insight into handling certain difficulties in the rehab process. For instance, lived experience and even strong feelings had come up and through the therapy the patients described how they had achieved a kind of tool to handle this. The cultural input in the care has the possibility to equip the patients with new strength as well as new self-insight, which promote well-being.

The meaning of the environment

In anthroposophic health care the ambiance of space is understood as having impact on the people using the space. The importance of including esthetic enhancements in attempts to reduce stress and anxiety and increase well-being is a central thought behind environmental design. The consciousness of creating and providing positive contexts to become actively healthy or salutogenetic is central. The meaning of such environment reaches the patients:

> "The architecture with soft deliberately designed shapes and forms, imagine I have beside my bed a window allowing me to view straight into the sky – quite amazing . . . being able to lie in bed with the nature getting in to you, the healing nature."
> "It is a kind of playfulness in the architecture, not always practically adequate as I am used to, but colors and form creates life, it becomes enlivened."

A central principle in anthroposophic care is the significance of warmth. Warmth mediated through the deliberate and consequent use of genuine materials as for instance in the bed linen and other textiles and furniture. Warmth is as well the mediating factor in many of the treatments such as foot baths and therapeutic baths, rhythmical embrocations of the body or as in an after-lunch coating with stimulating herbs followed by rest, in warmth. The constant use of hot-water bottles or millet cushions is central. Warmth is even mediated in the deliberate and consequent use of form and color on the wards.

> "The materials feels natural, it is really the basis that gives a feeling of natural warmth, the woolen blanket and the cover made of felt. And the treatments are all performed in heat, warmth . . . everything here is wrapped into something. There is hot-water bottles, the nurses are warming up their hands before they touch you. Then there is the heat wrappings, I have had a yarrow herb compress on the liver that has been affected by chemotherapy and radiation, and wrapped into the nice woolen carpet with a hot-water bottle on top."

The concept is the entirety of the healing milieu as it is experienced through the purity of the food, the moments of rest, the careful wrappings, the massages and embrocations, the colors and forms in the buildings and the genuine warmth. It is no coincidence that the windows are placed where they are or that the window recesses are angled the way they are or that the colors feel like being the necessary ones. The thought of a healthy existence is everywhere, according to the interviewees. In short, the environment has an influence on, and can support the health processes.

Green and white caring

Finally we want to describe some meanings that are originated from the patients' comparisons of the anthroposophic care with general care. In the interviews there are expressions such as "the green care" compared to "the white care".

> "The green care strengthens humans and cure on a more long term basis. The white care is fine, but above all – it does not see to the whole, even if it has become better in this respect."

"Previously, I have been through a whole range of treatments and become very crumpled up. // The white care should ask for help from the green care . . . when it is about helping people to be brought to order again after having been crumpled up."

As the anthroposophic caring focus is not on the illness per se, but on the individuals and their health and healing, there is no quick fix thoughts of for example giving a swift medication only to take away pain. Rather the concept is that of a slower edifying to strengthen and regenerate; to appeal to the body's own life power and recreative forces. This is noted and appreciated by the patients:

"Feels like I have been helped with finding back to the powers of my body and to build it up again – this is where I find conventional hospital care couldn't help me . . . and this is what this clinic has helped me out with."
"In conventional care, there is no awareness of how important every encounter is, and one is so terribly vulnerable in one's illness."

One of the interviewees, who suffers from breast cancer, had been in treatment several times and described how she had been very sad when she was about to leave a conventional care hospital after a period of inpatient care. A nurse sat down with her, but only for a few minutes, and then advised her to contact a counselor next week for further talking. But she needed something then and there. She didn't want to be reduced to a diagnosis, which treatment now had come to an end, but wanted to be seen and met as an individual who happened to be anxious about forthcoming time: "The white care claims that we are medically ready-made when the cancer cells are gone . . . but they don't realize that there is a whole lot to work through in the aftermath of the tough medical and surgical treatment".

"That someone really cares for you, that is not something one experiences in the conventional care, I'm afraid."

While "white care" is focused upon illness, "green care" is focusing upon health and it includes the notion of existence. "Green care" strengthens one's life power, vitality and life meaning. It is in this spirit we want to further explore the meaning of ecological in terms of the in-between caring, where we are inspired by the phenomenology of Merleau-Ponty.

In-between caring

For about four hundred years now, "the Western world" and not least North Europe have been directed by a positivistic view of how to gain scientific knowledge. For us within the area of health care this has been devastating. Without diminishing the value of medicine's successes it must be stated that the parallel development of a unified science approach to all research has become a serious obstacle to many good intentions of gaining knowledge about well-being. Positivistic approaches to research do not benefit projects with the aim of developing care practices that support and strengthen individuals' health processes and their participation in care processes.

It is not the focus upon mathematical and statistical research methods that is the worst impediment, even if critique of that single-eyed perspective must be challenged. In this context we instead want to direct the attention to dualism, atomism, reductionism and the frequent usage of categorization that is the essence and very foundation of positivism. Here hides an ontological view of the human world that seriously influences, even dictates, how we understand patients, their health situation and how they are best cared for. We can see it in how patients are being categorized, for example by the use of diagnoses, and in how the care planning system works, where the understanding of patients and their living contexts are being reduced into fragmented representations, sometimes sketches without any life at all. We can also see the positivistic ontology in the understanding of care as a one-way directed cause-effect driven idea.

We offer another option. As we can see in the data from the empirical investigation described above, as well as from other studies (cf. Dahlberg & Segesten, 2010) patients have a desire to be seen and recognized as individuals within a web of human relationships as well as a part of the natural world. They need care that addresses them as whole individuals, which sometimes is presented as body, soul and spirit. They need care that is embedded in environments that breathe health (cf. Seamon, 2015). They want to be acknowledged with their thoughts and plans for their life as well as with their emotions and hunger for what is meaningful, and they want to be cared for by warm hands in a joint event with health as the leading star. As we see it, individuals who become patients ask for ecological care.

In this section our aim is to deepen the notions of ecological health and caring in an excursive interpretation of the empirical findings, within the framework of phenomenology. In particular, we draw on Merleau-Ponty's philosophy.

Merleau-Ponty's philosophy displays an ontological understanding of human existence that is characterized by resistance against contemporary dualism, e.g. between body and soul, materialism and idealism, external and internal or movement and rest. Instead of seeing these aspects of life as radically separated categories he sees the dualities of them, how they belong together and define each other, as figure and background. Seeing these mentioned and other dualities as figures and backgrounds means that we outline areas of in-between; areas that don't belong to one of the two sides but are created by the interaction between them, between e.g. a person and his or her environment, or between persons.

Another way of understanding the duality (but not the dualism) of existence is through rhythm. Merleau-Ponty emphasizes the rhythms of existence, that belong to and characterize our existence because we are bodily creatures.

Take sleep as an example. Sleep is never absolute; it is the other side of wakefulness. Wakefulness thus always remains as a background and possibility for our sleeping state (Merleau-Ponty, 1995). In the same way, sickness is not absolute. Even if it interrupts our everyday world as well as the health that we had taken for granted, and places us in another world, one where we perhaps do not recognize ourselves and do not feel at home, our everyday (healthy) world will remain as a background for sickness, as a possibility that is always present. "[T]he sleeper is never completely isolated within himself, never totally a sleeper, and the patient is never totally cut off from the intersubjective world, never totally ill" (Merleau-Ponty, 1995, p. 164).

Seen this way we live in rhythm: we go in and out of sleep and in and out of relationships with other people and with the world. Even sickness and health can be seen as a rhythm of existence that we move between.

To understand this rhythmical movement of existence is to understand how it contains both active participation in the world and withdrawal from it, both movement and rest. Our existence has the power of directing us towards others, towards the living present and the future, but it also has the power of arresting this existential move, of shutting us up, of being "the place where life hides away" (ibid., p. 164). All this is because we are bodily, because it is, as Merleau-Ponty phrases it, the body that sustains "the dual existential action of systole and diastole".

> At the very moment when I live in the world, when I am given over to my plans, my occupations, my friends, my memories, I can close my eyes, lie down, listen to the blood pulsating in my ears, lose myself in some pleasure or pain, and shut myself up in this anonymous life which subtends my personal one. But precisely because my body can shut itself off from the world, it is also what opens me out upon the world and places me in a situation there. The momentum of existence towards others, towards the future, towards the world can be restored as a river unfreezes.
>
> (Ibid., p. 164)

Following Merleau-Ponty, one of the tasks of the caregiver, and an essential component of ecological caring, is to restore the patient's connection with the everyday world, to once again make possible the momentum of existence and, in this way, to create the opportunities for the river to unfreeze. It is the momentum of existence that opens up for possibilities.

Understanding the rhythms of existence and their importance for health can thus mean to bring an element of everyday life into the world of the sick patient, even in such subtle examples as seeing nature through the window of the hospital bedroom. It can also mean to awaken the patient's life power and life meaning by the use of an initial constraining action, by creating bounds for the patient, such as is done in the anthroposophic nursing care in e.g. foot baths and rhythmical embrocations. Such care and touch can be thought of as a way to constrain the world of the patient. But as our analysis shows, as well as a study by Ozolins (2011) it is rather the opposite that happens. To become aware of one's own boundaries through an attentive carer's touch makes room for acceptance and affirmation – for *letting be* – which, in its turn, makes it possible to look at oneself in a new light, and to see possibilities for change. This existential duality, or in other words, this in-between caring, where a limitation in fact opens up new possibilities, can be understood from Merleau-Ponty's ontology, where movement is not the opposite but the other side of rest, and where constraint is the other side of open possibilities.

In his last and unfinished work *The Visible and the Invisible*, Merleau-Ponty (1968) develops the ontology of flesh. He shows how it is not only the human body that can be understood as flesh, but being itself. The fleshy being is a being that consist of several layers or sides, and it is therefore never complete but always open, always changing (Dahlberg, 2013).

Think for example of your left hand touching your right. With your left hand you can feel your right hand; its shape and surface, and you can also turn this sensation around. Without switching the position of your hands, you can start to feel the left hand with your right hand. But there is a gap between the two sensations. The left hand cannot be both touching and touched at the exact same time. In other words, you can touch your own body, and in this way you stand in relationship with yourself, but at the same time you do not coincide with yourself. There remains an irreducible difference between the right and the left hand. In the same way, you can feel and know your personal self, but not completely. You cannot, for example, see the back of your head without the help of a mirror, and similarly, you cannot see the full source of your thoughts and feelings. Because we are fleshy creatures, our being is not complete; it remains open to relationships that define and change it.

Fleshy being thus carries a difference within itself in the same way that our human body never coincides with itself but stands in relation with itself, differs from itself. We can again think of this in terms of rhythms; the sleeper is never exactly one with his sleep, and the patient is never totally ill. There will always remain the other side, another possibility. We can also understand this irreducible difference within existence in terms of activity and passivity. Our active engagement in the world is never pure activity, but always also involves passivity.

In our everyday life, most of the time we are actively engaged in the world – seeing, hearing, touching. We are, in fact, engaged in the world already before we come to think of it. When we e.g. think about what it is that we see, we have already *seen*. Even if I decide to doubt what it is that I see, or what it is to see, the fact is that I see already. I am so much engaged in the world that I see more than I actually see: even if I only see the front of a house I have already seen and understood that it is a house.[3] We are thus constantly moving towards an understanding of the world, and in this way we are constantly ahead of ourselves. We are, as Merleau-Ponty chooses to phrase it, like the darkness in a theater salon, needed for the spectacle on the stage to be seen. In the same way, because I am bodily, I am already in a situation in the world before I come to reflect upon it. There is thus an engagement in the world that has already happened. Only afterwards can I come to reflect upon this engagement, often through the help of others.

The examples we use above are simple, but the activities where some things are visible and others invisible can be more complex, for example caring relationships. When carers meet patients there is always something that is hidden and invisible. The carers cannot, for example, read the thoughts of the patients or immediately grasp the feelings of the patient who a moment ago was told about a serious illness. What can be seen is maybe some movement in the look, an almost invisible trembling of the hand, which request from the carer to ask questions: How are you? How do you feel? What are your thoughts about (the examination) tomorrow? What do you need from the care and therapies to feel well again and to go on with your life projects?

Even though there are aspects of the patient's existential situation that don't present themselves, they must be acknowledged. When the urgent need of care emerges it is in general the biological body that presents itself and the rest of the patient's lifeworld is overseen or forgotten about. When the focus is on the illness or the diagnosis, the patient becomes a passivity, an object, and turns into a passive receiver of care in a way that allows for no movement, no duality, no activity. We call this suffering from care (cf. Dahlberg & Segesten, 2010; Todres et al., 2014).

To be existing, to be engaged in a world through one's lived body, thus means to overlook ourselves and the role we play when perceiving and understanding the world. In such ways we are passive and enacted by the world – *at the same time* as we are active, influencing and changing it. Like the darkness in the theater salon, our bodily perception brings the world to us, makes it visible, while remaining unnoticed, invisible. Or, when we look at for example a cat, we don't think that "now my eyes see a cat". The here and now, that place from which we see the world, that perspective from which the world becomes visible and meaningful for us, is itself invisible. We cannot see ourselves at the same time as we see the world. Only indirect, by self-reflection, or by another's look, can we turn around and see ourselves. And it is not only valid for seeing. We can easily take a bite from an apple, but cannot bite our own bite. Consequently, every activity means passivity – to be seeing means to not (completely) see oneself and to be seen by others' looks.

Being human, this corporeal being, thus means to not be one with oneself, to differ from oneself. When I look at the cat, for example, I cannot be completely contained within this looking – I am not *only* this look, I am also something else. I am also the back which I have forgotten about, but which my friend sees. I am also a body that soon will make its presence known when it is time for dinner. And I am also my past and my future; the possibility of maybe seeing something else, behind the cat. To exist means to be made anew in the interaction with others and the world.

What does this mean for illness, and for the meeting between patients and carers? The life crisis that comes with a (serious) disease demands a change, a new way of approaching one's existence. When my body has stopped functioning in the usual way, and the world has become a strange place, a special form of self-awareness is needed in order to find new possibilities, new ways of confronting my situation. This situation demands both rest from movement and movement from rest. The continuous movement of existence, where I engage with the world and at the same time forget about myself, needs to come to a momentary rest. And from this rest, a new movement has to be created. To meet and touch another's body – as e.g. when the carer lays a hand on the patient's body, can be such a brief pause, a rest in the space in between movements, as well as between bodies.

Because it is, as we have said, other people that help us to see and know ourselves. Even if we cannot see our own backs, we can ask a friend to look at it to see if there is maybe a bug with the intention to sting, or simply to tell us what the back looks like. Through others, we come to know ourselves, be it simple things as the look or shape of my body, or more complex things that have to do with our identity or health. Other people thus have the power to, in a way, make us more definite. Through the other, one experiences one's own contour, one's own border. That which is otherwise moving, engaging in the world, can come to a momentary rest, can rest with itself and discover itself. It is, however, important to note that we are not talking about a complete standstill, about a once-and-for-all definition (such as, for example, a diagnosis would be, or the experience of shame from a judging look). The meeting between the carer's hand and the patient's body instead offers a momentary pause, a possibility for self-reflection, a *space* in which the patient can discover her/himself and her/his possibilities.

How is this possible? Let us once again look at Merleau-Ponty's ontology and the difference that is inherent within existence. As human beings, our boundaries are not clearly and once and for all defined, but are constantly being drawn anew in our engagement with things and other human beings. It is in this relationship of connection and at the same time separation, that we find and develop our contours. When the patient meets with the carer, another human being, they are not completely the same, but also not completely different. The two bodies, e.g. the carer's hand on the patient's body, constitute each other's borders and thus create a new room between them. Between these two bodies, there is a common space opening up, a space that they share and that at the same time defines the border between them, their contours. It is an in-between space that also can offer a moment of rest, of just *being who I am*. This in-between space can also open up new possibilities, a *this is who I could be* (Dahlberg, 2013). In such light we can see how illness and care can open up for new forms of existence, new forms of being.

Concluding remarks

From the empirical exploration of ecological care we learned about how patients express their appreciation of caring concern that leads to both peacefulness and letting be as well as care that allows for their own life power to act in a way that strengthens their existential intentions and supports the realization of them. In such environment it is not about either-or, but both-and. Receiving and embracing such care could spontaneously be understood as care that fosters passive patients. What we find, however, is that care that includes peacefulness, rest, stillness and silence makes room for activity; it is the soil where active health processes grow. We can conclude that for patients in ecological care there is a steady movement between passively receiving caring concern and being active in their health processes. It is also the opposite: activity supports the experience of rest and recovery.

Drawing on both empirical data and philosophy (Naess, 1976; Merleau-Ponty, 1968, 1995), an essential feature of ecological caring seems to be that it addresses patients as whole lived beings in vivid contexts. They are not treated as "cancer patients", "the heart in room 3" or as "broken legs" but are cared for as persons with a living past and a future ahead of them. To be *whole*, consequently, does not mean, as one might think, to be in one piece, ready and definite, but rather the opposite. To be *whole* means to be involved in and belonging to contexts that surpass us as living existences. Contexts that we at once influence and are influenced by. The challenge to our thinking lies in the possibility to think of this *wholeness*, not as something closed in on itself, but as something open and changing. This is why we have chosen especially Merleau-Ponty's philosophy as the foundation for our conceptual understanding of ecological health and caring. Merleau-Ponty's ontology of the flesh explains precisely this wholeness that is there and at the same time is gaping open (Merleau-Ponty, 1968; Dahlberg, 2013). For example, the fact that I am constantly changing does not mean that I cannot have a clear sense of *who I am*, right here and now. The fact that one's experience of the world is continually altered does not mean that one cannot say what it is that one experiences right here and now. And even though one is never completely one with one's body, one can still perform actions (running along a rough forest path, jumping over a high fence) where it seems as though one is in complete harmony with oneself.

Ecological caring is caring that addresses human beings as continuously changing unities. It is care that can make the big world smaller, when so is needed, and equally make the small world bigger, by opening up new possibilities. It can offer a hiding place from a stressful life but it can also once again direct us towards our plans, our life meanings, our occupations, our friends and our memories. It provides rest from movement as well as movement from rest.

We argue that ecological in-between care addresses the whole person in her/his existential context, with focus upon the intentional lifeworld. Such care is the way to true well-being, first of all for patients but also for their professional carers.

We conclude that professional care would benefit from a change in favor of an ecological approach to health and care. Instead of being reduced to diagnoses, patients will be met as they are in the vibrating web of life. Such an approach includes a natural form of participation, where the patients are included in the caring processes as well in their health processes, contributing with their own experiences of what it is that brings well-being. Further, such approach includes both embracing care and care that supports the patients' own agency. We saw eloquent examples of such care in the interviews of patients in anthroposophic care, such as footbath, massage, embrocation and other treatment as well as the cultural inputs in forms of art, music, movement, etc. Not least our study gives more emphasis to relationships in caring, i.e. the patient-professional relationship as well as the relationship between humans and our environment. The development and improvement of all such relationships would support the well-being dimension of professional care.

Notes

1 This chapter is a reworked version of a paper in the *International Journal of Qualitative Studies on Health Well-being*, published as open access and republished here under Creative Commons License. *International Journal of Qualitative Studies on Health Well-being 2016*, 11, 33344. http://dx.doi.org/10.3402/qhw.v11.33344
2 We would like to express gratitude to Professor Karin Dahlberg who has inspired, supervised and made invaluable contributions to the process and the published work, including the previously published paper.
3 This is generally understood as the lifeworld theory or theory of intentionality within phenomenology, which we have previously described in Dahlberg et al., 2008; Ranheim & Dahlberg, 2012) and in several Swedish publications.

References

Arman, M., Hammarqvist, A. S. & Kullberg, A. (2011). Anthroposophic health care in Sweden – a patient evaluation. *Complementary Therapies in Clinical Practice, 17*, 170–178.

Arman, M., Ranheim, A., Rehnsfeldt, A. & Wode, K. (2008). Anthroposophical health care – different and home-like. *International Journal of Caring Sciences, 22*, 357–366.

Dahlberg, H. (2013). *Vad är kött? Kroppen och människan i Merleau-Pontys filosofi* (What is flesh? The body and the human in Merleau-Ponty's philosophy). Göteborg: Glänta produktion.

Dahlberg, K., Dahlberg, H. & Nyström, M. (2008). *Reflective lifeworld research* (2nd ed.). Lund: Studentlitteratur.

Dahlberg, K. & Segesten, K. (2010). *Hälsa och vårdande* (Health and caring). Stockholm: Natur & Kultur.

Dahlberg, K., Todres, L. & Galvin, K. (2009). Lifeworld-led healthcare is more than patient-led care: an existential view of well-being. *Medicine, Health Care and Philosophy, 12*(3), 265–271.

Merleau-Ponty, M. (1968/1963). *The visible and the invisible* (A. Lingis, Trans). Evanston, IL: Northwestern University Press.

Merleau-Ponty, M. (1995/1945). *Phenomenology of perception* (C. Smith, Trans.). London: Routledge.

Naess, A. (1976). *Ökosofi T. Ökosofi. Ökofilosofi* (Ecosophy T. Ecophilosophy). Oslo, Norway: Gyldendal.

Ozolins, L. (2011). *Beröringens fenomenologi i vårdsammanhang* (The phenomenology of touch in caring contexts). Linnaeus University Dissertations, nr. 62.

Ranheim, A. & Dahlberg, K. (2012). Expanded awareness as a way to meet the challenges in care that is economically driven and focused on illness – a Nordic perspective. *Aporia, 4*(4).

Seamon, D. (2015). The phenomenological contribution to interior-design research: place, environment, and architectural sustenance. Ch. 24. In J. Asher & N. Blossom (ed.) *The handbook of interior design*. London: Wiley-Blackwell.

Therkleson, T. (2005) Anthroposophical nursing. *The Australian Journal of Holistic Nursing, 12*(2), 43–50.

Todres, L., Galvin, K. & Dahlberg, K. (2007). Lifeworld-led healthcare: revisiting a humanising philosophy that integrates emerging trends. *Medicine, Healthcare and Philosophy, 10*, 53–63.

Todres, L., Galvin, K. & Dahlberg, K. (2014). "Caring for insiderness": Phenomenologically informed insights that can guide practice. *International Journal of Qualitative Studies on Health Well-being 2014, 9*, 21421. http://dx.doi.org/10.3402/qhw.v9.21421

15

A JUNGIAN CONTRIBUTION TO THE NOTION OF WELL-BEING

Chris Milton

Introduction

Jungian thinking (along with other theorists) has formed part of the early motivators of theory about well-being. The broad question which I seek to address in this chapter is does Jungian thinking have a role that is more than historical, more than simply a motivator, but does it contribute to our specific understanding of well-being?

Well-being, a word that first makes its appearance in English in the very early seventeenth century, can be taken to mean 'a good or satisfactory condition of existence; a state characterized by health, happiness, and prosperity; welfare' (Anon well-being, n.d.).

The above notwithstanding, the scholarly definition of well-being is problematic – the many attempts at articulating its psychological nature have primarily focused on dimensions of well-being, rather than on its definition (Dodge, Daly, Huyton and Sanders, 2012). Furthermore, scholarly attention has focused on two articulations of well-being: subjective well-being and psychological well-being.

Subjective (or hedonic) well-being, as a notion, refers to the experience people have of the quality of their lives. It is generally described as comprising of dimensions such as: happiness, satisfaction with life and the balance of positive and negative affect. Subjective well-being is considered to be stable over time and to be strongly associated with personality traits.

Psychological (or eudaimonic) well-being, as a notion, refers to processes of positive psychological functioning and human development. It was significantly contributed to by the theory and measurement scales designed and advocated for by Carol Ryff. Distilled from various theories, Ryff (1989, 1995) offered six dimensions in her model of psychological well-being: self-acceptance, purpose in life, autonomy, personal growth, positive interpersonal relationships and environmental mastery.

Many researchers currently believe that well-being is a multi-dimensional notion (Chen, Jing, Hayes & Lee, 2012). For instance Samman (2007) has attempted to integrate the notions of subjective well-being and psychological well-being into four aspects of general well-being: meaning of life, basic psychological needs (autonomy, competence and relatedness), life satisfaction (both domain specific and overall life satisfaction) and happiness.

Dodge et al. (2012, p. 230) propose that we define well-being generally as 'the balance point between an individual's resource pool and the challenges faced'.

Jung's thinking has played a contributory role in the construction of the notion of well-being. However, it does not seem to have been discussed as itself a theory of well-being. In her understanding of Jung, Ryff draws primarily on his 1933 work: *Modern Man in Search of a Soul*. She links Jung to the notions of personal acceptance (Ryff, 1989, p. 41), personal growth and autonomy (Ryff, 1995, p. 100).

In this chapter my argument will be that more detailed attention to Jung's thinking may well prove useful for scholars (and practitioners) operating within the field of well-being as a discipline. It offers some definite practical foci for understanding well-being: the importance of unconscious factors as well as conscious factors and a system of formulating the dynamics of psychological development in the achievement of well-being. Whilst I shall briefly remark on the former, I shall, in this chapter, explore the latter in more detail. In doing so I shall present the classical Jungian notion of individuation, a short case vignette that illustrates some of the processes and the way in which these may be discerned in fairy-tale. I shall conclude with a short phenomenological description of the way-of-being that is reflective of individuation.

Psychology of consciousness versus psychology of the unconscious

I would like to briefly address the notions of a 'psychology of consciousness' and a 'psychology of the unconscious'. Much of modern psychological thinking employs a psychology of consciousness. In clinical practice CBT is a case in point. It is assumed that what is needed to understand and change psychological life is consciously available. Likewise, the scholarly discussion of well-being seems to focus primarily on a psychology of consciousness. Chekola (1974), an earlier investigator in subjective well-being, in referring to the 'realizing of a life plan', seems to articulate happiness (a factor in subjective well-being) as a notion of a psychology of consciousness.

Jung's psychology is, however, not only a psychology of consciousness but also a psychology of 'that which is unconscious' (which I shall, for convenience and convention, call 'the unconscious' despite thereby reifying unconscious psychological processes). Jung believed that, through its encounter and interaction with the conscious attitude, the unconscious plays a necessary role in the development of the personality, a process he called individuation.

The classical Jungian notion of individuation

Jung believed that our, inevitably, one-sided psychological development is compensated for by a natural and progressive process. In particular, Jung became interested in the habitual *attitude* of the ego and how this is compensated for by unconscious material, e.g. dream images, symptoms and even psychosis.

Consistent with this arose the notion that whilst the ego is the centre of consciousness it is not the centre of the personality. The personality is understood to be the dynamic combination of both ego and the unconscious.

For Jung the unconscious consisted of both a personal unconscious, into which anxiety-generating impulses, affects, images and experience are 'repressed' and a collective unconscious, which has never before been conscious and from which compensating possibilities-of-being arise to challenge the ego attitude to change and develop, through differentiating, integrating and appropriating them.

These possibilities-of-being primarily find expression in images (or root metaphors) that are based in 'archetypes'. Archetypes are dispositions that structure our experience and behaviour.

The ongoing process of encounter between conscious and unconscious, the challenge this generates and, hopefully, its transcendence and integration, is called individuation.

When the ego attitude is challenged by the unconscious, great tension and defendedness may arise. There is, it seems, no way these quite different unconscious ways-of-being can combine with, and be appropriated to, consciousness. However, this *is* possible and Jung understood that there was a capacity, shared by all human beings, to transcend and incorporate something of both the conscious and unconscious. The product and means of this capacity is the symbol, which we may define as the 'best possible

description or formulation of a relatively unknown fact [i.e. a fact that is both conscious and unconscious]'
(Jung, 1971, CW 6, para: 814).

Jung understood individuation to be templated on and driven by the Self which is, *inter alia*, the ground
of the personality but also the central organizing archetype. The Self has also been defined as an

> archetypal image of man's fullest potential and the unity of the personality as a whole. The self
> (*sic*) as a unifying principle within the human psyche occupies the central position of authority in
> relation to psychological life and, therefore, the destiny of the individual.
>
> (Samuels, Shorter & Plaut, 1986, p. 135)

It is experienced as the centre of the personality (Brooke, 1991) and is implicated in individuation in that
it drives and shapes it. It is evident that the Self is paradoxically defined in many different ways and this is
an area of discussion and debate. Individuation can also be understood as the evolving relationship between
ego and Self. Whilst manifestly an intrapsychic process, individuation is also always manifest in the changing
shapes of our embeddedness in relationship to others and so is also interpersonal.

My personal and clinical experience has led me to develop a particular understanding of individuation. I have come to believe that, whilst traditionally the Self is seen as the centre of the personality,
it is more useful and meaningful to locate the relationship between ego and the Self as the functional
centre of the personality. I have come to understand that when we can live from out of a transcending
dialectic between ego and Self then we live relationally with true authority (author-ity), authenticity
and autonomy. In this sense analysis might be seen as the quest to become the true author of our own
existence.

I turn now to an illustration of some of these processes (particularly compensation through symptom
formation) by means of a case vignette.

Case vignette

Presentation and history

Robert is a man in his late thirties. He came to see me because of anxiety, claustrophobia and a disposition
to neglect his body because he privileged his tendency to think. In short he inhabited his mind rather than
his body. Around a decade previously he had seen a psychotherapist after he left his wife (whom he subsequently was divorced from). He had broken off the relationship and then experienced an intense period of
distress and anxiety much of which manifested in his body.

Robert is a successful commercial film director. He is the youngest, and only male, child of a fairly
large fundamentalist Christian family – a faith that he no longer follows. His ex-wife is also part of a fundamentalist Christian family. They had met whilst he was training in theology. Subsequently Robert has
maintained a relationship with another woman who is not of this religious persuasion.

Robert's father, a patriarchal figure, died when Robert was only 4 years old. Robert was idealized in the
family as the only male and also as manifesting a Christian spirituality – he was in a sense the replacement
of his father. Robert's mother withdrew into a natural grief and to an extent was unavailable to Robert as
a small boy. Robert himself withdrew into literal enclosed places seeking them out as refuges in which he
was able to give his thinking and imagination free rein.

Robert has seen me for a number of years. Gradually over that time he has become more and more
symptom free. We have explored the deep anxiety and guilt generated for a small boy whose father died and
who then quite concretely became a replacement for his father. This role as his father's idealized replacement promoted his intellectual, imaginal and spiritual capacities but at the same time truncated the development of his embodied awareness and presence, as well as his aggressive capacities.

What was less evident immediately was the way in which he had also suffered an attachment loss when his mother withdrew into her grief. This gradually emerged as an intense attachment to the land of his birth but also to his current female partner. Intense anxiety and grief started to emerge as the analysis progressed.

Another issue also gradually emerged: Robert was looking for a way in which he could more authentically and autonomously express his creativity. The main idea here was the development of a feature film. He also gained the sense of wanting to break with his profession as it was, travel to another country and be inspired to produce new creative works. He did this but after a short time suffered great distress and a grief-like reaction and needed to return home. Analysis continues.

Formulation

I understand Robert's presentation and work as layered. We might see these as: an Oedipal layer, a pre-Oedipal layer and an individuation layer. Whereas the former two dominantly refer to the stuckness of life, the truncated possibilities-of-being, the latter dominantly refers to the drive towards wholeness, towards well-being, and can be formulated, in Jungian terms, as individuation.

1   A deep Oedipal guilt that would have been generated for a boy whose father died as the Oedipus complex dawned and who quite concretely became a replacement for his rather spiritual and religiously knowledgeable father (Malan, 1979, pp. 60–61). Through healthy identification with his father, Robert developed his intellectual and spiritual capacities. However, there was another dimension to this – the defence against his aggression, and embodied awareness and presence. These would have been too dangerously close to a bodily Oedipal victory with its associated massive retaliatory anxiety and guilt. In Jungian terms we can understand this as a spiritual 'inflation'. In other words, there is a form of denial of his more chthonic competitive aggressive drives through an over-identification with spiritual and intellectual capacities (Neumann, 1954/1989, pp. 384–385). It is somewhat akin to Welwood's (1984) notion of 'spiritual bypassing'.

2   The pre-Oedipal layer is evident in his response to insecure attachment when his mother withdrew into grief. In attachment theory terms this was probably a form of anxious-avoidant insecure attachment (Ainsworth & Bell, 1970). Robert's withdrawal into literal enclosed spaces is more explicable in psycho-analytic terms; particularly in the form of what psycho-analyst Meltzer (2008) has called a 'claustrum'. This is a pre-Oedipal psychological retreat in which, typically, intense anxieties of loss and abandonment are held at bay by a complex binding of object relations through the use of projective identification. Meltzer describes three typical bodily locales for these psychological retreats: the anus-rectum, the genital and the head-breast. Robert's retreat is consistent with the head-breast: self-nurturance obtained by withdrawal into a retreat where he feeds on his own thoughts and leaves the drives and distresses of his body.

3   The layer of Robert's psyche that drives towards well-being, individuation in Jungian terms, is his impulsion to more authentically, and autonomously, express his bodily aggression and his non-intellectual creativity.

In particular the distress and anxiety, much of which manifested in his body, compensated for his defensive spiritualization and habitation of his mind rather than his body. The unconscious possibilities of chthonic aggression, bodylines, autonomy and authenticity were expressed through his anxiety and distress. After some time in analysis a deeper compensation emerged: a breakdown of his very identity as a commercial film director and his emerging desire to create a feature film that expressed his autonomy and authenticity. However, this individuatory task also provoked intense anxiety that is the remaining stuff of analysis.

Within all of this we see an old ego attitude confronted by a challenge, a challenge which augers the death of the old ego attitude. This configuration is also found reflected in fairy-tales of a certain sort.

Fairy-tales

Graça da Silva and Tehrani (2016) place certain folk- and fairy-tales as early as the European Bronze Age. They contend that such tales told in ancestral societies provide important insights into their culture, giving new perspectives on linguistic, genetic and archaeological reconstructions of human prehistory. Classical Jungians have long held that stripped as they are of more manifestly cultural elements fairy-tales reflect the structure and function of the human psyche. In particular it is an understanding of classical Jungian thinking that particular patterns of the individuation process are found echoed in fairy-tales. Von Franz (1970, p. 11) states that:

> Dr Jung once said that it is in fairy tales (*sic*) that one can best study the comparative anatomy of the psyche. In myths and legends, or any other more elaborate mythological material, we get the basic patterns of the human psyche through a lot of the cultural material. But in fairy tales (*sic*) there is much less specific cultural material, and therefore they mirror the basic patterns of the psyche more clearly.

We can take this further and say that fairy-tales, so to speak, reflect the structure and function of the individuation process. This may be set out somewhat as follows: there is an initial state (the ego attitude) which no longer works, there are attempts to repair this ego by using methods which rely on the existing ego attitude but which do not sufficiently respect the unconscious (usually imaged in fairy-tales by such as a fox, a dwarf or some other not-quite-human being). Only the unskilled part of the ego attitude (frequently presented as a foolish one, a Dummling) acts respectfully towards the unconscious and is provided with help. However, this character does not surrender to the representative of the unconscious but retains some autonomy. He thereby makes various mistakes that seem disastrous but also propel him on to the next stage of development. Once all the treasures of the unconscious are acquired the foolish one returns home but is somehow betrayed by the elements of the old ego attitude (frequently imaged by his brothers). However, the betrayal is overcome usually with the help of the representative of the unconscious (and also often the feminine figure who is part of the quest) and the foolish one is redeemed and becomes the new king – i.e. a new ego attitude is achieved.

I shall illustrate this process through the Grimm's fairy-tale, 'The Water of Life'.

Fairy-tale: The Water of Life

There was a King and he had three sons and the youngest was stupid. There came a time when the King fell ill and was dying. The sons came upon an old man who told them that the Water of Life would save him.

The eldest son begged that he might go in search of the Water of Life. The King gave in. This son hoped that if he fetched the Water of Life his father would make him the sole heir to the Kingdom.

He set out and came to a deep valley where he saw a dwarf. This dwarf asked him why he was in such haste and the Prince rudely refused to tell him and rode on.

The dwarf was enraged at this and cast a spell of ill-luck upon him. As the Prince rode into the mountain pass it grew narrower and narrower so he could not progress and he became trapped.

After a while the second son also asked his father if he could seek the Water of Life. The same pattern repeated itself with the second son and he too was rude to the dwarf and became spellbound.

And so the third son, who was stupid, asked his father if he could go. The King at first refused but the youngest son persisted and finally his father agreed. When the dwarf asked him too where he was going, the stupid Prince told him. The dwarf then said to the Prince that the Water of Life was in a castle, and gave him an iron wand with which to open the castle gates and also gave him two loaves of bread with which to feed to the lions he would find inside. The dwarf said to the Prince that he must have the Water of Life before midnight, for then the gates would shut fast. Thanking the dwarf he set off again.

Finding the castle, the Prince opened the gate with the iron wand and fed the lions the bread. He then came to a hall where he found several knights in a trance. He pulled off their rings and put them on his own fingers. He also found a sword and a loaf of bread on a table and took these. He then came upon a beautiful Princess who sat upon a couch. She welcomed him joyfully, and said that if he set her free from the spell that bound her, the kingdom would be his if he returned in a year and married her. Then she told him where the well with the Water of Life was. He went on, but feeling weary lay down on a bed lay down and slept. When he woke, it was quarter to midnight. He sprang up, fetched the Water of Life, and escaped but not before the closing gate had taken the heel of his boot off.

He again met the dwarf who told him what happened to his brothers. He begged the dwarf to release his brothers. The dwarf did so but warned the Prince that his brothers had evil hearts. Reunited, the three brothers came to a kingdom that was plagued by war and famine. The youngest Prince killed the foes with the sword and fed the people with the loaf that gave abundantly. The brothers then came to two more kingdoms in the same bad situation, and the same was done. Finally they found a ship in which to cross the sea and go home. During the sea voyage the two older brothers stole the Water of Life and filled his bottle with seawater.

On arriving home the seawater made the King even more ill. The older brothers said that the youngest son had tried to poison the King and they then gave him the Water of Life. The King had the youngest son and a huntsman go into the woods where the huntsman was to kill the youngest son. This the huntsman could not bring himself to do so and told the Prince all. The Prince and the huntsman then swapped clothes and the Prince fled.

Treasure then arrived from the three kingdoms that the youngest Prince had saved. The King regretted having his son killed. The huntsman then confessed that he had not killed the Prince. The King made a proclamation that the Prince could return.

Meanwhile the Princess waited the return of the Prince who was said to be stupid. She had a road of shining gold up to her palace. She told her courtiers that whoever rode straight up to the gate upon it, was her true lover and should be granted entry. However, whoever rode on one side of it was not the right one and should be sent away.

The time soon came when the eldest brother thought that he would go to the Princess. Coming to the golden road he thought, 'I cannot ride up this beautiful road'. So he rode only on the right-hand side of it. When he came to the gate, the guards would not admit him and sent him away. Likewise, the second brother rode up the left-hand side and he too was sent away.

When a full year had passed, the stupid Prince left the forest in which he had hidden and went in search of the Princess. Thinking only of her he did not even see what the road was made of, but went with his horse straight up the middle. So the gate was opened and the Princess welcomed him with joy. The Princess told him that his father had forgiven him and wished him to return home. He returned home and told his story. The king was very angry with his brothers but they escaped and were never seen again.

The old king invited all his court and his people to celebrate the wedding of his son and the Princess. And the wedding was held, bells were rung, all the people danced and sang and feasted. *The End*

In short we see the fairy-tale reflect the process of compensation and the relationship between the ego and the unconscious. The old ego attitude represented by the King and the older sons no longer functions well and is unadapted to the rejuvenating elements of the unconscious. We notice that no Queen, no feminine element, is mentioned at the beginning. The stupid Prince, i.e. the one who does not have the 'cleverness' of the old ego attitude engages with the elements of the unconscious: the dwarf, the iron wand, the bread, the lions, the knights, the Princess and the Water of Life. In doing this he almost slips up but just manages. The outcome is a new, adapted, ego attitude which has a different relationship with the unconscious, and most particularly the feminine.

The phenomenology of individuation – pointers to well-being

I have described the individuation process in terms of theory, of a case study and as reflected in fairy-tale. However, whilst this gives some sense of how a Jungian might approach and even translate the notion of well-being it does not give a sense of what the phenomenology of individuation might indicate of well-being. I shall try to give some sense of this (although this is probably the proper subject of a much more comprehensive study). Although not generally a sound phenomenological practice, I will in places use Jungian terms to give a Jungian sense of this phenomenology.

Individuation is an ongoing process so it is not strictly correct to speak of the 'outcome' of individuation. Nonetheless there is a way-of-being that the individual comes to when a reasonably functional relationship exists between the ego and the Self. This way-of-being has its own phenomenology. I shall describe some aspects of this.

When a reasonably functional relationship exists between the ego and the Self there is a knowing of one's 'place' in the world; of one's unimportance but also how that being unimportant is itself unimportant. At the same time there is a heightened awareness of what one's conscious sense-of-self, or ego, does and, especially, does not contribute to activities one is engaged in. One is conscious of an Otherness, mostly, within oneself (what Jungians call the Self). A feeling of partnership and dialogue with this Otherness provides a deep and mysterious source. (For myself, I mostly experience this source as a deep black pool out of which actions, ideas and feelings unexpectedly emerge. I am able to observe and accept these. In another, possibly more everyday way, I experience the givenness of certain abilities, such as the speed and accuracy of 'my' reflexes or 'my' capacity to sing as not belonging to my sense-of-self/ego but to the deep source, although mediated by my ego.)

Without claiming them as one's own there is an awareness of, and an openness to, receiving ideas, feelings and creative impulses, which emerge from this deep source that is other than the ego itself. (This appreciation expands to include a sense and respect of other people – so there is a parallel between the ego–Self relationship and sense-of-self–other interpersonal relationships.) The ego is not only receptive of but collaborates with the deep source of ideas, feelings and creative impulses but it still knows that it is not itself the source of them. Furthermore, the ego surrenders some (but not all) of its willpower and direction-taking to the deep source. Working together with the deep source the ego becomes the co-author of psyche's activities.

With the relativization of the ego there is somewhat of a decrease in anxiety and an increase in letting-be-ness. Along with these processes there is also an increase in one's self-confidence and an increased sense of autonomy, authenticity and authority. However, the autonomy is not individualistic, the authenticity is more than egoic and the authority is true authority not authoritarianism.

The ego's encounter with the Self is frequently marked through the experience of a numinous and awesome symbol.

Ryff has linked Jung's thinking to the notions of personal acceptance, personal growth and autonomy. More generally she has offered six dimensions in her model of psychological well-being: self-acceptance, purpose in life, personal growth, positive interpersonal relationships, environmental mastery and autonomy. These are, I feel, all echoed in the way-of-being that is individuation but are more nuanced and with an extra dimension to their meaning. The first, self-acceptance includes Self-acceptance, i.e. acceptance of generative otherness. Purpose in life and personal growth are more like a sense of directionality and a felt sense of meaning which may not be cognitively articulated but which are flavoured with numinosity. Positive interpersonal relations are an extension of acceptance of otherness and its contribution to one's life. Environmental mastery is not mastery by the ego alone but is contributed to by the deep Otherness and is more of a collaboration with the environment. As mentioned above, autonomy is not individualistic. In addition, there is a sense of authenticity that is more than egoic and an author-ity that stems from the collaboration of ego and Self. Furthermore, the experience of numinosity has a place in articulating well-being.

Deriving from the phenomenology and theory given above, well-being can be considered a way-of-being that emerges from the individuation process. The individuation process itself is the capacity to live out of a transcending dialectic between ego and deep Other (or Self). Individuation thus means that we live relationally with true authority (author-ity), authenticity and autonomy thereby being the true author of our own existence flavoured with numinosity.

Conclusion

In this chapter my argument has been that more detailed attention to Jung's thinking proves useful within the discipline of well-being. It offers some definite foci for processes that may lead to well-being: the importance of unconscious factors as well as conscious factors and a system for articulating psychological development, or individuation, in the achievement of well-being. I have presented the classical Jungian notion of individuation, a short case vignette that illustrates some of the processes and also how these may be discerned in fairy-tale. I have concluded with a short description of the phenomenology of individuation and how this provides a more nuanced and meaningful articulation of well-being.

I believe that Jungian thinking can make a number of significant contributions to the discipline of well-being:

1   A psychology of the unconscious in addition to a psychology of consciousness.
2   Individuation (and particularly compensation) as autochthonous processes and a system for articulating psychological development in the achievement of well-being.
3   A more nuanced and less individualistic articulation of the experience of well-being that includes the flavour of the numinous.

Further research might include the phenomenological mapping of the individuation processes and the development of well-being and what the phenomenology of individuation might indicate of well-being.

References

Ainsworth, M.D. and Bell, S.M. (1970). Attachment, exploration, and separation: Illustrated by the behavior of one-year-olds in a strange situation. *Child Development*, 41: 49–67.

Anon. well-being. (n.d.). *Dictionary.com Unabridged*. Retrieved December 26, 2015 from Dictionary.com website http://dictionary.reference.com/browse/well-being

Brooke, R. (1991). *Jung and Phenomenology*. London: Routledge.

Chekola, M. (1974). *The concept of happiness*. Unpublished Dissertation, University of Michigan. worlddatabaseofhappiness.eur.nl/hap_bib/ . . . /chekola_mg_1974.pdf

Chen, F.F., Jing, Y., Hayes, A. and Lee, J.M. (2012). Two concepts or two approaches? A bifactor analysis of psychological and subjective well-being. *Journal of Happiness Studies*. Retrieved January 29, 2018 from http:/midus.wisc.edu/findings/pdfs/1350.pdf

Dodge, R., Daly, A., Huyton, J. and Sanders, L. (2012). The challenge of defining wellbeing. *International Journal of Wellbeing*, 2(3): 222–235. doi:10.5502/ijw.v2i3.4

Graça da Silva, S. and Tehrani, J.J. (2016). Comparative phylogenetic analyses uncover the ancient roots of Indo-European folktales. *Royal Society Open Science*, 3: 150645. http://dx.doi.org/10.1098/rsos.150645S

Jung, C.G. (1971). *Psychological Types (CW 6)*. Princeton, NJ: Princeton University Press.

Malan, D.H. (1979). *Individual Psychotherapy and the Science of Psychodynamics*. London: Butterworths.

Meltzer, D. (2008). *The Claustrum: An Investigation of Claustrophobic Phenomena*. London: Karnac Books Ltd.

Neumann, E. (1954/1989). *The Origins and History of Consciousness*. London: H. Karnac (Books) Ltd.

Ryff, C.D. (1989). Beyond Ponce de Leon and life satisfaction: New directions in quest of successful ageing. *International Journal of Behavioral Development*, 12(1): 35–55.

Ryff, C.D. (1995). Psychological well-being in adult life. *Current Directions In Psychological Science*, 4(4): 99–104.

Samman, E. (2007). *Psychological and Subjective Wellbeing: A Proposal for Internationally Comparable Indicators*. Oxford: Oxford Poverty and Human Development Initiative.

Samuels, A., Shorter, B. and Plaut, A. (1986). *A Critical Dictionary of Jungian Analysis*. London and New York: Routledge & Kegan Paul.

Von Franz, M.-L. (1970). *Interpretation of Fairy Tales*. Dallas, Texas: Spring Publications, Inc.

Welwood, J. (1984). Principles of inner work: Psychological and spiritual. *Journal of Transpersonal Psychology*, 16(1): 63–73.

16

A NEW STANCE ON QUALITY OF LIFE

Lennart Nordenfelt

Quality of life à la mode

"Quality of life" has since a long time been an expression *à la mode*. It is much used in the public debate and it is influential in the field of commerce. It has been claimed that this or that measure or this or that product will enhance our quality of life. But "quality of life" has also become a technical term in social science and medicine. One can ask: what lies behind this development? And how come that quality of life has become a technical concept also in scientific research?

To some extent there was a political demand. The politicians in the Western world wanted to know what has been the result of their input into social and medical welfare. What had happened to all the people who had been the target of various social experiments and what had happened besides the construction of schools, hospitals and day care centers? Had the quality of life of these people been raised?

It became clear to politicians at all levels that one had to set up goals for people's welfare in a broader sense than had previously been stated. A person no less than President Lyndon Johnson talked about these matters already in 1964 in the US. He is claimed to have been the first person who advocated the term "quality of life". In his campaign for president in 1964 he said the following about his political goals:

> These goals cannot be measured by the size of our bank balance. They can only be measured in the quality of the lives that our people lead.
>
> (See Rescher, 1972, p. 60)

The sociologists and the social researchers in the world now faced gigantic tasks, among others to define concepts such as welfare and quality of life and also to devise instruments for the measurement of these phenomena.

But as is well-known it was not only social research that was affected by the expression *à la mode*, viz. quality of life. It affected also health care and medicine to a high degree. The goal of health care became no longer just to eliminate disease and create health. It should also entail the quality of life of the patient. This change of attitude became visible all over the Western world. In my own country Sweden it gained official status through the revision of the Swedish Health and Medical Services Act from the year 1997. There it is explicitly said that quality of life together with health is a primary goal for the official health care of the country.

Several factors have contributed to this ideological change. One of these factors is of course the technological development of medicine. In a few decades medicine had acquired impressive technological tools to save and prolong such lives as had hitherto been impossible to treat, for instance in connection with serious accidents. In some cases the use of these technologies could result in amazing results, even restoration of full health. In other cases the treatment could save lives but the life to follow could be miserable, a life in great suffering and disablement. The question could be put this life was worth living, in short, if it had a reasonable quality.

Another crucial factor behind the medical discussion about quality of life was the anthropology adopted in much modern medicine. What I have in mind is the view that is implicitly put forward in many medical textbooks, viz. that a human being is a mechanical machine, whose defects could in principle be mended through mechanical manipulations of the body. Many critics, also many medical doctors, have protested against this. They have claimed that it is fatal if medicine forgets that the human being is a person with a mind who is living in complex social relations to other human beings. Medicine and health care must recognize this fact. If medicine has the purpose of helping and healing a person and not just a mechanical body then it must recognize the quality of the life of the person. This means taking into account facts that concern the whole person and not just facts concerning details in the person's body.

Dimensions of the good life

Quality of life must have to do with the goodness of life. And the topic of the goodness of life has been in the foreground in the philosophical debate ever since antiquity. In spite of this it is astonishing that there is so little consensus about the nature of the good human life. It is equally interesting but also disturbing that this lack of consensus also holds for the modern scientific notion of quality of life. The situation is particularly problematic since the notion of quality of life is so well established both in the health sciences and the social sciences. There is now a whole industry producing "instruments" for the evaluation of quality of life and these instruments are used for a variety of purposes.[1] But the instruments differ very much. And the difficulty is not that they differ in details and in focus, which could indeed be expected when they are used for such a variety of purposes. The problem is that they reflect different views about how the basic notion of quality of life should be understood.

This fact has been known to philosophers and theoreticians in this field for ages. And although much has already been written to clarify the topic, rather little has happened in the arena of application. Much production of instruments for the measurement of quality of life is still going on as if this discussion had not existed. There is then good reason for pursuing the philosophical analysis of the topic and also for reminding ourselves of the ethical consequences of assessing the quality of people's life, not least in a situation where this kind of assessment is being made in different ways in different settings and in different parts of the world. In the present situation there is hardly a fundament for comparing results about people's lives. But if such a comparison is nevertheless made, the result can be disastrous.

A first observation in our analysis is of course that we must concentrate on a dimension pertaining to human beings. The people who request assessments of quality of life, for instance politicians, researchers within medicine and the social sciences, as well as clinicians, are asking for the quality of the life of a *human being*. Moreover, the quality should concern the human being as a whole. Still, the quality of life, when we focus on medicine and social affairs, does not concern all aspects of a person. The questions asked within these discourses do not, for instance, concern the moral value of the person in question. Nor does one ask about the aesthetic or intellectual values of the life of this person. I think it is salient that the concern is rather about what could at least vaguely be called the *welfare* of the person. Central in the quality-of-life discussion are questions about how life (in the form of external and internal events) is treating the person, and less central are questions about how the person lives his or her life, in the sense of how the person plans life and makes choices in life. The latter kind of questions would of course be particularly pertinent if the discourse were to concern moral or intellectual aspects of life.

By narrowing the scope in this way we seem to exclude the classic Aristotelian analysis of the good life. Aristotle's had an all-encompassing idea about the good life and this had a very strong moral foundation. Its basic tenet was that *eudaimonia*, the perfect life, mainly consisted in the person's virtuous activity (Aristotle, 1934).

But even if we focus on welfare in the modern sense we are left with a broad concept. And we can still dispute about what is the ultimate welfare. We can wonder whether it primarily has to do with the possession of certain objective things such as money, a job, freedom from political suppression or indeed freedom from disease, and we can wonder whether it primarily has to do with the individual's judgment of his or her situation in these respects, or, finally, we can wonder whether it has to do with the presence of pleasant mental states in the subject, partly resulting from certain external facts.

Observe that the answer to the conceptual question concerns whether welfare *consists in* certain objective things, or in things preferred by the subject, or in certain pleasant mental states of the subject. To take a definite stand on this issue does not preclude that one observes the variety of empirical connections between the three ontological categories. Two obvious such connections are that certain external states of affairs, such as money and a good job, are normally preferred by the subject, and that they normally contribute causally to his or her happiness. In such cases there is a congruence in practice between the three main ideas. A judgment of the subject's quality of life would in such a case be similar from whichever platform we judge. But, of course, it is also easy to see when the three platforms can part company.

Much of the present discussion in medicine and social affairs on quality of life focuses on choices between the three theoretical platforms. There seems to be a reasonable consensus, however, in particular in health care, that one should not ask for a purely objectivist measure. This is easy to understand when we consider the rationale for the introduction of the quality-of-life concept. The concept was introduced in medicine, as I have just said, as a supplement to ordinary medical "objective" judgments of people's health. The doctors and the researchers now want to know whether the alleged improvement of a heart or a lung had really improved the life of the individual. The objective anatomical and functional measure had always been there. Now there was a desire for information that surpassed this basic biological knowledge. The new knowledge might still contain certain objective features, but then on the molar level of the person. It could concern his or her abilities, such as the ability to walk or use one's hands. But the new knowledge must also include certain mental features of the person such as his or her preferences, attitudes and emotions. This story entails that the shift within medicine into talking about the quality of a person's life (from roughly a welfare point of view) meant a step away from an exclusively biological objectivistic position.

There is an interesting *ethical* argument for adopting a subjectivist notion of quality of life. It is clear that there is an anti-paternalist potential in a subjectivist notion. It is much more in line with respecting the autonomy of the patient to ask how the patient finds a particular treatment to be or how the patient in general judges his or her state of health to be. It is indeed difficult to involve the patient in decisions about treatment, as the principle of autonomy requires, unless the patient has made his or her own self-assessment with respect to health and quality of life.

I myself have for a long time supported a subjectivist idea of quality of life, an idea where life basically is in accordance with the subject's wants or preferences with regard to his or her life. This can also be interpreted as a life in happiness. Let me attempt to explicate this by making a brief digression into my proposed analysis of happiness.[2]

The basic notion of happiness

We normally understand happiness as a kind of feeling, or sometimes as a disposition for having a feeling. It is a very positive feeling. Many would say it is the best feeling that one can have. But it is not so easy to characterize the particular qualities of this feeling. We often have to use metaphors in describing the nature of happiness as a feeling. One may say that it is elevating, liberating or overwhelming or such things. One may conclude that the qualities of happiness can vary somewhat from individual to individual. A reasonable characterization of happiness should therefore take a different route. This route is based on the significant fact that happiness is a feeling *about* something. One can be happy about recent developments, one can be happy about the situation of one's family, and so on.

The crucial question then is: What in general can we be happy about? A classical answer to this runs in the following direction: Happiness is conceptually connected to the wants and goals of human beings. One is happy about the fact that one's wants and goals are realized or are becoming realized. One is happy about being able to do what one intends to do; one can be happy about an academic achievement or an achievement in sport; or one can be happy about some external event which contributes to the realization of some of one's goals. One may inherit a fortune which makes a journey to Australia possible.

If one's life as a whole is characterized by the fact that one's most important goals are fulfilled or are in the process of becoming fulfilled, then this life is – with great probability – a life of great happiness. It is important to emphasize that the goals talked about here need neither be conscious to the individual nor be the result of a personal achievement or even constitute a change. One of our most important goals may be to maintain the *status quo*, to keep our nearest and dearest with us, to keep our jobs and in general maintain our most fundamental conditions in life.

With this reasoning as a background I shall now give a preliminary characterization of the concept of happiness (see Nordenfelt, 1993 and 1994):

> P is happy with his life as a whole, if and only if P wants his conditions in life to be just as he finds them to be.

A more formal and abstract way of expressing this thought is the following:

> P is completely happy with his life as a whole, if and only if,

    (i)   P wants at t that $(x_1 \ldots x_n)$ shall be the case at t,

    (ii) $(x_1 \ldots x_n)$ constitutes the totality of P's wants at t,

    (iii) P finds at t that $(x_1 \ldots x_n)$ is the case.

Another more general way of expressing this intuition is to say that there is an equilibrium between P's wants and the reality as P finds it to be. The concept of happiness which I characterize here could therefore be called *happiness as equilibrium*.

It follows from this characterization that happiness must be a dimensional concept. P can be more or less happy with life according to the degree of agreement between the state of the world as P sees it, and P's wants. Moreover P can be completely happy with life only if his conditions in life are exactly as he wants them to be. Similarly, P is completely unhappy with life, only if nothing in P's life is at all as P wants it to be. There is then a continuum from complete happiness to complete unhappiness. This continuum of happiness must be distinguished from any particular state of happiness.[3]

A question

Now, is this understanding of quality of life universal in the discussion about quality of life in health care? We can hardly say that. Although there has been a tendency in the subjectivist direction it is far from clear in most instances how this subjectivism should be interpreted. One reason behind this obscurity is the lack of a thorough theoretical discussion about happiness and quality of life in health care. Please don't misunderstand me. There is not a lack of theoretical analysis of these concepts within philosophy or sociology. The lack is noticeable within the health sciences. Most constructors of instruments for the measurement of quality of life in health care do not take the time or do not make the effort to analyze the basic concepts. They have preferred different routes, mainly relying on questionnaires and interviews with a sample of people. Another source of confusion is that some instrument constructors prefer the term, and perhaps also the notion, "health" to the notion quality of life. It is thus unclear whether the constructor measures health or quality of life. I will return to this issue and discuss it more thoroughly below.

Thus, many instruments used, in particular for measurements in health care, are not as clear as could be hoped for in their conceptual underpinning. It is striking that many of them seem to collect elements from both the subjective and the objective side. They normally contain a substantial element of subjective assessment. But in addition to this one can often also find elements of an objective kind within them, for instance in terms of objective symptoms or disabilities.[4] It is indeed true that it is normally the subject who is asked to make the "objective" assessments about his or her symptoms or abilities. On the other hand, the subject is rarely asked to evaluate the impact of this symptom or disability. The person is not in general asked whether the symptom or disability is particularly disturbing for his or her way of living.

One can then wonder what the constructor of such an instrument thinks that he or she is doing. Does the constructor believe that it is not necessary to be clear about the basic concept? Or, does he or she think that there is a merit in "mixing" concepts in one and the same instrument? Or, is there a more sophisticated answer like the following? There is one basic (subjective) concept of quality of life reflected in the instrument. The questions in the instrument must however sometimes be formulated in semi-objective terms in order to catch the relevant judgments of the subject. I leave these questions unanswered here.

Health, quality of life and health-related quality of life

But let me now somewhat scrutinize the concept of health that seems to lurk in the backyard of the quality-of-life discussion. What is the relation between health and quality of life? Is there even a partial identity? Or, are the concepts very different? There is a lot of confusion on this point, which is mirrored in the instruments purporting to measure health and/or quality of life. Let me just illustrate this by pinpointing one example. The famous health economist Alan Williams (1995), who has been a pioneer in the theory of measurement in health care, in his publications explicitly talks about measuring *health*, but the unit for measurement used is called *qualy*, which is commonly taken as a unit for measuring quality of life in health care. (Note that Williams and his colleagues [Kind et al., 1982] sometimes also use the term "health-related quality of life".)

The answer to our 10 million dollar question about the relation between health and quality of life of course lies in how we define the basic concept of health. And unfortunately there are in the literature different definitions that give different answers. Let me go into this issue to some extent here. So what is health?

Two main streams of theories of health and disease have appeared in the arena. One main stream is sometimes called the bio-medical one. In modern discussion it has been specified and made precise by the American Christopher Boorse. In this version the theory has become known as the bio-statistical theory of health. What is typical of philosophers within this stream is that they claim that the concepts of health and disease and their allies – there is a whole network of medical concepts including illness, injury, impairment, defect, disability and handicap – are, or can be treated as, biological, or in certain cases psychological, concepts. "Health" and "disease" are biological concepts in the same sense as "heart" and "lung" and "blood pressure" are biological concepts. In particular, there is, according to this position, nothing evaluative or subjective about the concepts of health and disease.

The other main stream in the philosophy of health involves a completely opposite position regarding these basic matters. According to these philosophers, who are often called normativists or holists, health and disease are intrinsically value-laden concepts. They cannot be totally defined in biological or psychological terms, if these terms are supposed to be value-neutral. To say that somebody is healthy partly *means* that this person is in a good state of body or mind, the holist claims. And to say that somebody has attracted a disease is to say that this person has attracted something which is bad for him or her.

What I have done so far is just to give a superficial and rough demarcation of two lines of thought within this subject. It is very complicated to spell out and disentangle the different versions of these lines of thought. At least on the holistic side there are a number of versions. What I shall do here is rather to simplify matters and concentrate on a specific version of each line of thought and analyze them in more detail.

Boorse's bio-statistical theory of health and disease

The choice of theory on the biological side is very easy. The articles by the American Christopher Boorse (for instance 1977 and 1997) have been completely dominant in the arena. They have also been the target of most of the normative counterclaims. In presenting Boorse's theory I shall mainly use the formulations made by Boorse himself in his long defensive article, published in 1997, called *A Rebuttal on Health*. He has not abandoned the ideas expressed there in his later writings.

The aim of Boorse's bio-statistical theory of disease (*BST*) is to analyze the normal-pathological distinction. In order to capture the modern Western concept of disease Boorse proposes an explication of the ancient idea that the normal is the same as the natural in saying that health is conformity to species design. In modern terms, Boorse says

> species design is the internal functional organization typical of species members, viz.: the interlocking hierarchy of functional processes, at every level from organelle to cell to tissue to organ to gross behavior, by which organisms of a given species maintain and renew their life.
>
> (p. 7)

All conditions which are called pathological by ordinary medicine are disrupted part-functions at some level of this hierarchy, he says.

With this general description as a background Boorse presents the following definitions.

> 1 The *reference class* is a natural class of organisms of uniform functional design; specifically, an age group of a sex of a species, such as the human being.
>
> 2 A *normal function* of a part or process within members of the reference class is a statistically typical contribution by it to their individual survival and reproduction.
>
> 3 A *disease* is a type of internal state which is either an impairment of normal functional ability, i.e. a reduction of one or more functional abilities below typical efficiency, or a limitation on functional ability caused by environmental agents.
>
> 4 *Health* is the absence of disease.
>
> (1997, pp. 7–8)

An action-theoretic theory of health and disease

Some of the theories on the holistic side also focus on goals, but they do so in a very different way. They do not refer to biological goals but to goals in the ordinary human sense, viz. goals of intentional actions. When we intend to do something or achieve something we automatically intend to achieve a goal. Such a goal is not a goal of just a particular organ. It is a goal of the whole human being. Thus, these theories are often called holistic theories.

It is significant that most holistic theories consider the concept of health to be the primary one and disease as a secondary concept. Health has its basis on the level of the whole person. It is the person, not the individual organs, who is healthy. Let me put this general idea of health in the old way once expressed by Galen, the famous Roman physician and philosopher from 200 AD: *Health is a state in which we neither suffer from evil nor are prevented from the functions of daily life.*[5] Let me then introduce my own presentation of this general idea:

> A person *A* is completely healthy, if and only if, *A* is in a mental and bodily state, given accepted [or standard] circumstances, which is such that *A* has the second-order ability to realize all his or her vital goals, i.e. the states of affairs which are necessary and together sufficient for *A*'s minimal happiness in the long run.
>
> (2000, p. 93)

(Observe, however, that the concept of vital goal, in my terminology, need not be a consciously intended goal by the subject. For a detailed scrutiny of the notion of a vital goal and its place in the analysis of health, see Nordenfelt, 1995 and 2007.)[6]

According to my version of a holistic theory a person is to some extent ill when he or she does not fully possess such ability. A state of illness can have various causes within the person's body or mind. Such causes of ill health as are common or typical are what we designate as diseases. Thus, diseases, according to my theory, are such bodily and mental states of affairs as tend to lead to their bearer's ill health.

Two kinds of phenomena have a central place in traditional holistic accounts of health and illness. First, a certain kind of feeling, of ease or well-being in the case of health, and of pain or suffering in the case of illness; second the phenomenon of ability or disability, the former an indication of health, the latter of illness. These two kinds of phenomena are in many ways interconnected. There is first an empirical, causal connection. A feeling of ease or well-being contributes causally to the ability of its bearer. A feeling of pain or suffering may directly cause some degree of disability. Conversely, a subject's perception of her ability or disability greatly influences her emotional state.

In my own analysis I make an assumption of a strong connection between suffering and disability, where suffering is taken to be a highly general concept covering both physical pain and mental distress. A person cannot experience great suffering without evincing some degree of disability. But the converse relation does not always hold: a person may have a disability, and even be disabled in several respects, without suffering. There are, for instance, paradigm cases of ill health where suffering is absent. One obvious case is that of coma, when a person does not feel anything at all.

These observations indicate that the concept of disability must have a more central place in the *defining* characterization of ill health than the corresponding concept of suffering. If one of these notions is essential to the concept of ill health it must be disability. This conclusion does not deny the extreme importance of pain and suffering – as experiences and not just as causes of disability – in most instances of ill health. But it does not make suffering a part of the definition of ill health.

On subjective health

There is a further concept which is crucial for health care. It is the concept (or concepts) of *subjective* health. So far I have introduced some variants of objective health. What then is the meaning of subjective health? I have earlier (1993) discerned two primary senses of subjective health and ill health.

There is first a purely epistemic sense. A person is healthy in the subjective sense if, and only if, the person *is aware of* his or her health or *believes* that he or she is healthy. And the person is ill in the subjective sense if, and only if, he or she is aware of or believes that he or she is ill. This epistemic sense of subjective health and ill health can of course be applied to both the bio-statistical and holistic variant of health and ill health.

In another use of subjective health or ill health one refers to the typical set of mental states associated with health or illness. Some of them have already been mentioned above, when I introduced the concept of holistic health. When a person feels ill, he or she is not only aware of some illness. The person also has a number of experiences, for example feels pain, tiredness or anguish. These are examples of sensations, perceptions and moods which we typically associate with ill health.

Thus, a person is subjectively healthy or ill in this second sense, when he or she is in one of these mental states. From this it follows of course that in the holistic case, objective ill health and subjective ill health normally go together. The person who is ill in the sense of being unable to reach his or her vital goals is normally also a person who is suffering to some extent.

The relation between health and quality of life

What then is the relation between the concepts of quality of life and health when specified in this way? Let me put the various interpretations of the concepts between each other. First, I mention quality of life as welfare, the person's objective life situation. Second, we have the person's evaluation of his or her life situation. Third: the person's happiness with life. On the health side: first the person's bio-statistical health. Second, the person's holistic health. Third, the person's subjective bio-statistical or holistic health. These notions are all clearly quite different. They have different definitions. Some of these notions are very far from each other. A person's welfare in the sense of his or her objective life situation, for instance, is something very different from the person's subjective health. Some of the concepts, however, are much closer and can sometimes be difficult to separate. We could perhaps in particular scrutinize the relation between quality of life as happiness and the concept of subjective health in the mental state interpretation. Subjective health in this interpretation entails the subject's well-being of a certain sort, and subjective ill health entails a kind of ill-being. When a person is in pain because of a disease, then this person is feeling poorly and is normally unhappy with his or her life at that moment. Here is then a close relation. Can these notions then be differentiated at all?

Indeed they can. Subjective health cannot entail, pace the famous WHO definition of health (1948), all kinds of human well-being. It entails only sensational well-being and parts of emotional well-being. In general, it entails such well-being as is directly dependent on the state of the body and the psyche. Other kinds of well-being or ill-being, for instance a depression following the loss of a loved person, do not directly belong to the ill health of this person. (However, they may be causal factors behind a person's ill health.)

Assume now for a moment that we have been able to distinguish fairly clearly between the mentioned concepts of quality of life and health. How crucial is this exercise for the field of health care? Does it matter very much for how care should be organized? Should, for instance, one consequence be that health care should only deal with health matters in a more restricted sense and that considerations with regard to quality of life (in some of the senses specified above) should be directed to other kinds of carers, such as psychologists and priests?

This seems at first sight to be a reasonable demarcation. Within health care we should not seek to measure or affect people's total quality of life, at least not with means outside the sphere of medical competency, it might be contended. We must, according to this line of thought, instead focus on the strictly disease-related quality of life, that which has chiefly to do with pain, mobility, ability to sleep, etc., phenomena which are directly related to the disease in question.

On care and rehabilitation

However, there are problems with such a radical resolution. I shall only mention one such problem here. It has to do with the demands of really humane care and rehabilitation. Care and rehabilitation involves – *must* involve – taking into account of the patient's entire situation, including things that lie outside the strictly medical area. There are two important reasons for this. The first is that there is a causal feedback loop from quality of life to health. If a person feels in harmony with life and has a high degree of satisfaction with life in a broad sense, he or she will be better able to cope with illness, at the same time as – and for this there is a great deal of evidence – the healing process, on the purely medical plane, will be facilitated. The second reason has to do with our common humanity. Public health and health care are ethical institutions. They exist to help people in need. It would be absurd if within such institutions, at least in the emergency type of situation, a distinction were to be made between different causes of people's need. Suppose that a nurse has before her a person in a state of the deepest personal crisis – a person, that is, with a very low general quality of life. Will she refrain from helping this person until she has first found out whether or not the crisis has a medical cause? No, of course not: she will regard the encounter as being with the *whole* person before her, and not care whether the crisis has a strictly medical cause or not.

This argument, which I should like to call *the care argument*, is of great importance in the context of clinical prioritization, and thereby of importance with regard to our view of the clinical use of instruments for measuring quality of life.

The care argument put to use

We can imagine a very common situation in care, particularly in the care of the gravely ill and the terminally ill. You have before you a person – call her Jill – who has, and who is aware that she has, a grave and incurable disease. You have done a thorough measurement of her health and of her quality of life. We assume that the latter measurement was done with a disease-specific instrument, an instrument that in principle takes account only of the presence or absence of symptoms of the disease, for instance pain and mobility.

The disease being incurable, Jill has no care need on the health scale. Let us further assume that she has no major symptoms either. She is not in pain and has full mobility. Also according to a specific quality of life scale, she has no great need of care; this despite having an incurable disease.

Let us now assume that Jill is filled with anxiety about her life situation. She knows that she is soon going to die, and she finds this difficult to bear. She is a person in the greatest of need according to our common intuition. It would be wrong to call the anxiety a symptom of her illness: it is not an automatic consequence of a particular disease process, but the result of her *reflection* on her condition. In this sense it has the same status as the anxiety a woman can feel when her husband or child has disappeared and cannot be found. The anxiety can be severe or almost unbearable, but it is not a symptom of a physical illness.

Anxiety in this case falls within the person's general quality of life. But shall such anxiety be of no concern in public health and health care? Is it not rather the case that helping the person filled with anxiety shall be a hallmark of good care? And is it not nursing staff and paramedics that should lead the way here?

There is enough good sense in most clinical settings, not least among nurses, to fulfil also this general kind of care. All I want here is to offer a reminder that one can hardly expect to be able to set priorities, least of all care priorities, just on the basis of technical measurements of health and health-related quality of life.

In public health and health care there is not only the ethical rule whereby staff shall seek to achieve the general objectives of care, health and health-related quality of life. There are also general ethical considerations. Staff should of course, as the aforementioned example illustrates, show general compassion and attempt to reduce a person's suffering even if this has nothing directly to do with medicine or, in the strictest sense, nursing. An ethical attitude like this can require resources, as the example indicates. Thus it has consequences regarding prioritization in public health and health care.

One can here be reminded of a crucial passage in the Hippocratic oath. There is mention here of in what respects the doctor shall do good. The doctor shall if possible cure or alleviate, but always *comfort* the patient. The concept of comfort or consolation is rarely used these days, either generally or in the discussion of medical ethics. There is perhaps a new role for it in the discussion of prioritization in health care.

Notes

1 For a classical overview of instruments, see Bowling (1991).
2 See my publications (1993, 1994, 2000 and 2006).

3 For recent elaborate analyses of the concept of happiness, see Brülde (2007) and Feldman (2004, 2008).
4 See, for instance, Hunt and McEwen (1980) and the modern much-used instrument *EuroQuol* (Williams, 1995).
5 Galen: *De sanitate tuenda*, I, 5, reproduced in Temkin (1963, p. 637).
6 Another theory in the action-theoretic tradition has been developed by Fulford (1989).

References

Aristotle. (1934): *The Nicomachean Ethics*. The Loeb Classical Library. Cambridge, MA: Harvard University Press.

Boorse, C. (1977): Health as a Theoretical Concept. *Philosophy of Science*, 44, 542–573.

Boorse, C. (1997): A Rebuttal on Health. In: J. Humber and R. Almeder (eds.) *What Is Disease?* Totowa, NJ: Humana Press, pp. 1–134.

Bowling, A. (1991): *Measuring Health: A Review of Quality of Life Measurement Scales*. Milton Keynes: Open University Press.

Brülde, B. (2007): Happiness and the Good Life: Introduction and Conceptual Framework. *Journal of Happiness Studies*, 8, 1–14.

Feldman, F. (2004): *Pleasure and the Good Life – Concerning the Nature, Varieties, and Plausibility of Hedonism*. Oxford: Calderon Press.

Feldman, F. (2008): Whole Life Satisfaction Concepts of Happiness. *Theoria*, 74, 219–238.

Fulford, K.W.M. (1989): *Moral Theory and Medical Practice*. Cambridge: Cambridge University Press.

Hunt, S.M. and McEwen, J. (1980): The Development of a Subjective Health Indicator. *Sociology of Health and Illness*, 2, 231–246.

Kind, P., Rosser, R. and Williams, A. (1982): Valuation of Quality of Life: Some Psychometric Evidence. In: M.W. Jones-Lee (ed.) *The Value of Life and Safety*. Amsterdam: North Holland.

Nordenfelt, L. (1993): *Quality of Life, Health and Happiness*. Aldershot: Avebury.

Nordenfelt, L. (ed.) (1994): *Concepts and Measurement of Quality of Life in Health Care*. Dordrecht: D. Reidel Publishing Company.

Nordenfelt, L. (1995): *On the Nature of Health: An Action-Theoretic Approach*. Second edition. Dordrecht: D. Reidel Publishing Company.

Nordenfelt, L. (2000): *Action, Ability, and Health: Essays in the Philosophy of Action and Welfare*. Dordrecht: Kluwer Academic Publishers.

Nordenfelt, L. (2006): *Animal and Human Health and Welfare: A Comparative and Philosophical Analysis*. Wallingford: CABI Publishers.

Nordenfelt, L. (2007): The Concepts of Health and Illness Revisited. *Medicine, Health Care and Philosophy*, 10, 5–10.

Rescher, N. (1972): *Welfare: The Social Issues in Philosophical Perspective*. Pittsburgh: University of Pittsburgh Press.

Swedish Health and Medical Services Act (1982): revised 1997, 1982:763. Stockholm: Ministry of Health and Social Affairs.

Temkin, O. (1963): The Scientific Approach to Disease: Specific Entity and Individual Sickness. In: A.C. Crombie (ed.) *Scientific Change: Historical Studies in the Intellectual, Social and Technical Conditions for Scientific Discovery and Technical Invention from Antiquity to the Present*. New York: Basic Books, Inc, pp. 629–647.

WHO. (1948): *Official Records of the World Health Organization*, 2, 100. Genève.

Williams, A. (1995): *The Measurement and Valuation of Health: A Chronicle*. York: Centre for Health Economics.

17

"WHAT CAN'T BE CURED MUST BE ENDURED"

Living with Parkinson's disease

Virginia Eatough

Introduction

This hermeneutic-phenomenological study offers an understanding of what it means to be a person living with Parkinson's disease. It does so through a close examination of the lifeworld of a woman with Parkinson's whom I call Elsa. The lifeworld or *Lebenswelt* is "the realm of immediate human experience" (Halling, 2008: 155) which is constituted out of shared human structures or fractions which are implicated in all our experiences. These fractions include our embodied natures, our relationships with time, the various activities we are committed to and care for, our moodedness or attunement and the fact that we inhabit a world with and of others (Ashworth, 2016). They can be seen as heuristics, links in the existential chain (Van Der Bruggen & Widdershoven, 2004) which elucidate and clarify lifeworlds. Furthermore, "Each fraction is there for any phenomenon whatsoever, though some fractions may be weightier for the meaning of a given phenomenon than others" (Ashworth, 2016: 23).

The central argument presented here is that understanding the lifeworld of someone with Parkinson's can strengthen and enrich relevant healthcare practices and policies in order to improve peoples' well-being. (Van den Berg, 1972; Svenaeus, 2000; Toombs, 2002). First, this requires broadening our ideas of what constitutes evidence to include detailed research-based descriptions of people's lifeworld experiences rather than simply service users'/patients' views about healthcare services (Todres, Galvin & Dahlberg, 2007).

Second, it involves making use of phenomenological concepts and phenomenologically inspired theories to help develop a form of care and attention to well-being which has at its centre this lifeworld; that world which *matters* to the person and which an exploration of can illuminate their lived experiences. One such example is the existential theory of well-being proposed by Todres and Galvin (2010, also Chapter 8, this volume), which aims to reach beyond more traditional understandings of well-being (equating with health but not illness for example). They suggest that specific forms of well-being such as physical, emotional, economic and so forth presuppose a fundamental experiential structure of well-being, at the heart of which lies what they call a "unity of dwelling-mobility" (2010: 5). This dwelling-mobility is the deepest experiential possibility of well-being, one which contains within it multiple possibilities of well-being within a person's lifeworld:

> The essence of mobility lies in all the ways in which we are called into the existential possibilities of moving forward with time, space, others, mood and our bodies. The feeling of this "moving forward" is one of energized flow.

> The essence of dwelling lies in all the ways that we existentially "come home" to what we have been given in time, space, others, mood and our bodies. The feeling of this "coming home" is one of acceptance, "rootedness" and peace.
>
> (Todres & Galvin, 2010: 5; Chapter 8, this volume)

In what follows, I hope to illustrate the value of a lifeworld approach and of phenomenological theories and concepts. Moreover, I hope to achieve this through a focus on *one* person's lifeworld. There is a discussion to be had on the merits (or not) of this form of idiographic methodology which will not be discussed here. Suffice to say, that the view held here is akin to John Bayley's (2012) view of Tolstoy's characters which is that people are both completely particular and completely general.

A lifeworld

At the time of the interviews, Elsa was aged 82, lived alone and had been diagnosed with Parkinson's three years previously. Her experience is no longer one of a taken-for-granted world, a world of often unthinking engagement with her body, other people, objects, activities and so on. Rather the disease has and is transforming Elsa's lifeworld and to illustrate this change, I focus on four lifeworld fractions, namely embodiment, relations with others, self-understanding and project because they carry weight in Elsa's descriptions of her life.

The embodied presence of Parkinson's

Phenomenologists are concerned with the body as it is lived (*Leib*) rather than the body of physiological mechanisms and chemical interactions (*Körper*) (Merleau-Ponty, 1962) and *Leib* is "one's animate body with its 'inner life' and 'point of view'" (Hanna & Thompson, 2003). Elsa's embodied perspective is now shot through with the pervasive presence of Parkinson's, which she describes as "constantly in my head" – a significant phrase pointing to how cognition is a deeply embodied and situated activity. Tremor is one such bodily presence which moves in and out of Elsa's awareness:

> If I get cold the tremor is more pronounced. There are times when I'm not aware of the tremor at all, perhaps I'm engrossed in a film or a play or a book, lovely escape route all of them. So, I've had that sort of relief, perhaps that's what you meant. There are times when I would not know that there's anything wrong with me, and that's lovely.

Tremor is accentuated when Elsa is cold but diminished or even disappears when engaged in pleasurable activity. Most of us will have experienced when the pain or inconvenience of a minor injury, headache or toothache, for instance, fades into the background when focused on a task and the pleasure or relief it can bring.

In contrast, other aspects of Parkinson's do not so much fade or hover in and out of Elsa's awareness; rather they are stubbornly present. Housework requires her to "be conscious of every move" and getting dressed is no longer an effortless daily activity:

> I can tell you that getting dressed is a burden unlike what it used to be. You seem to be fighting everything. I think my very early experience of Parkinson's is when I discovered I was quarrelling with buttons. It [*sic*] wouldn't do what I wanted then you get suits that don't do what you want to and shoes that don't lace up the way you want. So you have a running battle with all these inanimate objects, you see? So getting undressed is an adventure, getting undressed at night is a bigger one still, because you are hopping about, one leg into the pyjamas, yes, that's great, how about the other leg, oh yes.

Elsa invokes a battle metaphor which highlights the meaning these struggles have for her. In a very real sense, inanimate objects such as buttons and laces are experienced as animate and purposive. Similarly, Elsa's "tottering" requires mindfulness:

> But that is my biggest fear that I will totter, because that's one of the difficulties at night struggling into the pyjamas and then finding myself suddenly stuck up against the cupboard because I am trying to get the other leg in.

This tottering is more than a symptom of Parkinson's; rather it is an expression of how Elsa *lives* the disease. It has become her way of being-in-the-world (Phinney & Chesla, 2003).

Elsa's body has been rendered obtrusive by the disease and constant vigilance and concentration is required as she goes about her daily life:

ELSA: Well, I have learnt to be very careful, especially in the kitchen and I have got rid of a pair of slippers with smooth soles and now have these.
INTERVIEWER: Those slippers have got grip I can see.
ELSA: That's right, because that I think it's what enabled me to totter and fall, that was in the kitchen you see and it's a blow to one's pride, it takes you by surprise you know, if you're not in control, it's a bit daunting.

The natural decline of motility means that greater awareness is needed to carry out mundane household tasks. Such restrictions are part of aging and are typically met with acceptance that one's body will increasingly impose unwelcome limitations. However, Parkinson's disease makes the task of aging more arduous because in a very real sense the disease renders one's body unknowable. Both old age and Parkinson's have rendered Elsa's bodily movements slow and tentative, making her body visible in contrast to the invisible and 'absent' body (Leder, 1990) we enjoy in health. Her body can no longer be taken-for-granted; rather it is experienced as something she *has* rather than something she *is* (Van Der Bruggen & Widdershoven, 2004).

By wearing slippers with grips, Elsa attempts to regain some sense of unreflective movement, to experience her body as less conspicuous. Those involved in the care of people with Parkinson's can assist in these attempts to become at ease with one's changing body, to develop strategies which make it more familiar again and which encourage flow and restrict over-thinking.

For Elsa, pleasurable activities, which in some way define who we are, are integral to our projects and connect us to the world, are no longer harmoniously embedded daily practices:

> I used to walk – well, it wouldn't mean much to you – but from here to my mother's at X. That's quite a few miles, it would take me an hour to get there. And I did that for the sheer joy of doing it, I did all my best thinking when I was walking. But now my thinking is restricted to the next paving stone.

Undoubtedly, Elsa's age has limited her ability to walk long distances. Nonetheless, Parkinson's disease not only restricts how far she can walk but has removed the joy and sense of freedom it brought. Walking is a source of deep enjoyment for many people; it can feel elemental, evoke a sense of positive well-being and is beneficial to maintaining good health. These aspects are diminished because of Elsa's need to focus on a reduced microscopic world – the next paving stone. This vigilance is existentially charged because it highlights how the freedom to engage in fundamental life-enhancing activities is severely curtailed.

The changing nature of Elsa's body is characterized by what Svenaeus (2000) calls "unhomelikeness", a sense of no longer inhabiting seamlessly a familiar world. Her body has become conspicuous and in doing so it is no longer capable of skilled flow of action. Elsa has lost what Heidegger (1962) describes as our typical way of being-in-the-world: unreflective "ready-to-hand" coping and engagement in smooth habits and practices. This is similar to accounts of people with dementia when dementia is understood as a deeply embodied breakdown and not simply as a disease of the brain: "The everyday grace of engaged activity is lost . . . what has in the past been transparent, seemingly 'thoughtless' activity is now revealed as a reflective act" (Phinney & Chesla, 2003: 296). One consequence of these bodily changes is the imposition of unwanted aid objects into Elsa's home giving rise to distress, resentment and helplessness. These feelings are most keenly experienced over "a bath which sat in the bath":

INTERVIEWER: Are you ok? You look as if you are in a bit of pain there.

ELSA: No, I'm just reliving, this is painful to me because she's a nice person [healthcare professional] and she was doing her best for me, so we get this thing attached to the bed, which I hate, still hate it, bang the head on it now and then. Hmmn . . . she sent someone in to put in a rail. That is really the best thing she did, I mustn't detract from her kindness. And I had this lavatory guard (laughs) but the worse [sic] thing that happened was that she sent Mediquip with a bath which sat in the bath. That arrived one Friday, hard on its heels came X, that's the name of the rehabilitation officer. She wanted to demonstrate to me how it worked. She did. And as the demonstration proceeded I got more and more uneasy, that's why I'm looking like this.

INTERVIEWER: What was your unease about?

ELSA: Having that thing sitting in my bath and turning the place into a nursing home rather than a home.

Although this event happened some time before the interviews, it has the power to evoke negative feelings still, so much so that Elsa was perceived to be in pain. The new and unwanted bath was experienced as invasive, transforming her *home* into something impersonal and unfamiliar.

The relational presence of Parkinson's

Halling (2008: 1) succinctly reminds us "To live is to live with other people." Living with Parkinson's has had a profound effect on Elsa's relations with others, and as with the physical world there has been a corresponding diminishment of her social world. To a large extent, Elsa has withdrawn from her relationships with family and friends because of a perceived imbalance between what they can do for her and what she can do for them. For example, she no longer accepts invitations to dine with friends: "The fact that I no longer feel I can entertain and then I don't like accepting hospitality because I can't reciprocate. I'm told that's not relevant, you know, but I feel it is." Not being able to contribute to the easy exchange of 'give and take' in the way she once did is a significant loss for Elsa and points to a shortfall in the relational duality which is at the heart of meaningful human relationships.

In part, Elsa's social world is shrinking because she is on her guard against "pitying looks" and friends "feeling sorry" for her. She says clearly, "I just don't like the idea of being labelled, as that's the person who has Parkinson's." Recognition that friends wish to help gives rise to uncomfortable feelings:

INTERVIEWER: And what's that like for you, knowing that people do things that they probably wouldn't have done in the past?

ELSA: Well, I accept it but inside myself I think it's a pity that they feel obliged to do that. I have more sympathy with the disabled, the blind and the deaf, I am one of them now, I'm not normal anymore, and that's a blow to one's pride.

Having Parkinson's has led to a tangible shift in how Elsa perceives herself. Its persistent presence has led to unwanted and negative changes in Elsa's most significant and enduring relationships; to such an extent that the fleeting company of strangers/acquaintances is experienced as more enjoyable. With strangers, she can experience the value of feeling equal which arises from not knowing about her condition:

ELSA: That's all right; I can meet them on equal terms because they don't know about my condition. And I kid myself; I hope that it's not obvious. Although people are very kind to me.
INTERVIEWER: Strangers are kind?
ELSA: Yes. (laughs)
INTERVIEWER: In what way?
ELSA: I never, I keep my fingers crossed on this, I never get on a bus that's full without somebody leaping up and giving me their seat. Now, I know I look feeble or I look old, I don't know which it is but I'm very grateful for the kindness of strangers.

Elsa embraces the kindness of strangers with a real sense of warmth and gratefulness. She is able to accept this level of generosity because she believes it has been given because of her elderly appearance and associated infirmity and not her Parkinson's. She shows her ease at being an elderly woman who is accepting of a societal act, which represents respect to those who are aged and inevitably less able-bodied.

Many studies report the importance of good social relationships for the maintenance of health and well-being (Antonucci, 1990; House, Landis & Umberson, 1988). Graham and Bassett (2006: 345) point to how "The tender balancing of acts, needs and intentions can make reciprocity difficult to negotiate. Some have difficulty receiving, especially those with a past history characterized as 'giver' rather than 'receiver'." This appears to be true for Elsa. Moreover, there is growing evidence that receiving nonreciprocal support is harmful because of feelings of indebtedness, lowered self-esteem and loss of self-respect (Väänänen, Buunk, Kivimäki, Pentti & Vahtera, 2005). Thus, family therapy and counselling which draw attention to how throughout one's life there are 'inevitable dependencies' (Fineman, 1995) which reflect our deep interconnectedness with others would seem one way to help people like Elsa whose struggle to maintain independence has meant a withdrawal from those most dear to her.

Elsa's relationships with healthcare professionals are characterized by tensions reflecting Elsa's changing, less powerful agentic sense of self and her evolving status as a 'patient'. Despite this, it is notable how Elsa's relationships with caring professionals are alive and meaningful for her in contrast to those with family members and longstanding friends which appear increasingly distant. The former is characterized by an emotional richness and involvedness suggesting that, at least in part, Elsa is more at ease with them.

Within this highly specific relational context, Elsa alternates between being grateful and yet resentful of the help she receives. At times, these feelings almost completely straddle one another:

I think that all that is being done for me, is with the aim of improving my quality of life. If you saw B [physiotherapist] you'd feel the same I think. He's very positive and he makes me feel like I am doing alright – I know I am not – but he assures me that I am. So I try and hold onto that. . . . He's played havoc with my life, I can tell you. The whole of this year I haven't been able to call my soul my own because he comes on Wednesdays and Fridays, so there's not much I can do either side of his visits.

The tone is light-hearted but clear: Elsa appreciates the support but this is set against a discernible resentment of its invasiveness which is especially directed towards the various assessment processes involved. Elsa experiences these as things that are 'done' to her and she is left feeling undignified and vulnerable:

"Can you get on the bed?" So I got on the bed on top of the duvet, I was like a stranded whale then. I couldn't get off. The result of that was that she got a fitment for the bed, which I didn't want. I told her I didn't want it. "Well, just try it" she said. Very nice person. "Just try it" she said. I had to do it out of decent feelings and there it remained.

Being asked to demonstrate her physical skills is experienced as being asked to 'perform':

ELSA: I would say there are times when I resent having to perform, walk to the wall, come back, walk backwards, walk sideways . . . it's a bit demeaning.

INTERVIEWER: What do you mean by that?

ELSA: I mean that I don't like having to do things to please other people.

INTERVIEWER: I see.

ELSA: You know, that's the first thing they want you to do, it's to walk. And unless they are exceptionally sensitive, that can be something you'd rather not do.

Elsa's descriptions speak of a complex mix of humiliation, umbrage, respect and a wish to please and these relationships are characterized by delicate negotiations:

We're doing tai chi together. He's [physiotherapist] doing his best to restore my balance. But that other bit of me says "you can do as much as you like but if my balance is going, it's going. However, I'll do anything you tell me dear, because you're a nice fellow and I don't want to hurt your feelings." (laughter)

Tension is palpable and fluid and tempered with a wry humour as Elsa navigates between valuing advice and 'knowing what is best for her'. Her age and generation may account, at least in part, for her need to please and be respectful when faced with those 'in authority'. In the attempt to determine 'what is best', acknowledging the *experiential expertise* of the person with Parkinson's can contribute much to the development and maintenance of positive relationships with the healthcare professionals they encounter.

Fine and Glendinning (2005) suggest that dependency in old age is perceived as shameful in some way, a personal attribute to be alleviated. They propose that 'care' and 'dependency' be seen as multi-faceted intertwined phenomena rather than as a relationship of opposites signifying power/powerlessness respectively. This involves thinking about seeking and receiving care as a positive adaptation strategy (Baltes, 1996) one which involves an ethic of care that establishes a relational practice, and which supports the notion of a "complex, life-sustaining web" of connectedness between caregivers and those being cared for (Tronto, 1993). Caring practices founded on reciprocity and mutual obligation with some sense of 'equivalence' cannot be overestimated; in their absence people like Elsa experience a severely weakened sense of belonging and shared interdependence (Graham & Stephenson, 1992; Lewinter, 2003) which shrinks further their already diminished lifeworld.

Self-understanding and projects in a Parkinsonian lifeworld

As one gets older one becomes all too aware of unwanted shifts and changes in our lives and which have an indelible effect on oneself and the people, activities and things we care for. Previous care and commitments to these projects have to be revised and our lives refashioned or even transformed. Elsa's changing body and relationships are testimony to how the 'double whammy' of old age and Parkinson's disease means that her taken-for-granted "being able to be" (Carel, 2008) is challenged. She has to work out a new way of being-in-the-world and those involved in her care face the task of helping her to do this and to envision new possibilities for living. Elsa has been thrown into the world of Parkinson's and this thrown-ness requires her to seek its significance, to make sense of it, so that she might continue to pursue projects that are meaningful for her.

One way Elsa does this is to actively reflect and *place* Parkinson's in the context of her life. For instance, she is reluctant to attribute loss of energy and balance solely to the disease:

INTERVIEWER: So you have noticed a change in the level of your energy?

ELSA: Oh yeah, not half. But then you see, when you get to 80, you don't know if it's because you're 80 or because you've got a condition. (laughs)

INTERVIEWER: Right.

ELSA: I tried that with the Parkinson's nurse but she didn't seem to agree with me.

INTERVIEWER: Right, what would she have said?

ELSA: Well, she more or less conveyed that any troubles that I've got are Parkinson's. . . . I tried to convince her that if I go off balance that's the sort of thing that happens when you are 80 anyway, she wouldn't buy it.

There is clear resistance in the phrases "I tried to convince her" and "she wouldn't buy it" which indicates something is at stake in terms of Elsa's perception of herself. Impression management is fundamental to our relations with other people and requires sensitive handling especially by those in the caring professions. Elsa wants to be and to be seen to be *more than* the disease; she does not deny the disease rather she is attempting to integrate it into her life and acknowledge that change is inevitable:

ELSA: I'm sure they [her sons] must be quite sad to see me now compared to that dragon that used to run up and down the stairs. I'm just a different person and that's what illness and old age can do to you, it seems to me. I think you go through different phases all through your life, you are the child, and you are the sulky adolescent, and you might be the young bride, or the mother, or the grandmother, you know, each phase becomes a different person in you.

INTERVIEWER: How would you describe the phase you are in now?

ELSA: (Laughs) Grumpy old woman.

INTERVIEWER: You say that with a smile.

ELSA: Yeah, well, I think you need to take these things like that. I've done very well. That is one of my attitudes. I have done very well to get to 80 with so very little to bother me.

The metaphor *dragon* suggests that Elsa perceives her younger self as a formidable personality that illness and old age has eroded. Yet, the description of herself as a "grumpy old woman" retains vestiges of this resilient tough self. It echoes a television programme in the UK, *Grumpy Old Women* in which older female celebrities discuss topical issues. Invariably, the women are feisty and spirited. If Elsa is aware of this she might be (un) consciously identifying with such women, helping her to manage this late life stage with resilience.

Acceptance and "gritted teeth" is another way Elsa manages her Parkinson's. Elsa was a teenager during WW2 and it is perhaps not surprising that her way of thinking about the disease is stoical:

What can't be cured must be endured. That was a constant saying of my mother's. She lived to 98 and a half and I pray to God I don't. Accept. I think that's the only way to deal with challenges, accept and do what you can about them.

Of course, Elsa's acceptance could be taken to signify that she is resigned in the face of the disease; however it seems to me that the better interpretation is that it reflects the accumulated awareness of a life that is being lived and reflected on.

Finally, old age and chronic illness bring the future into sharp focus. A diagnosis of Parkinson's disease dramatically changes any future one might have envisaged:

179

Oh I cried because I know it's (pause) one of the things that seem to be underlined, is that it's progressive, so I was frightened at what the future might be, living alone. I've got two sons but I don't want to be a burden to them – who does?

As Elsa correctly identifies, elderly people do not want to become a burden. This phrase is so commonplace that all too often we fail to appreciate what it *means* to the person who fears becoming one. As already noted, relationships and roles are no longer founded on a taken-for-granted give and take; rather they are perceived as skewed and characterized by a one-sided dependency. Feeling an inconvenience means that one's *worth* is eroded, that one's existential legitimacy and self-belongingness is under threat (Craig, 2013).

For Elsa, and other people living with Parkinson's, the range of existential possibilities is pared down; one has to come to terms with unwanted limitations and unrealized projects and develop new ways of being. Understanding what it means to inhabit this world of diminished possibilities is a crucial aspect of their care. This care includes support and guidance for how to make room for and accept vulnerabilities, involves thoughtful actions and encouragement to try and restore well-being possibilities so that their lives, as far as is possible are not impoverished:

> To help restore well-being for a person whose physical movement is very limited, a helper may focus on the well-being possibilities of facilitating contact with greater spatial horizons through accessing beautiful and expansive sights, smells and sounds; to help restore well-being in an ill person isolated in intensive care, a mere human touch or voice may be the intersubjective welcome that is needed to invite the person out of their sense of isolation.
>
> (Todres & Galvin, 2010: 5; Chapter 8, this volume)

One does not need to be ill to understand how, for example, the experience of walking through woodland, up mountains or on a beach is an expansive one that deepens our embodied connections to the world and others. As we saw for Elsa, walking has always been a source of pleasure, a "sheer joy" which enabled her "best thinking". If someone concentrated on the next paving stone for her, her world could and would expand again. An awareness and understanding of Elsa's loss can lead to a form of care which aims to enable an enhanced experience of well-being. After all, there is a reason we bring flowers to those whose worlds have literally shrunk, whether to a hospital bed, a living room or a front gate.

Concluding comments

In this chapter I have engaged in a hermeneutic-phenomenological reflection of one person's experience of living with Parkinson's disease. Hopefully I have conveyed, at least in part, how Elsa has made sense of this experience, and in turn, how I have interpreted this meaning-making. In my view, understanding something of Elsa's lifeworld can be insightful for the understanding of other people in similar predicaments. I have suggested that there is a need to develop caring practices which conceive of well-being as the multiple possibilities described by Todres and Galvin at the outset of this chapter. For example, carers of people with Parkinson's disease can reflect on how to magnify their contracted spatial horizons by bringing the outside world to them – perhaps bringing beautiful and scented flowers or placing a favoured armchair by a window. Such things aim to *enable* people like Elsa to grasp their existential possibilities so that well-being might flourish and a sense of existential legitimacy be maintained (Craig, 2013). In the face of old age and Parkinson's disease which inevitably looks towards death, many things can be done to help access well-being possibilities which render life more liveable and meaningful. In other words, we should aim to bring "our ways of knowing into closer harmony with our ways of being in the world" (Buttimer, 1976).

References

Antonucci, T. A. (1990). Social support and social relationships. In R. H. Binstock & L. K. George (Eds.) *Handbook of Aging and the Social Sciences* (3rd ed.) San Diego, CA: Academic Press, pp. 205–226.

Ashworth, P. (2016). The lifeworld-enriching qualitative evidence. *Qualitative Research in Psychology*, 13, 20–32.

Baltes, M. (1996). *The Many Faces of Dependency in Old Age*. Cambridge: Cambridge University Press.

Bayley, J. (2012). *Iris. A Memoir of Iris Murdoch*. London: Gerald Duckworth & Co.

Buttimer, A. (1976). Grasping the dynamism of the lifeworld. *Annals of the Association of American Geographers*, 66, 277–292.

Carel, H. (2008). *Illness: The Cry of the Flesh*. Durham, NC: Acumen Press.

Craig, E. (2013). One-ing and letting-be. *The Humanistic Psychologist*, 41, 247–255.

Fine, M. & Glendinning, C. (2005). Dependence, independence or inter-dependence? Revisiting the concepts of 'care' and 'dependency'. *Aging & Society*, 25, 601–621.

Fineman, M. (1995). *The Neutered Mother, The Sexual Family, and Other Twentieth Century Tragedies*. New York: Routledge.

Graham, J. E. & Bassett, R. (2006). Reciprocal relations: The recognition and co-construction of caring with Alzheimer's disease. *Journal of Aging Studies*, 20, 335–349.

Graham, J. E. & Stephenson, P. (1992). Ethnography and the study of aging: A critical evaluation of ethnographic description, theory, data and metaphors in social gerontology. *Santé, Culture, Health*, 8, 55–76.

Halling, S. (2008). *Intimacy, Transcendence, and Psychology: Closeness and Openness in Everyday Life*. New York: Palgrave Macmillan.

Hanna, R. & Thompson, E. (2003). The mind-body-body problem. *Theoria et Historia Scientiarum: International Journal for Interdisciplinary Studies*, 7, 23–42.

Heidegger, M. (1962). *Being and Time*. San Francisco: Harper & Row. (Translated by J. Macquarrie & E. Robinson).

House, J. S., Landis, K. R. & Umberson, D. (1988). Social relationships and health. *Science*, 241, 540–545.

Leder, D. (1990). *The Absent Body*. Chicago: University of Chicago Press.

Lewinter, M. (2003). Reciprocities in caregiving relationships in Danish elder care. *Journal of Aging Studies*, 17, 357–377.

Merleau-Ponty, M. (1962). *The Phenomenology of Perception*. London: Routledge (Translated by C. Smith).

Phinney, A. & Chesla, C. A. (2003). The lived body in dementia. *Journal of Aging Studies*, 17, 283–299.

Svenaeus, F. (2000). *The Hermeneutics of Medicine and the Phenomenology of Health: Steps Towards a Philosophy of Medical Practice*. London: Kluwer Academic Publishers.

Todres, L. & Galvin, K. (2010). "Dwelling-Mobility": An existential theory of well-being. *International Journal of Qualitative Studies on Health and Well-being*, 5, 5444. doi:10.3402/qhw.v5/3.5444

Todres, L., Galvin, K. & Dahlberg, K. (2007). Lifeworld-led healthcare: Revisiting a humanizing philosophy that integrates emerging trends. *Medicine, Health Care and Philosophy*, 10, 53–63.

Toombs, S. K. (Ed.) (2002). *Handbook of Phenomenology and Medicine*. (Series: Philosophy and Medicine, Vol 68). London: Springer.

Tronto, J. C. (1993). *Moral Boundaries: A Political Argument for an Ethic of Care*. London: Routledge.

Väänänen, A., Buunk, B. P., Kivimäki, M., Pentti, J. & Vahtera, J. (2005). When it is better to give than to receive: Long-term health effects of perceived reciprocity in support exchange. *Journal of Personality and Social Psychology*, 89, 176–193.

Van den Berg, J. H. (1972). *A Different Existence*. Pittsburgh: Duquesne University Press.

Van Der Bruggen, H. & Widdershoven, G. (2004). Being a Parkinson's patient: Immobile and unpredictably whimsical. *Medicine, Health Care and Philosophy*, 7, 289–301.

18

THE DISTRIBUTION, DETERMINANTS AND ROOT CAUSES OF INEQUALITIES IN WELL-BEING

Eleonora P. Uphoff and Kate E. Pickett

An introduction to the terminology of inequalities

An exploration of inequalities in well-being could focus on various types of inequalities. This chapter will start with an overview of inequalities in well-being *between* countries and move on to inequalities *within* countries, particularly in developed countries. We will touch upon change in these inequalities over time, for example under the influence of changes in macroeconomic circumstances, and discuss theories used to explain inequalities in well-being. The chapter finishes with a reflection on directions for future research, including recommendations on producing evidence relevant to policy makers by making better use of existing data sources and methodologies across disciplines.

There is a distinction between inequality and inequity, with inequality referring to the difference in well-being between different people or groups of people, and inequity referring to those inequalities viewed as unfair and unjust (WHO, 2008). Inequalities in well-being between young adults and the elderly, or between men and women, are to some extent the result of unchangeable biological factors. However, these inequalities in gender and age are inequities if they are the result of the way we shape our society, for example in case of the stigma related to seeking help for mental health problems. Men and young people are more likely to be faced with the prejudice associated with mental illness, and the gender gaps in health-seeking behaviour and receiving appropriate treatment grow as a result (Oliver et al., 2005). The inequalities discussed in this chapter are inequities, as these are the differences in well-being we can actively reduce through action on the social determinants of health; the circumstances in which people grow, live, work, age and deal with illness (WHO, 2008).

Research on inequalities within countries studies differences between groups of people, with groups defined by gender, ethnicity, socioeconomic position, age, geographical location, sexual preference, disability status or any other characteristic that results in one group of people being more disadvantaged than another group. Most examples provided will be of spatial inequalities (geographical location), social inequalities (socioeconomic position) and ethnic inequalities in well-being, with well-being predominantly measured through indicators of health and illness.

Although most research into inequalities in health and well-being involves adults for reasons of practicality, much of the literature cited in this chapter will explore inequalities in child well-being. First and foremost, the injustice of some having greater chances of 'being well' than others is undeniable when it concerns children. Second, child well-being shapes lifelong trajectories which influence adult well-being and the well-being of subsequent generations, making early childhood a crucial stage of life in which to intervene effectively. The Early Intervention Foundation estimates that nearly £17 billion per year is spent in England and Wales on intervening after problems have arisen instead of preventing them, such as costs associated with the care for looked-after children, domestic abuse and young people who are not in education. This financial and social burden is heaviest in the most deprived areas (EIF, 2016). We will highlight how these inequalities in child well-being are affected by the context of the society, the neighbourhood we live in and our family and social networks.

Describing inequalities in well-being *between* countries

Child mortality

The mortality rate for children under the age of 5, perhaps the starkest measure of child well-being, shows large variation between countries. In 2015, UNICEF estimated that 6 per 1000 children born in developed regions of the world die before the age of 7, compared to 47 per 1000 children in developing regions, which includes Sub-Saharan Africa with 83 under-5 deaths per 1000 live births (UNICEF, 2015). The leading causes of death for under-5-year-olds in 2013 were complications associated with preterm birth and labour, and pneumonia, diarrhoea and malaria (Liu et al., 2015). The inequality in child mortality indicates that many of these deaths are preventable.

Fortunately, inequalities in child mortality are decreasing, largely due to a reduction in deaths caused by pneumonia, diarrhoea and measles in developing regions (Liu et al., 2015). The Millennium Development Goals (MDGs) were agreed in 2000 to measure and promote progress in indicators including child mortality. The reduction in child mortality goal was met for several regions of the world in 2015. Most progress was found in Eastern Asia, driven by a sharp decrease in child mortality in China (UNICEF, 2015). Oceania on the other hand had a MDG target of 25 per 1000, but only achieved a small reduction since the year 2000 with a child mortality rate of 51 per 1000 in 2015. However, the choice of presentation of statistics greatly influences the interpretation of these results. To paint a complete picture of inequalities in child mortality, both relative and absolute inequalities between countries ought to be considered. For example, if absolute counts are used rather than percentages, Sub-Saharan Africa is clearly at the bottom of the league table with nearly 3 million child deaths in 2015, compared to 80,000 in the developed world and 13,000 in Oceania (UNICEF, 2015).

Telling the story of inequalities in well-being between countries

The growing availability of freely accessible data in online databases creates opportunities to explore these differences in well-being between countries, as well as providing information on progress over time. Non-profit web server Gapminder hosts data on global development trends which is presented graphically to make public health information more accessible (Rosling and Zhang, 2011). Figure 18.1 shows that, in 2010, it was less likely for women to give birth at a young age if they lived in wealthier countries, and this is true for all regions of the world. Sliding the time bar back on the horizontal axis shows that teen fertility rates display a downward trend over the last few decades, while inequalities in these rates continue to exist.

Another way to visualise data on inequalities in health and well-being is by reshaping maps, so that the size of countries or regions is a representation of their performance on key indicators, rather than a representation of their surface area. The map in Figure 18.2, along with many others, is freely available through the Worldmapper website, and shows the size of countries according to the number of people living in

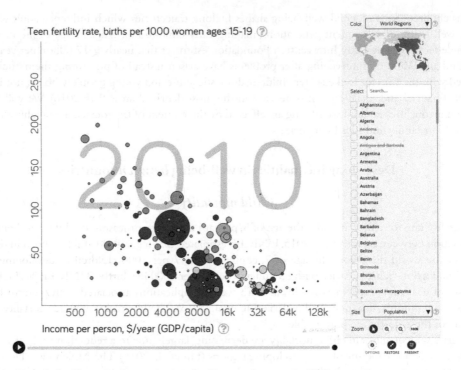

Figure 18.1   Gapminder illustrates the gap in teen fertility rates by country GDP per capita

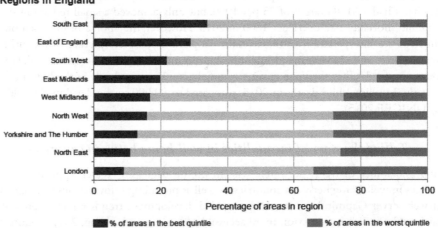

Figure 18.2   Regions in England with their best and worst scoring child well-being areas

This graph was re-created from figures presented in the original report (Bradshaw et al., 2009).

urban slums. Northern Africa and large parts of the Asian continent have ballooned, driven by estimates of 158 million people living in slums in India, 178 million in China and 42 million in Nigeria (World-mapper.org, 2005). This is in sharp contrast to 'only' 6 million people living in slums in Japan, out of their population of 128 million. These powerful visualisations may help to inform the public on inequalities in well-being between countries.

Describing inequalities in well-being *within* countries

Inequalities in well-being within countries are found in societies across the world. A study comparing adults with different income levels found inequalities in self-rated health in 45 out of 48 countries, including low-, medium- and high-income countries (Beckfield et al., 2013). These social gradients in health, with outcomes being consistently better for those closer to the top of the social ladder, have been found for various measures of social position, such as income, education, employment and perceived financial situation (Wilkinson and Marmot 2003; Marmot 1991; Uphoff et al., 2016).

Social gradients have been demonstrated for a wide range of health outcomes, with only a few notable exceptions. Skin cancer (melanoma) has historically been more common for those higher up the social ladder who could afford to visit sunny holiday destinations, although the prognosis is worse for people lower down the social ladder (Mackie et al., 1996; Shack et al., 2008). A more puzzling reversed social gradient is apparent for allergies. Possibly due to limited possibilities for building up the immune system in a very hygienic childhood environment, various allergies are more commonly found in children and adults of higher socioeconomic status (Uphoff et al., 2015).

Child well-being

UNICEF published a league table of inequality in well-being for children in high- and middle-income countries in 2016 (UNICEF, 2016). Four main aspects of child well-being addressed in this report card are: income for households with children, educational achievement at age 15, self-rated health for 11- to 15-year-olds and life satisfaction for 11- to 15-year-olds. Inequality is operationalised by measuring how far disadvantaged children fall behind the country's 'average' child.

The league tables demonstrate large inequalities in child well-being between developed countries. In Norway, at the top of the income league table, there is a difference of 37% between the median income of families with children and the income of those with an income lower than 90% of families (the 10th percentile). In Romania, at the bottom of the income league table, families with children at the bottom fall 67% behind the average. Life satisfaction scores show that Dutch children at the bottom score 24% lower than average on life satisfaction, while Turkish children at the bottom score 36% lower than average. Overall, there has been limited progress in reducing these gaps since a similar study by UNICEF was published ten years ago. As the report states, "ten years might seem too short a time frame . . . but for the individual child this covers most of their childhood" (UNICEF, 2016).

Striking inequalities in child well-being are found between regions within countries. In England, an index has been developed to assess inequalities in child well-being between local areas (Bradshaw et al., 2009). Figure 18.3 shows that, in the London region, 34% of areas are among the 20% of areas in England with the lowest child well-being scores, followed by 28% of areas in the bottom fifth for Yorkshire and The Humber. This is in contrast to the South East of England, where 35% of areas are among the highest scoring 20%, and only 8% are in the bottom fifth.

Ethnic inequalities in well-being

In societies across the world, some ethnic groups have a higher social position than others. Socially disadvantaged ethnic groups are labelled 'ethnic minorities', a term which is used to refer to a minority in numbers but also to a lower position in the social hierarchy. Ethnic minorities may derive health benefits from belonging to their ethnic group, for cultural reasons affecting health behaviours, or because of the strong social connections within some ethnic groups hypothesised to provide beneficial types of social support (Pickett and Wilkinson, 2008). More common, however, is that the lower socioeconomic position of ethnic minorities in combination with discrimination and reduced access

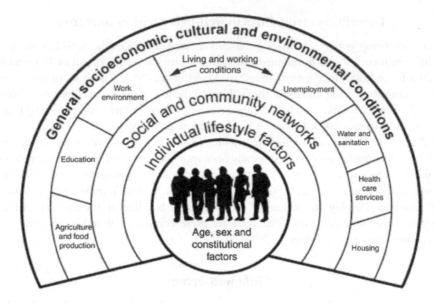

Figure 18.3 Rainbow diagram by Dahlgren and Whitehead (1991)

to services leads to poorer outcomes for a range of health and well-being indicators (Bartley, 2017a). These ethnic inequalities in health and well-being are widespread and have enormous consequences for children and adults.

In Niger, under-5 child mortality rates are 1.4 times higher in ethnic minority groups than for the dominant ethnic group (Brockerhoff and Hewett, 2000). In the UK, ethnic minority children have been found to experience more socio-emotional difficulties, with potential negative effects on opportunities for well-being later in life (Zilanawala et al., 2015). In the US, racial/ethnic inequalities were found for nearly all of the 17 included indicators of child health, even when the lower socioeconomic status of ethnic minority groups was statistically controlled (Mehta et al., 2013). There was little evidence of reductions in these inequalities in child health, and for some indicators, inequalities grew between 1998 and 2009. Ethnic inequalities in health and well-being provide evidence that a lower position on the social ladder is harmful, and these differences are not explained by socioeconomic indicators such as a lower income or lower level of education alone. In the next section we will explore the frameworks most commonly used to explain inequalities in health and well-being.

Theories of inequality in well-being

Ever since social gradients in health and well-being were first demonstrated, epidemiologists have studied what causes socioeconomic inequalities within societies. Whereas researchers were originally preoccupied with finding the right explanation and proving others wrong, it is now recognised that multiple explanations must be considered simultaneously. These multi-faceted social determinants of health, interacting with each other on different levels from the individual to the societal sphere of influence, give research on population health and well-being its complexity. From an epidemiological point of view, there are very few illnesses or states of health and well-being which are the result of a single cause, and exploring inequalities in health and well-being therefore requires a framework rather than a single explanation.

Reverse causality

As true experiments are rare in population health research, causality of relationships is often assumed rather than proven. Although we assume that a multitude of risk factors associated with socioeconomic position leads to poor health and well-being, it cannot be ruled out that the opposite may be true. Especially in the case of long-term illness and disability, poor well-being may lead to a lower socioeconomic position. However, social gradients in child well-being, based on parents' position on the social ladder, indicate it is unlikely that 'reverse causality', also called 'social selection', is the only important explanation for socioeconomic inequalities in well-being (Marmot, 1997).

Material deprivation

It was initially assumed that the main explanation for the poorer health and well-being of poorer people was that they were deprived of the tangible key ingredients for a healthy life. This may be a lack of nutritious food, poor quality housing with damp and mould, a lack of suitable clothing for all seasons, fuel poverty or limited access to healthcare due to limited financial means. The contribution of material deprivation to socioeconomic inequalities in health seems more prominent in the Western world since the 2008–2010 Global Financial Crisis. There has for example been an enormous rise in people dependent on food banks in the UK; more so in councils where larger budget cuts were made (Loopstra et al., 2015). Across the European Union, child poverty has risen in this period, particularly in the countries most affected by the financial crisis, such as Iceland and Greece (Chzhen, 2014).

Health behaviours

A third explanation for socioeconomic inequalities in health and well-being, and one upon which most public health policy is based, is that people of lower socioeconomic status display health behaviours which are more likely to lead to ill health (Bartley, 2017a). People lower down the social ladder are more likely to smoke, less likely to meet recommendations on daily levels of physical activity, more likely to eat and drink energy-dense food rich in sugar and saturated fats and less likely to meet recommendations on daily minimum intake of fruits and vegetables. These health behaviours are influenced by cultural factors varying within society, which for example explains the low rates of smoking during pregnancy in the UK South Asian population.

The cluster of health behaviours and related indicators consisting of tobacco use, high blood pressure, high cholesterol, alcohol use and high BMI are estimated to be responsible for 47% of the burden of disease in developed regions of the world (Ezzati et al., 2002). What causes these health behaviours to display stark social gradients is more difficult to quantify. The 'causes of the causes' are often described using the rainbow diagram developed by researchers Dahlgren and Whitehead in 1991 (Dahlgren and Whitehead, 1991). In this diagram (Figure 18.3), health behaviours are shown to be influenced by the wider societal determinants of health, which impact on health and well-being throughout life.

The last two decades have brought major advances in statistical methodology used to study determinants of health on multiple levels and the interactions between them. In theory, it is now possible to determine the influence of area-level factors such as neighbourhood crime, availability of nutritious food in the local area, the demographic composition of the neighbourhood, air pollution and the walkability of neighbourhoods on inequalities in health and well-being, while controlling for the influence of individual and family socioeconomic status on this relationship. In practice, disentangling these factors is near impossible and multilevel statistical models offer a simplified version of a complex reality at best.

What has brought nuance to the behaviour explanation of socioeconomic inequalities in health is the availability of research designs not relying on simple correlations between risk factor and outcome alone.

Comparing health behaviours in the same person over time, rather than comparing health behaviours between people of different socioeconomic status at one point in time, not only strengthens the evidence of causal relationships but enriches a debate which often results in blaming the victim.

The ever-popular idea that poorer members of society lack the willpower, stamina, understanding or intelligence to choose healthy over unhealthy behaviours is simply not supported by evidence. Health behaviours change as context changes. In a large birth cohort of families living in a deprived city in the North of England, we have shown that health behaviours worsened during the 2008–2010 UK recession (Uphoff et al., under review). Women who were recruited into the study during – as opposed to before – the recession were more likely to smoke during pregnancy, especially if they reported their financial situation had deteriorated over the last year.

Both the initiation and continuation of addictive health behaviours, such as tobacco use, are affected by the social and socioeconomic environment. For those lower down the social ladder, circumstances of life involve substantial financial, social and emotional distress, and this is often combined with the knowledge that these circumstances are unlikely to improve in the future. Whereas a relaxing weekend away, a spa treatment, comfort eating or a movie night are generally considered acceptable ways of coping with stress, tobacco smoking is judged and has become increasingly unacceptable as it has become a behaviour less commonly displayed by those higher up the social ladder. While there are declining trends in smoking across the developed regions of the world where the smoking prevalence has been high, smoking is now associated with the weakness and lack of motivation of the poorer part of the population (Farrimond and Joffe, 2006). Whereas most people recognise how life circumstances shape their own behaviours and well-being, interventions aimed at reducing inequalities in well-being too often focus on achieving individual behaviour change, with limited impact as a result.

The outer layer of the rainbow diagram

The higher up we move in the rainbow diagram (Figure 18.3), and the further away from the individual, the larger the opportunities for influencing other social determinants of health at multiple levels. Here we find the socioeconomic, cultural and environmental characteristics of a society.

The explanations for socioeconomic inequalities in health and well-being discussed above may explain differences in health and well-being between the rich and the poor, but they do not fully explain why every step up the social ladder is associated with slightly better outcomes. We need to look to the outer layer of the diagram, to the way we structure our society, to complement other explanations of social gradients in health. At the heart of this explanation is the nature and size of the social ladder itself.

Income inequality and well-being

In higher income countries, a rise in average wealth is no longer associated with a rise in population health. Instead, the differences in income between individuals seem to drive poorer well-being (Wilkinson and Pickett, 2009). The first empirical tests of this theory date from 1975 and 1979, and focus on the relationship with mortality (Preston, 1975; Rodgers, 1979). In 1992, Richard Wilkinson provided evidence for a relationship between income inequality and life expectancy, with life expectancy being higher in more equal countries (Wilkinson, 1992). These findings have since been replicated for different indicators of health and well-being including crime levels, school bullying and educational attainment (Wilkinson and Pickett, 2009; Pickett and Vanderbloemen, 2015). Similar results were found for different sets of countries and regions including the US (Lynch et al., 1998), for various measures of income inequality and for differences in income inequality over time (Kawachi and Kennedy, 1997; Pickett and Wilkinson, 2015b). In societies which are more socially unequal, population averages for different indicators of health and well-being are consistently lower. Countries which have experienced the largest increases in income inequality between 2007 and 2013 showed the greatest decline in child well-being (Pickett and Wilkinson, 2015a).

In more unequal societies, the social ladder is steeper and climbing the steps is harder (Figure 18.4). In the US, the pay for the average CEO was 354 times more than the pay of the average employee in the same company (Kiatpongsan and Norton, 2014). A study into perceptions of the public regarding pay ratios found that American respondents greatly underestimated the 354:1 ratio of pay for CEO to unskilled worker at 30:1, while the ideal rate was viewed to be somewhere between 20:1 and 2:1 depending on the respondent country. Across the world, and regardless of political affiliations or views on inequality, respondents favoured smaller pay gaps (Kiatpongsan and Norton, 2014).

Income inequality has been growing in the US and UK but also in countries undergoing rapid economic development such as China. Those at the bottom of the social ladder are less likely to climb up in more unequal societies; social mobility is low (Corak, 2013). The most ironic example is the American dream, which for most Americans remains just that, a dream. The best chances of making the 'American dream' come true are found in the most equal countries.

Associations between income inequality and poorer health and well-being are driven by the nature of the socially unequal society as well as the effects on its population. Some have argued that capitalist societies are more individualistic and less likely to implement generous welfare policies, since there is no public mandate or political aim to support more disadvantaged members of society, leading in turn to greater social inequality (Coburn, 2015). This means social mobility is not facilitated, and the health benefits of a higher socioeconomic position are only enjoyed by a minority.

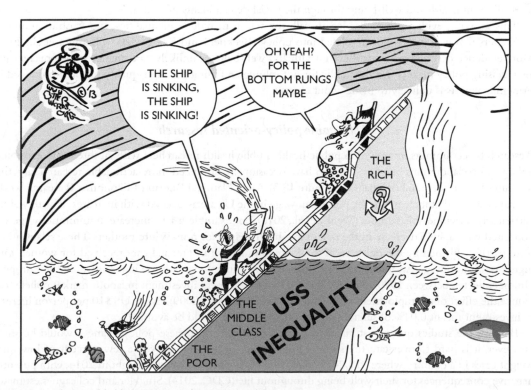

Figure 18.4 The social ladder on the US ship on inequality

Source: www.otherwords.org, by Khalid Bendid for Other Words

The social fabric is thought to benefit from connections between people of different socioeconomic status, so that relationships help you not just to 'get by' but to 'get up'. The perception that people are very different from yourself, as is the case with an insurmountable social ladder, prevents you from connecting with others and leads to lower levels of general trust (Rothstein and Uslaner, 2005). Some believe there has been a decline in 'social capital' in recent years (Putnam, 1995), while others suggest declines in social capital are related to increased social inequality and poorer well-being (Knack and Keefer, 1997; Kawachi, 1997; Kennedy et al., 1998; Layte, 2012).

Lastly, it seems that in highly unequal societies one's position on the social ladder is more important than in more equal societies. The social pressure to climb the social ladder or to at least 'keep up appearances' of a respectable social position, also described as 'status anxiety', is associated with a wide range of contemporary phenomena and health problems (Wilkinson and Pickett, 2009). Consciously or unconsciously, our ideas about how others perceive and judge us influences what we buy, which jobs we aspire to, what we do in our spare time, whom we spend time with and increasingly, how we provide evidence of all this on social media. It is feared the desire and need to fit in has led to an increase in illness, including common mental disorders, as well as a lower level of well-being for those not on the clinical end of the spectrum (Layte, 2012).

Future directions for research on inequalities in well-being

Inequalities in well-being are well established, we have a good understanding of the drivers of these disparities, and there is growing recognition that the way we shape modern society creates an environment which promotes and maintains social inequality between people, contributing to the persistence of unfair inequalities in health and well-being through the social determinants of health.

This growing evidence base has led to calls for action to reduce inequalities, and frustration among researchers that evidence is not translated into policy (Beckfield and Krieger, 2009; Bambra et al., 2010). More evidence describing inequalities in health and well-being is unlikely to convince policy makers, just as criticising policy makers and the public for not valuing and using the high-quality research produced by academic experts is unlikely to bring about change.

Actionable policy-oriented research

Research by economists interested in public health, public health researchers with an interest in economic policy and collaborations between the two have occasionally produced more actionable research targeting the outer layer of the rainbow diagram (Figure 18.3). A US National Bureau of Economic Research working paper shows that increases in the minimum wage in the US are associated with increases in birth weight, particularly for vulnerable families (Wehby et al., 2016). For example, a 10% increase in minimum wage was associated with a 4.6% decrease in the rate of low birth weight for non-White mothers. These relationships were partly explained by the decrease in smoking and increase in prenatal care received for women on a higher minimum wage. Another study using data on government expenditure in countries in the European Union collected between 1970 and 2007 showed that government investment in labour market policies can reduce the effect of unemployment on suicide risk (Stuckler et al., 2009). Every US $10 per person increase in investment meant 0.04% of suicides due to unemployment could be avoided.

Both of the studies quoted estimated that the size of effects of these policy changes would be small. However, it is hard to overstate the societal implications of preventing even a few percent of low birth weight cases in a country where 318,847 babies were born with a low birth weight in 2014, with potential negative consequences for their well-being throughout life (CDC, 2014). Stuckler and colleagues estimated that a spending of US $190 per person on labour market programmes would mean that unemployment has no adverse effect on suicide rates. In other words, the average 310 excess deaths following a 1% rise in unemployment could be prevented entirely in future periods of economic turmoil (Stuckler et al., 2009).

Similarly, there is evidence that governmental policies to protect the welfare system in Iceland after the collapse of major banks may have prevented negative impacts on child well-being (Gunnlaugsson and Einarsdóttir, 2016).

The realisation that economic and social policies are also *health* policies, even if not intended to impact on the distribution of health and well-being (Schoeni et al., 2009), should bring together researchers across disciplines including epidemiology, sociology and economics. There is room for improvement regarding the data and methodology available to provide evidence of policies effective in improving well-being and reducing inequalities. However, many methodologies have been used in the confinement of one scientific discipline, while much of the available data remains underused. Cohort studies tracking participants' well-being over time provide rich individual-level data, which could be used to compare outcomes for countries with different social and economic policies. Natural experiments have been used in epidemiology and economics to assess the impact of a societal change in exposure, for example showing a link between Scotland's smoking ban and a reduction of pregnancy complications (Mackay et al., 2012), and this methodology could be applied to inequalities in well-being. Taking advantage of existing methods, data sources and structures for data collection and cooperation could lead to advancements in research on inequalities in well-being and increase its usefulness for policy.

Conclusions

It becomes less and less credible to keep targeting individual behaviours related to well-being, when major improvements throughout the centuries and across the world have not come from telling people to live healthier. In a key textbook on health inequalities, Mel Bartley warns against this 'lifestyle drift' in policy and politics, and states: "There is no reason to think that lectures on healthy behaviour will be more effective when concentrated in poor communities than when they are targeted at the whole population" (Bartley, 2017b, p. 197). Population health will no longer be dramatically improved through advancements in medical technology. The same could be said for behavioural interventions. If the environment we live in is not conducive to good health and well-being, actions taken to prevent poor well-being through individually targeted behavioural interventions already represent secondary rather than primary prevention. The social and socioeconomic environment has become the elephant in the room, leaving a large potential for improvements in well-being and especially reductions of inequalities in well-being. Rather than investing in short-term solutions to reduce the detrimental effects of social disadvantage on well-being, we should readdress at least some of our efforts to the underlying causes of inequalities in well-being, and shape our society to provide equal chances of well-being for all.

References

Bambra C, Gibson M, Sowden A, Wright K, Whitehead M, Petticrew M. Tackling the wider social determinants of health and health inequalities: evidence from systematic reviews. *Journal of Epidemiology & Community Health*, 2010; 64:284–291.

Bartley M. Ethnic inequalities in health. Chapter in: *Health inequality: an introduction to concepts, theories and methods*. 2017a, 2nd edition. Cambridge: Polity Press. pp. 151–161.

Bartley M. *Health inequality: an introduction to concepts, theories and methods*. 2017b, 2nd edition. Cambridge: Polity Press.

Beckfield J, Krieger N. Epi + demos + cracy: linking political systems and priorities to the magnitude of health inequities – evidence, gaps, and a research agenda. *Epidemiological Reviews*. 2009; 31:152–177.

Beckfield J, Olafsdottir S, Bakhtiari E. Health inequalities in global context. *American Behavioral Scientist*. 2013; 57(8):1014–1039.

Bradshaw J, Bloor K, Huby M, Rhodes D, Sinclair I, Gibbs I, Noble M, McLennan D, Wilkinson K. *Local index of child well-being: summary report*. 2009. London: Communities and Local Government.

Brockerhoff M, Hewett P. Inequality of child mortality among ethnic groups in Sub-Saharan Africa. *Bulletin of the World Health Organization*. 2000; 78(1):30–41.

CDC. *Births: final data for 2014.* National Vital Statistics Reports, 64(12). Atlanta, GA: Centers for Disease Control and Prevention. 2014.

Chzhen Y. Child poverty and material deprivation in the European Union during the Great Recession. Innocenti Working Paper No. 2014–06. Florence: UNICEF Office of Research. 2014.

Coburn D. Income inequality, welfare, class and health: A comment on Pickett and Wilkinson. *Social Science & Medicine.* 2015; 146: 228–232.

Corak M. Income inequality, equality of opportunity, and intergenerational mobility. *The Journal of Economic Perspectives.* 2013; 27(3):79–102.

Dahlgren G, Whitehead M. *Policies and strategies to promote social equity in health.* 1991. Stockholm: Institute for Future Studies.

Early Intervention Foundation [EIF], (Eds) Chowdry H, Fitzsimons P. *The cost of late intervention: EIF analysis 2016.* 2016. London: Early Intervention Foundation.

Ezzati M, Lopez AD, Rodgers A, Vander Hoorn S, Murray CJL. The comparative risk assessment collaborating group. *The Lancet.* 2002; 360(9343):1347–1360.

Farrimond HR, Joffe H. Pollution, peril and poverty: a British study of the stigmatization of smokers. *Journal of Community & Applied Social Psychology.* 2006; 16(6):481–491.

Gunnlaugsson G, Einarsdóttir J. All's well in Iceland? Austerity measures, labour market initiatives, and health and well-being of children. *Nordisk välfärdsforskning| Nordic Welfare Research.* 2016; 1(1):30–42.

Kawachi I, Kennedy BP. The relationship of income inequality to mortality: does the choice of indicator matter? *Social Science & Medicine.* 1997 Oct; 45(7):1121–1127.

Kawachi I, Kennedy BP, Lochner K, Prothrow-Stith D. Social capital, income inequality, and mortality. *American Journal of Public Health.* 1997; 87(9):1491–1498.

Kennedy BP, Kawachi I, Prothrow-Stith D, Lochner K, Gupta V. Social capital, income inequality, and firearm violent crime. *Social Science & Medicine.* 1998 Jul; 47(1):7–17.

Kiatpongsan S, Norton MI. How much (more) should CEOs make? A universal desire for more equal pay. *Perspectives on Psychological Science.* 2014; 9(6):587–593.

Knack S, Keefer P. Does social capital have an economic payoff? A cross-country investigation. *The Quarterly Journal of Economics.* 1997; 112(4):1251–1288.

Layte R. The association between income inequality and mental health: testing status anxiety, social capital, and neo-materialist explanations. *European Sociological Review.* 2012; 28(4):498–511.

Liu L, Oza S, Hogan D, Perin J, Rudan I, Lawn J, Cousens S, Mathers C, Black RE. Global, regional, and national causes of child mortality in 2000–13, with projections to inform post-2015 priorities: an updated systematic analysis. *The Lancet.* 2015; 385(9966):430–440.

Loopstra R, Reeves A, Taylor-Robinson D, Barr B, McKee M, Stuckler D. Austerity, sanctions, and the rise of food banks in the UK. *BMJ.* 2015; 350:h1775.

Lynch JW, Kaplan GA, Pamuk ER, Cohen RD, Heck KE, Balfour JL, Yen IH. Income inequality and mortality in metropolitan areas of the United States. *American Journal of Public Health.* 1998; 88(7):1074–1080.

Mackay DF, Nelson SM, Haw SJ, Pell JP. Impact of Scotland's smoke-free legislation on pregnancy complications: retrospective cohort study. *PLoS Medicine.* 2012; 9(3):e1001175.

MacKie R, Hole DJ. Incidence and thickness of primary tumours and survival of patients with cutaneous malignant melanoma in relation to socioeconomic status. *BMJ.* 1996 May 4; 312(7039):1125–1128.

Marmot M, Ryff CD, Bumpass LL, Shipley M, Marks NF. Social inequalities in health: next questions and converging evidence. *Social Science & Medicine.* 1997 Mar; 44(6):901–910.

Marmot MG, Smith GD, Stansfeld S, Patel C, North F, Head J, White I, Brunner E, Feeney A. Health inequalities among British civil servants: the Whitehall II study. *The Lancet.* 1991 Jun 8; 337(8754):1387–1393.

Mehta N, Lee H, Ylitalo KR. Child health in the United States: recent trends in racial/ethnic disparities. *Social Science & Medicine.* 2013 Oct; 95:6–15.

Oliver MI, Pearson N, Coe N, Gunnell D. Help-seeking behaviour in men and women with common mental health problems: cross-sectional study. *The British Journal of Psychiatry.* 2005; 186(4):297–301.

Pickett KE, Vanderbloemen L. *Tackling social and educational inequality.* 2015. York: Cambridge Primary Review Trust.

Pickett KE, Wilkinson RG. The ethical and policy implications of research on income inequality and child well-being. *Pediatrics.* 2015a Mar; 135 Suppl 2:S39–S47.

Pickett KE, Wilkinson RG. Income inequality and health: A causal review. *Social Science & Medicine.* 2015b Mar; 128:316–326.

Pickett KE, Wilkinson RG. People like us: ethnic group density effects on health. *Ethnicity & Health.* 2008 Sep; 13(4):321–334.

Preston, SH. The changing relationship between mortality and level of economic development. *Population Studies*. 1975; 29(2):231e248.

Putnam, R. Bowling alone: America's declining social capital. *Journal of Democracy*. 1995; 6(1):65–78.

Rodgers, G. Income and inequality as determinants of mortality: an international cross-section analysis. *Population Studies*. 1979; 33(3):343–351.

Rosling H, Zhang Z. Health advocacy with Gapminder animated statistics. *Journal of Epidemiology and Global Health*. 2011 Dec; 1(1):11–14.

Rothstein B, Uslaner EM. All for all: equality, corruption, and social trust. *World Politics*. 2005; 58(1):41–72.

Shack L, Jordan C, Thomson CS, Mak V, Møller H. UK Association of Cancer Registries. Variation in incidence of breast, lung and cervical cancer and malignant melanoma of skin by socioeconomic group in England. *BMC Cancer*. 2008;8:271.

Schoeni RF, House JS, Kaplan GA, Pollack H, eds. Social and economic policies as health policy: moving toward a new approach to improving health in America. Policy Brief #18, National Poverty Center. 2009 May.

Stuckler D, Basu S, Suhrcke M, Coutts A, McKee M. The public health effect of economic crises and alternative policy responses in Europe: an empirical analysis. *The Lancet*. 2009; 374(9686):315–323.

UNICEF. *Fairness for children: a league table of inequality in child well-being in rich countries*. Innocenti Report Card 13. 2016. Florence: UNICEF Office of Research–Innocenti.

UNICEF. *Levels and trends in child mortality*. 2015. New York: United Nations Children's Fund.

Uphoff E, Cabieses B, Pinart M, Valdés M, Antó JM, Wright J. A systematic review of socioeconomic position in relation to asthma and allergic diseases. *European Respiratory Journal*. 2015 Aug; 46(2):364–374.

Uphoff EP, Pickett KE, Wright J. Social gradients in health for Pakistani and White British women and infants in two UK birth cohorts. *Ethnicity & Health*. 2016 Oct; 21(5):452–467.

Wehby G, Dhaval D, Kaester R. Effect of the minimum wage on infant health. NBER Working Paper No. 22373. June 2016. Cambridge, MA: National Bureau of Economic Research.

WHO. *Closing the gap in a generation. Health equity through action on the social determinants of health*. Commission on the Social Determinants of Health Final Report | executive summary. 2008. Geneva: World Health Organization.

Wilkinson RG. Income distribution and life expectancy. *BMJ*. 1992 Jan 18; 304(6820):165–168.

Wilkinson RG, Marmot M. *Social determinants of health: the solid factos*, 2nd edition. 2003. Copenhagen: WHO.

Wilkinson RG, Pickett KE. Income inequality and social dysfunction. *Annual Review of Sociology*. 2009; 35: 493–511.

Worldmapper.org [website]. United Nations Statistics Division; Millennium Development Goals Indicators: Slum population in urban areas (UN-HABITAT). Data last updated on 24 Feb 2005. Date accessed: 01/11/2016.

Zilanawala A, Sacker A, Nazroo J, Kelly Y. Ethnic differences in children's socioemotional difficulties: findings from the Millennium Cohort Study. *Social Science & Medicine*. 2015 Jun; 134:95–106.

19

AGENCIES OF WELL-BEING

Stephen Wallace

While ancient oriental cultural practices such as Buddhism, meditation and Yoga have long been widely recognised as significant and enduring purveyors of well-being over history, it wasn't until the 4th century BC that Greek philosophers like Epicurus and Aristotle turned their attention to the 'good life', a topic which marks out the modern Western attitude to well-being which continues to the present day (see Francesconi, Chapter 29, and Jørgensen, Chapter 24, this volume).

Yet it is only since the last half millennium that westerners have considered human well-being the result of anything other than God's will, random fates or deserved destinies. Indeed the concept of well-being itself is quite a modern Western invention. One of the signal arrogances of the modern humanist project asserts, as many do, that the powers of science and knowledge may allow (even require) modern man to reverse, avoid, correct and indeed ameliorate details of God's designs, if not the vagaries of fate and chance.

Over the same period various public/private enterprises and rationales for the progressive application of suffering upon other sentient co-habitants on the planet moved forward, and became socially and culturally embedded on a global scale (see *inter alia* Weapons of Mass Destruction, torture, sacrifice, entertainment, vivisection, witchcraft trials, rites of passage and executions).

As the modernist enlightenment continued to thrive in western Europe from the 17th century, it was only from the 1800s that thinkers like JS Mill and Henrik Ibsen recognised the potential (and thereby moral imperative) of the new scientific knowledge to contribute to social well-being. One of the most popular treatises which linked well-being, politics, economics and the media sprung in the 1800s from the pen of dramatist Henrik Ibsen, whose *Enemy of the People* perhaps laid an analytic template for understanding the modern program of amelioration. By the turn of the 1900s American William James had codified what might later be seen as the pragmatic roots of the Modern Ameliorist Program (hereafter MAP).

Whereas the concept of 'wellness' found various expressions in the early 20th century, much of the history of this activity and enterprise has been either dismissed or compartmentalised as way too religiously inspired to be considered under the MAP. In fact it wasn't until 1935, when physician Halbert Dunn became chief of the National Office of Vital Statistics in Washington, that wellness finally fell under statistician's gaze, and started to thrive at an official political level. It is indeed interesting to wonder how the companion projects of well-being research and statistical and demographic methods have played synergic roles in each other's historic fates.

Recent political interest in well-being has taken hold of some public imaginaries, and considerable public funding now is invested in all kinds of disparate investigations and measures of well-being (Davies 2015). Whereas Eastern philosophies have always asserted the primacy of the individual in well-being-enhancement, nowadays agencies as modest as local governments and august as the UN and WHO now are attempting to locate themselves centrally within this discourse. In fact wellness was at the heart of the WHO's 1947 Constitution. What is perhaps surprising is that official public attention (e.g. through the 1952 Magnuson Report) upon the centrality of food, shelter and employment has received such little emphasis in the following decades when compared to the psychological elements which now dominate the professional literature, and much of government enterprise. It might equally surprise some to learn that Thomas Jefferson explicitly argued that any violation of the inalienable right for the pursuit of happiness might itself justify the overthrow of government.

In 1990 the United Nations Development Programme published its Human Development Report including its first annual *Human Development Index*. This was an attempt to progress greater human well-being partly by providing country-level data for a wide range of well-being indicators. Unsurprisingly the HDI has been the subject of significant criticism since that time, for all kinds of reasons, including its misleading correlation with per capita GDP. Yet in spite of these criticisms Stanton (2007) continues to see virtue in analysing global well-being using a variety of economic metrics.

While the modern program of amelioration, resting upon its solid foundations of science and rationality, perhaps has under-delivered its promissory manifestos, other cultural programs of well-being have emerged over the last century, (such as health psychology, self-help literature, personal development programs), which retain a certain cachet of credibility even in the most sceptical quarters. So in short it seems that well-being has become a topic of considerable scholarly interest and public investment, particularly over the last three decades, and as such deserves some fresh attention in this light. I confess, at the outset, a biased reading of Anglophone literature, and a modern occidental appreciation of such matters, which can only be enhanced by other appreciations such as offered in this volume (see Takenouchi, Chapter 4 and Inahara, Chapter 12).

But the question of what animates all this activity across all these domains and periods remain a central and perennial issue which I would like to address in this chapter: what are the agencies of well-being? And this title specifically resonates in a number of ways. It asks about the kinds of agents of well-being-enhancement which may be involved; and it asks how well-being itself produces effects which might be described and measured in future times. In such a chapter as this I will have only the opportunity (and indeed resources) to provide the merest sketch of an answer to these questions, but an answer which is informed both by historic and recent enterprises.

Embedded in each of these questions of course are nests of implicated questions such as: who/what are the ultimate arbiters of well-being, and how might they be interrogated, let alone recorded, assembled and analysed? And rather than delaying the reader with a careful circumlocution about definitions etc., I will try to commence with a rough and robust review of enterprises which have been most helpful at least in clarifying these questions for me.

There have been many public trends arising out of the modern ameliorative program (MAP) including the professionalization of public health, the sciences of caring, the importance of the patient voice, the significance of scale, and primary unit of analysis. One of the most important tools of well-being literature is the statistical method of modern science. Keys, Shmotkin and Ryff (2002) suggest that first attempts to measure subjective well-being started in the 1950s as part of a scientific trend seeking to quantify life quality. The recent fetish for all things surveyable and self-reported cannot be underestimated in importance. At the same time, well-being has decentred from an essentially individual matter to a matter almost of everybody's business.

On a related front, the much-hated body/mind dualisms often attributed to continental philosophers have also been decolonised and secularised by such terms as 'subjective' and 'objective' measures of well-being, but little resolution of the fundamental philosophical problem is leveraged by such attributive stratagems. In fact the well-being arena has now been successfully colonised by an active industry of enterprising researchers with interests and investments in all things molecular and genetic. It now seems that fMRI brain scans can be used to determine mood states.

Some researchers estimate that a large percentage of well-being is due entirely to heredity, which in turn invites the evolutionary analysis of well-being. One can only imagine the delight of the research team who claimed to have identified 5-HTT as the 'happiness gene'. On the other hand, evidence has recently emerged to suggest that environmental/external conditions rather than innate dispositions are the factors more responsible for human unhappiness (Kinderman 2014) and other empirical studies have also shown how adversity may foreshadow positive life experiences for some individuals (*Counselling Psychology Review* 2015)

There is no shortage of arenas to study well-being and its enhancement in the modern world, which makes the analytic focus even more problematic. The empirical record suggests that well-being can be investigated productively through any and all of the lenses of philosophy, economics, gender, family relationships, memory, education, trauma, criminology and religion/spirituality (Davies 2015).

Our clinical language has saturated public discourses, and *doppelgangers* and proxies of well-being surround and assail us from every direction at every moment – *Take care, have a good day, you'right? Howya garn?* The study of civility has assumed a respectable place in cultural studies as well. Our putative well-being has shaped the telephonic design which attempts to assuage our impatience and insignificance through updated electronic prompts of imminent service, soothing electro-music and reassuring greetings, security checks and clearinghouse questions. The very embodiment of presenting well-being is the imperative to 'smile' for the now ubiquitous camera.

More ironically, in this period of increased investment in well-being, it is almost the greatest stigma to report low levels of well-being without a corresponding external cause or diagnosis appending. While Durkheimian anomie (or even existential anxiety) may have passed as reasonable human dispositions up to the last few decades, there seems very little acceptable space now available for unexplained low levels of well-being. In fact the MAP may well be responsible for the seductive chimera that well-being is not only a basic (Jeffersonian) human right, but moreover a readily achievable, and indeed normative, human state available for all those enrolled in the MAP. The rise in a plethora of enhancement movements such as humanistic psychology, self-actualisation, career counselling, personal coaching and positive psychology evidence both emerging occupational opportunities and demonstrable (consumer) demand for all kinds of analogues of self-improvement. Mainstream researchers (see Special Edition of *Counselling Psychology Review* September 2015) are now warming to the idea of a 'positive psychology' which seems to follow in the underexplored footsteps of theorists such as Abraham Maslow and Carl Rogers.

Positive psychology is one of the most distinctive, vibrant and potentially influential fields of psychology to have emerged in recent times. Originating with the empirical work of Martin Seligman, and theoretically developed by Mihali Csikzentmihalyi, has developed a significant theoretical corpus and empirical tradition over the last 25 years. Unsurprisingly, research activity in positive psychology has found applications everywhere from well-being/happiness, mindfulness, personal coaching and professional skill training.

Aside from the obvious hedonic virtues of well-being, positive psychology has produced evidence that (even if there seems to be gender differences in happiness) happy people may live longer, have more children, be more extroverted, be able to diffuse happiness through a social network, be more politically conservative (as they are less troubled about inequalities in society), enjoy more protection against illness (of both cardiovascular and mental kinds) perhaps through improved immune system functioning, show higher resilience to adversity, and demonstrate improved work performance. What's not to like?

While the pro-modern enthusiasts (yep even the famous rational-moral bounty-hunter Alan Sokal has had a swing at the 'non-science' of well-being research) would have hoped that by now all rational humans would have signed up to the MAP, they too recognise there are still a few minor details to clear up. While still insisting that the internal meltdown of modernism at the hands of its highest priests Bertrand Russell, Kurt Godel, Ludwig Wittgenstein, Willem van Orman Quine and Werner Heisenberg probably hasn't happened yet, they pursue what they see as pseudo-scientific outlaws attempting to enter the homeland of science (all in the name of truth, justice and myth-busting). But like traditional dragon-slaying, the beast simply refuses to die, and simply grows more offensive wings and organs. And well-being is a very flourishing dragon indeed; despite the slings and arrows of infidels it has cultivated, welcomed and embraced its loyal opposition, and has become a thriving body of scientific activity for all (pre-, pro- and post-) modern kinds. Well-being has become an emerging and vital locus of scholarly activity characteristic of a young and promising science. While everyone seems to agree that it is an important topic of study, there is much less agreement about its definition, factor structure, metric adequacy and appropriate methodology.

While I profess a thoroughgoing agnosticism to all such claims/programs, I am convinced however that failure to believe in the heaven of eternal happiness in the hereafter (life) in no way relieves us of any ethical obligation to work against the prospect of anybody enduring a life of hell here and now on earth (*contra* Genghis Khan). In saying this, I am aware of my relative cultural insensitivity and failure to appreciate any cultural view which suggests that happiness may cause bad things to happen. While few well-being theorists dared to venture into the battlefield of universal/cultural capabilities of well-being, Martha Nussbaum has notably investigated cultural norms through the analytic of well-being, and insisted that the imperatives of individual well-being trump particular cultural/moral norms, especially in those concerned with bodily integrity and health (see Calder, Chapter 9, this volume).

It may also be pertinent, in such a volume as the present, to consider just what companion programs the well-being agenda may carry along in its wake. Those most critical of the Cartesian axiom – 'I think, therefore I am' may not be reassured by this millennium's cyber axiom – 'iphone, therefore I am'. While 15 minutes of fame (or even talk/data time) may no longer suffice our well-being needs, it now seems pretty obvious that a minimally comfortable solo public performance (e.g. on subway, in the street, waiting space) is afforded by the ostensive use of some kind of smart-phone device. And it may not be unwise to assume that differential experiences of reported well-being may flow from one's choice and manifestations of consumer products in this regard. In fact, contemporary marketing strategies seem to have mined this vein of consumption motivation more and more explicitly over the years, with very little resistance from the target audience. So it is unlikely that such global enterprises in well-being will not produce effects other than those intended or expected, especially in the well-being arena. Or to put it another way; what has well-being ever done for us?

Wouldn't it be ironic if the space and opportunity to investigate (and even unfold) well-being at all is available only for those whose lives are sufficiently invested with this now much-valued human resource? In a recent film titled *The Trouble With Being Human,* Zygmunt Bauman describes two related primary challenges to human well-being: on one hand is what he describes as consumer capitalism, whereby consumer 'goods' rely increasingly less on human production; and on the other where the increasing demands upon human labour allow little time for anything (like analysis or discussion) other than the labouring and its enframing.

Some academics of a certain age are very fortunate in that they consider they were paid to live a contemplative life. And while such contemplations can assuredly elicit very dysphoric mental states, one of the most rewarding academic activities for me has been the thinking-through, drafting and editing of scholarly articles; this legitimate academic activity has produced substantial periods of well-being for all sorts of reasons. But in the present case I find myself ironically facing an historically congenial activity while still reeling from considerations of the mundane, quotidian life of Ebola epidemics, airline disasters, armed conflict, civil rights infringements, *et al.* One of the adaptive consequences of close attention to complex matters is that human cognition generally needs to 'alternate' difficult cognitive tasks such that one finds it very difficult to empathise with disadvantaged and set-upon black youth in American cities while attempting, at the same time, to locate and store a bibliographic data-base using a desktop computer. This wonderful feature of human behaviour (which has been described as 'reciprocal inhibition' by behaviourists, or 'flow' by the wellness psychologists) goes some way to explaining how some compassionate and clever people spend much of their waking hours supposedly absorbed (even obsessed) with the academic minutiae of bibliographic conventions and statistical calculations. It sure makes life a lot easier when faced with the contemplative alternative of considering how one could harness one's considerable talents and skills to address the pressing and urgent human problems which continually assail the perception of anybody claiming any contemporary awareness or knowledge of the state of their world. Successful academic performance thereby relies upon a certain degree of 'suspension of awareness' or required selective focus upon professedly trivial, menial matters while attempting to produce some opus of social significance. Even the term 'academic' seems to capture some of the ambivalence of this occupational role. While many agree that disinterested theorising and rigorous critiquing of current explanations underlying the treatments of certain haemorrhagic diseases has become an issue of global urgency and importance, few appreciate just how mindless adherence to the mundane occupational routines of plasmid-preparation taking place daily in many biochemical laboratories across the world could relieve the suffering of thousands of people. But I would argue that the enhancement of well-being for all actors in this lifeworld functions as both driver and network effect.

Further contemplation also leads the academic to consider the relativities of such circumstances – a job well-practised by most academics. While it is hard not to prefer the modern Western cushion of stable climate, cheap and accessible sources of energy, nutrition and waste-disposal and immunity to the adversities faced by most of the world's populations, many scholars will be quick to remind any attentive audience just how difficult and deprived are their circumstances (e.g. heavy workloads, impossible grant expectations, ungrateful students, impoverished teaching resources and conditions) when compared to their more fortunate ivy/ivory-league/tower colleagues (who seem to have/avoid it all).

It should be apparent that the modern Western way of life for a privileged minority of the world's population is doing pretty well. But enjoying privilege, welfare and happiness in no way affords us in recognising our good fortune, its provenance and its rather fortuitous and special circumstances. Indeed some may argue that it is just such an undeserved and long-lasting state of well-being that immunises one from less fortunate circumstances, whether deliberately or otherwise. It certainly predisposes most people to ignore unpalatable and uncomfortable criticisms which might disturb their *status quo*. So a current state of well-being may produce a global scotoma, or at least myopia, which may imperil the security of our current fortunate status of well-being. I accept that this is an argument writ large, but I suspect then any discussion of well-being, is a good opportunity to tackle topics on the larger scale, even at the cost of detailed and documented empirical evidence to support each claim.

It seems that a relatively modest state of well-being may be sufficient to enable us to survey our circumstances and appreciate our immense good fortune. Conversely, exposure to protracted and widespread circumstances of ill-being is never far from the minds of its sufferers. Even our own highly self-interested media assure us that our status is relatively comfortable on a daily basis. The modern Western community (in some parts of the Western world) overall has become a herd of contented cows, whose relative affluence is largely taken for granted, expected for the future, and seen fundamentally as an exemplar of the 'just world hypothesis'; you get what you deserve, and we deserve exactly what we have. Even though the economic theory of marginal utility (or Easterlin/Happiness-Income Paradox as it has been labelled) fails to explain how those Western media icons who seem to have achieved everything that everybody else aspires to, still seem to live such widely documented miserable lives, often leading to a premature demise.

But it also might be argued that the relative indifference to its good fortune, and the relative ill-fortune of its neighbours identifies the modern Western world as the self-serving, complacent and inconsiderate global neighbour, whose icons and values now become a legitimate target for a range of fundamentalist activist groups. It well may be that the kind of smug, congratulatory well-being, coveted so vigorously by the West, has blinded us to our position in the world; especially in so far as we enjoy so much of its benefits, comforts, securities and pleasures. Without going into the details of the regrettable history of accelerated inequality, which most Westerners are now recognising (at the very least on a descriptive level), it appears that massive increments in well-being for some sectors of the world community have been accompanied by corresponding declines for increasing numbers of the world community; in short our (modern Western) well-being has grown just as the well-being of others has deteriorated. Whether one calls this a problem of distribution, Justice, or simply global politics, it seems that well-being seems to flow upstream – as it flourishes for some, so it diminishes for most. And while this is not terribly shocking to any reasonably well-informed scholar of world events, what at the very least now emerges as a threat to our well-being, is the question of which group do we belong now, and in which group may we belong in the future.

And such discussions of the distribution of well-being are unwelcome on many fronts. For if we were to follow the logic of principled discussion, it may well be that ongoing arrangements for our material welfare may need some re-evaluation and even reconfiguration. While classroom discussions of global injustice may seem to be innocuous and inconsequential, any serious discussion of well-being which has large-scale political implications is unlikely to be welcomed by the current custodians of authority. The rise of secularism in the modern West is no accident; the famous fact/value distinction, and evacuation of all ethical content from discussions of economic and operant utility, characterises most popular and political discourse, especially amongst those enjoying the highest standards of well-being.

We can see that well-being has created a large and seemingly exponentially growing body of scholarly activity and output, which may in the long run come to be embedded in our language. This has been a result of the burgeoning numbers of academics and others who are always scanning for the next career opportunity; not to mention those in industry and government who seek to learn and profit from using the fruits of such labours. The history of psychology reveals how opportunities for applying empirical and practical applications of psychological theory have flourished over times of conflict and war. And one of the largest recipients of such enterprise was the psychometric movement, and its specialists in factor analysis. Unsurprisingly, well-being has provided psychometric researchers with new opportunities, new factors, new rotations and promising research corrections. Humans are one species who demonstrate time and time again that they are unable to resist any vanity project which reinforces their special status in the animal kingdom. And the well-being project could well qualify as just another demonstration.

But perhaps more disturbingly, it is becoming increasingly obvious how the empirical corpus of knowledge of well-being has been applied to purposes other than intended by the original researchers. And it says nothing of those whose work is funded to investigate the drivers and circumstances to produce states of dysphoria said to produce useful government and military intelligence.

It is axiomatic in the modern Western capitalist world that growth is good, especially growth in well-being. But this must be tempered by the marketing maximum that although uncertainty is said to be a 'bad' in the world of markets and investments, it can be (and certainly has been) quite useful as a primer for consumption behaviour. Indeed anxieties of all kinds (which may lead to reduced states of well-being) have been well documented as fundamental and reliable drivers of consumption, the satisfaction of which seems to result in reported escalations of well-being. Simply put, temporary and strategically implemented circumstances of threats to well-being can be remedied by otherwise unmotivated consumption behaviour, which restores and resets the well-being of many of the actors. When the going gets bad, the good go shopping.

From a similar perspective, it is fairly obvious that the spectacular growth of psychoactive remedies developed by big Pharma since the 1950s has in part benefited from a growth in all kinds of anxieties. It would not be difficult to imagine that high and sustained rates of popular well-being would augur poorly for the sales but more importantly for the development of new pharmaceuticals which have dysphoria-defeating potential. Again it seems obvious that widespread well-being is bad for anxiolytic sales. And were it not the case that so much activity and profit in big Pharma derives from these well-being remedies, increased well-being may not present such a problem.

On a most final note, the last paper published by visionary social theorist Ulrick Beck (2015) presents us with his usual provocative, and perhaps most paradoxical challenge. While discussions of well-being may seem a little academic and arcane for most readers, (even if the enjoyment it confers is a highly desired and universal good) the condition of human survival as a *sine quae non* for a life of well-being should command our urgent and singular attention. And it is to this very prospect of human survival in the face of future catastrophe, perhaps through global warming, that Beck turns his attention. While Beck's work is considered as canonic when discussing the negative side of worldly 'goods' through his theorising of the 'world risk society', he turns in his final piece to a detailed consideration of what he calls 'emancipatory catastrophism'; that is how thoroughgoing discussion about the imminence of global catastrophe (bottom line 'bads') might produce a host and range of public 'goods'. In brief he argues that catastrophe may well end badly; but in the current circumstances (which I call the pre-catastrophic period) we enjoy sufficient well-being and indeed strategic resources which theoretically may avert, avoid or even mitigate such anticipated catastrophe. While I'm sure humans have faced and recognised many periods when catastrophe seemed both imminent and unavoidable, Beck argues that the crisis he anticipates sometime in the future is unprecedented in at least two ways: in the first instance, it may well be the ultimate crisis for well-being, as annihilation, extinction or simply environmental intolerance take their toll on the human race; in the second instance, some human beings believe that humans have the capacities and resources which, if implemented in time, may forestall such a catastrophe. And one of those cardinal resources is time for strategic consideration and preparation.

Conclusion

In a funny sense, Beck seems to be arguing that the MAP, which he considers may be the cause of our ultimate demise, may well be turned around to see afresh our dysphoric future, and present itself as the weapon of choice to once again render our salvation. In starkly dramatic terms Beck sees that humanity's future rests urgently upon a thoroughgoing 'rational' consideration that all future human well-being may be a thing of the past. Indeed Beck is asking us to fully attend to that kind of dystopic future unimaginable before now. He wants us to fully consider how bad life might become, but further he argues that such dystopic focus (which of course is the antithesis of the MAP) may be the ultimate positive driver to avoid catastrophe. Could it be that well-being is so essential to being human that the mere prospect of its absence is sufficient to motivate enough humans to change their ways of living, so well-being may be even available for all in the unforeseeable future? It may well turn out that the prospect of any human life at all may depend on some humans living some now unimaginable version of 'the good life'.

References

Beck, U. (2015) Emancipatory catastrophism: What does it mean to climate change and risk society? *Current Sociology* 63(1): 75–88.

Counselling Psychology Review (2015) Vol 30, No 3, September, BPS.

Davies, W. (2015) *The Happiness Industry: How the Government and Big Business Sold Us Well-Being*, London: Verso

Keyes, C.L.M., Shmotkin, D., & Ryff, C.D. (2002) Optimizing well-being: The empirical encounter of two traditions. *Journal of Personality and Social Psychology* 82(6): 1007–1022.

Kinderman, P. (2014) *A Prescription for Psychiatry: Why We Need a Whole New Approach to Mental Health and Wellbeing*. London: Palgrave Macmillan.

Stanton, E.A. (2007) *The Human Development Index: A History*, Working Papers, Political Economy Research Institute, University of Massachusetts at Amherst.

WHO (1947) Off. Rec. Wld Hlth Org., 2, 100.

20
EMBODIED ROUTES TO WELL-BEING

Horses and young people

Ann Hemingway

Introduction

A key element of well-being is connection, social connection through knowing and being together. Animals left to their own devices will make and work to maintain and enhance emotional relationships and connections with others and as human animals we are lucky that this proclivity also extends to us . . . provided we behave in an 'acceptable' way for that animal and that species remembering who we are as human animal hunter gatherers. This article will focus on strategies in partnership with animals through which we may promote well-being in young people and will expand on Hanlon et al.'s (2011, p. 34) articulation of a current need to "discover a new image of what it is to be human" to begin to promote well-being (Eckersley, 2004; Lane, 2000). This chapter will consider humans as part of nature, one element within our ecology (Bateson, 1972), and will consider ways to promote well-being which tap into our nature and our ability to learn to be well using our bodies and our emotions; the underpinning philosophy of which focuses on inter-dependence, intersubjectivity and cooperation with each other and with other species (Hemingway, 2011).

This chapter will consider two areas in relation to the current knowledge base, learning to be well (All Party Parliamentary Health Group & The Health Foundation, 2016), and the contribution of animals to this. It begins with a consideration of what is meant by well-being and then proceeds into the evidence to date on how animals in general and then specifically horses can contribute to our well-being. The chapter will then go on to consider in detail research developments relating to young people and horses and this growing area of study, focused on learning to be well.

Well-being

Understanding well-being and its determinants allows for a whole new endeavour, that of well-being promotion, that builds on the work of the positive psychology movement (Csikszentmihalyi, 2004). This movement is concerned with enabling people and communities to see well-being as achievable and something that they can influence. The well-being of a person can be seen in terms of the 'well-ness' of the person's being. A person consists of his or her 'beings' and 'doings' (Sen, 2002); the elements of this can vary from being adequately fed, in good health and escaping early morbidity and mortality, to more complex achievements such as having security, self-respect, potential, happiness and love (Nussbaum, 1988). These complex achievements can also be articulated in existential terms as 'dwelling' or feeling peacefully at home and 'mobility' relating to one's potential thoughts, experiences and actions (Todres & Galvin, 2010; Chapter 8, this volume). It is important to note however, that problems of social justice and inequities in health relate strongly to extensive disparities in well-being, including the freedom to achieve or strive for increased well-being or 'wellbeing freedom' (Sen, 2002).

Since the mid-19th century UK public health policy has progressed from immediate threats to health (water and sanitation) to longer-term issues such as housing standards and health care provision. Most recently it has been interested in the habits of individuals, such as smoking and diet, and since the early 2000s in promoting well-being and Quality of Life (QoL) at the individual and societal level (Hanlon et al., 2011; Hemingway, 2011). These concerns have been reflected in national and international public health strategy, which has similarly begun to move from a treatment paradigm to a consideration of how to build the well-being and QoL of individuals and communities (Anderson et al., 2010; Local Government Improvement and Development, 2010; All Party Parliamentary Health Group & The Health Foundation, 2016). These developments mirror those in a number of other developed countries. In the UK, important practical outcomes of this have been the development of cycle ways and hiking routes, and the promotion of sports and outdoor activities of all kinds, including the concept of 'green' and 'blue' gyms (Cresswell, 2010; Birch, 2005) to encourage us to exercise and crucially engage with nature.

Well-being can be measured as satisfaction with life in general (uni-dimensional measurement) or satisfaction with different aspects, or domains, of life (a multi-dimensional approach) (Nawijn, 2010). Subjective well-being differs between individuals (Camfield & Skevington, 2008). It depends upon socio-political, economic, cultural and geographical contexts and changes, all of which influence people's perceptions of well-being (Bohnke, 2008; Ferriss, 2010). Well-being has been closely correlated with life and job satisfaction (Wu et al., 2009); however, subjective well-being has a hedonic element, concerned with maximising the pleasant effects of life and avoiding unpleasant experiences and their consequent negative feelings and also a eudaimonic element, concerned with self-development, self-actualisation and making a contribution to the lives of others (Le Masurier et al., 2010; McMahan & Estes, 2010; Francesconi, Chapter 28, this volume). While the hedonic aspect is mainly concerned with the self, the eudaimonic perspective tends to be socially and pro-actively oriented, and together they represent the richness of human life satisfaction and happiness in a holistic way (Le Masurier et al., 2010).

Animals and well-being

In a review of animal assisted therapy (Kamioka et al., 2014) which included only randomised controlled trials, a potential positive impact on well-being was seen in individuals with mental and behavioural disorders, and the need for more research was articulated in order to better identify longer-term impacts and effectiveness in different groups along with more detail being offered of the intervention itself. Animals included in the papers within this review as partners for humans were dogs, dolphins and farm animals. In a recent review of animal assisted therapy for young people the authors found that interventions which had been studied and published in order to measure outcomes have primarily included dogs and horses as human partners although there is also a fewer number of studies including diverse animals such as dolphins and cats (May et al., 2016). This review found that although research approaches to this area have become more rigorous in recent years more funding for evaluation is needed and that the description of interventions is still limited in published work. In addition the review found that research funders, policy makers and consumers need to gain confidence in being influenced by the positive findings of some studies so far.

Background to Equine Assisted Interventions (EAI)

In the broader equine intervention related literature there have been studies showing positive impacts on well-being through equine assisted therapy with individuals suffering with disabilities (Gabriels et al., 2015;

Del Rosario-Montejo et al., 2013; Benda et al., 2003; MacPhail et al., 1998; McGibbon et al., 1998; Brogen et al., 1996; Haehl, 1996), chronic illness, physical or mental (Dabelko-Schoeny et al., 2014; Lasa et al., 2013; Araujo et al., 2011; Hakanson et al., 2009) or individuals with eating disorders (Haumery, 2010; Hakanson, 2009; Christian, 2005). In addition, the potential benefits of equine assisted psychotherapy or experiential therapy have also been studied although the outcomes have been mixed in terms of the effectiveness of the interventions with some studies showing positive results and some no effect (Rothe et al., 2007; Klontz et al., 2007; Shambo, 2008; Selby & Smith-Osborne, 2012; De Villers et al., 2013; Yorke et al., 2013; Alfonso et al., 2015; Kendall et al., 2015).

The key difference emerging from the literature between equine facilitated learning interventions (EFL) and equine assisted psychotherapy (EAP) seems to be that EFL focuses on participants learning key social and communication skills with EAP focusing on finding ways to solve participants' emotional problems. However the evidence base is not well developed or defined at this stage.

Exploratory qualitative research has identified particular insights and emotions that may be experienced from interaction with horses and these include trust, motivation, patience respect and empathy (Hemingway et al., 2015; Schultz et al., 2007). Furthermore, some research suggests that horses may be able to reduce anxiety (Lessick et al., 2004) and help individuals develop mental and emotional self-control (All et al., 1999). Further qualitative research with young vulnerable adults has found improvements in disruptive behaviour, relationships with others and self-esteem (Trotter et al., 2008), while research by Burgon (2011) explored the experiences of 'at-risk' young people who participated in a therapeutic horsemanship program, finding improved feelings of self-confidence, self-esteem, self-efficacy and a sense of mastery and empathy.

In addition, research by Dell (2011) focused on equine assisted education (as opposed to psychotherapy) and captured through a qualitative study, the enhanced communication skills and sense of pride which the young participants experienced through their ability to communicate with the horses. Hemingway et al. (2015) gained qualitative insights into the positive impacts of an Equine Assisted Intervention (EAI) with prisoners in a young offender's institution who reported feeling calmer, and more positive about education and who also experienced marked improvements in behaviour in prison. In addition, a qualitative study in Guatemala focused on developing natural horsemanship techniques in order to reduce violent behaviour which produced positive results, particularly in relation to calmness (Gibbons et al., 2015).

Pendry and Roeter (2013) published a randomised controlled trial (undertaken in the US) focused on evaluating the effectiveness of an EAI using natural horsemanship techniques on improving child social competence. Their findings reported moderately significant improvements in the social competence of 5th to 8th grade children following the intervention. Further research is required however to gain other insights than the participant's parents into potential improvements such as teachers or social workers.

Social competence is an outcome of interest in relation to EAIs as it is considered a key domain of development that plays a critical role in mental health and overall well-being (Shonkoff & Phillips, 2000). Lower social competence is positively associated with the development of anti-social behaviour which also impacts on those communities in which the young person is living (school, home, neighbourhood; Sorlie et al., 2008). Depression (Rockhill et al., 2009), substance use (Griffin et al., 2001) and lower educational attainment (Wentzel, 1991; Sorlie & Nordhal, 1998) have also been linked to lower social competence. Young people with lower social competence are more likely to experience difficulty regulating negative emotion and arousal, which can interfere with initiating and maintaining positive peer interactions, leading to peer rejection (Dodge & Somberg, 1987), relationship problems with peers and adults, difficulty with emotion regulation; behaviour and attention challenges contribute to the development of mental health issues and poor well-being.

Interestingly a systematic review of equine assisted interventions on psychological outcomes found that the quasi-experimental design studies included in their review (n=7) tended to find no outcomes in relation to self-control, satisfaction and interpersonal trust. However all these studies showed improvements in social and behavioural outcomes thereby suggesting a potential role for equine assisted interventions in developing socially appropriate responses (Kendall et al., 2015).

Overall the papers included here have been primarily from a psychological or sociological perspective focused on either psychological changes in mood or behaviour or capturing the emotions and responses of participants and have been primarily qualitative in nature. Two recent reviews of animal assisted therapy for youth have highlighted the need for studies in this area to offer detailed insights into the description of the intervention offered and to use reliable measures as well as detailed qualitative exploration (May et al., 2016; Selby & Smith-Osborne, 2012). The systematic review reported above (Kendall et al., 2015) also concluded that the differences between equine assisted interventions themselves were substantial in that some courses offered four sessions whereas others offered 40. Interestingly the study which provided 40 sessions reported reductions in the negative symptoms of schizophrenia (Cerino et al., 2011) which are traditionally hard to treat (McGlaskin & Fenton, 1992).

Learning to be 'well'

To date there have been attempts to develop programs for young people which focus on building resilience which one could argue begins to get us thinking about teaching well-being to youngsters (Seligman, 2011; All Party Parliamentary Health Group & The Health Foundation, 2016), such as the Penn Resiliency Program in the US. Many studies have been undertaken on this program including several randomised controlled trials including over three thousand youngsters aged 8–22. This program teaches about how to handle every-day problems common for teenagers. It teaches relaxation, assertiveness, decision making and other coping skills (Seligman, 2011). However for those youngsters disengaged from traditional education and for whom talking therapies do not work learning these important skills may need to be tackled another way, possibly using an embodied route for learning.

Despite its growth in international popularity little is known currently about how inter species equine facilitated interventions may impact on human beings emotionally and physically during and after the learning experience (Selby & Smith-Osborne, 2012; Hemingway et al., 2015). The project now considered in this chapter provides a unique opportunity to begin to understand and develop this area of research, with the overall aim being to improve the well-being of young vulnerable people. The EAI (www.thehorsecourse.org/) is a charity which operates across counties in Southern England and in London and refers over 200 people every year (the majority of whom are aged 8–18 although all ages appear to benefit) by Schools & Pupil Referral Units, Children's Services, NHS Mental Health Services, Troubled Families, Offender Services and other specialist agencies (such as charities working with Domestic Violence or Drug and Alcohol Services). These people have typically more than four issues from the list below and they are referred because they are 'stuck' or disengaged from talk-based support.

- Attention Deficit Hyper-activity Disorder
- Autism Spectrum Disorder
- Anxiety diagnosis
- Not attending school (training, work)
- Relationship difficulties
- Mood swings/impulsivity
- Highly disengaged
- Self-harm
- Bullying, aggression, anger management issues
- Being bullied
- Risk taking behaviour

- Drug and alcohol misuse
- Eating disorder
- Offending
- Domestic violence
- Neglect/abuse
- Parents with mental health problems, offending or drug and alcohol issues
- Living in care or leaving care
- Conduct disorder

The course teaches, rehearses and repeats key resilience skills in an intensive five-day course with feedback in-the-moment from specially trained horses and 1-to-1 facilitator support. Thus far this intervention has been evaluated using qualitative (Hemingway, 2015) and quantitative methodologies (before and after measures) and currently a one year follow-up is being undertaken to gain insights into any possible longer-term impacts of the program. The before and after and two month follow-up score results thus far show that more than 80 per cent of participants:

- are less anxious,
- have reduced problem behaviours,
- improve attendance/engagement at school,
- have better relationships and
- increase self-belief.

(THC 2015)

Details of the Intervention (EAI)

The intervention uses the principles of the Parelli Natural Horsemanship program as its philosophical basis and structure (Parelli, 2011). Although this program has existed for 30 years its use with this group of vulnerable young people is innovative. This approach is based on cooperation and partnership development. At this introductory level this involves 'playing' with horses, inviting them to respond to requests with the young person on the ground and the horse on a loose rope. The learning is facilitated by the course instructor and the students are taught how to play the seven 'games' (Parelli, 2011) with the horses. The course takes place over seven two-and-a-half hour sessions. The games taught are:

1) *The friendly game* (creating relaxation through touch, grazing, grooming, hanging out).
2) *The porcupine game* (moving the horse's feet through using steady pressure, touching the horse).
3) *The driving game* (moving the horse's feet through rhythmic pressure, not touching the horse).
4) *The yo-yo game* (moving the horse backwards and forwards).
5) *The circling game* (asking the horse to travel around you on the circle).
6) *The sideways game* (asking the horse to move sideways).
7) *The squeeze game* (asking the horse to go through, under or over something; Parelli, 2011).

Although the students are learning, the horses are highly trained but will only comply if the young person can gain the horse's trust through appropriate actions and behaviour. These games help to establish a simple yet comprehensive communication between horses and humans. However in order to be effective the human needs to use clear, phased assertive communication and control their body language and energy in an assertive, non-aggressive way. Rather than using the horse as a passive adjunct or emotional 'mirror' to a therapeutic intervention as in many other EAIs these horses teach the human participants through their responses while playing these games. A horse which has been developed to communicate with humans in this way is able to be an active participant in the development of the young person. They will respond appropriately only when the human succeeds in developing these essential embodied skills.

The approach used in this program enables the students to make progress with the horses without direct physical management by another person. Students spend the majority of their time on the course rehearsing the skills of empathy, communication and calm assertiveness, rather than talking about them. This rehearsal process gradually enables the human to become an effective partner and leader for the horse. Interestingly the interactions between the facilitator and the student in this intervention are guided by the same principles used for teaching horses, which focus on reading body language and responding appropriately in the moment. The course teaches through simulation rather than explanation and uses non-verbal methods (through rehearsal) to positively impact on the thoughts and emotions of the students. The course facilitator allows the students to try and aims to help them achieve excellent horsemanship skills from the start of the program.

The course facilitator also takes a ten-minute video of the student playing with a horse which is submitted to the Parelli organisation who assess the performance of the human (Parelli, 2011). All the students who have undertaken this program so far have achieved their level 1 natural horsemanship qualification with some achieving level 2 or components of level 3 of the program. At the end of the course the students will be able to demonstrate their new skills with horses to the course facilitator and invited guests, normally their social workers/teachers, parents, as appropriate.

Emotions and learning

The relationship between emotions and learning is well established in theory (Carter & Smith Pasqualini, 2004; Damasio, 2010); however, it has not been tested in real-world applications focused on behaviour change. Indeed research has suggested that stronger autonomic responses produce better learning, indeed that somatic marking facilitates learning (Carter & Smith Pasqualini, 2004). A growing body of literature suggests that somatic states related to emotion are involved in cognitive processes, including learning (Lo & Repin, 2002). An example of this development is Damasio's somatic marker hypothesis (SMH) which states that for every life event, somatic consequences are marked and then reproduced when that event recurs. These somatic consequences are strongly connected with the emotion systems of the brain; according to the SMH the prefrontal cortex coordinates external stimulus information with internal information about emotion-based body states provided by brainstem nuclei, somatosensory and insular cortex and the amygdala. When this loop is activated by the recurrence of an external event it can take the form of a complete reproduction of the body experience or a weaker reproduction which bypasses the bodily experience. This reproduction of an emotional state assists in distinguishing the merits of one option over another; therefore somatic marking enables us to make decisions based on previous learning quickly. This would suggest that emotional marking of experiences as either rewarding or punishing enables us to learn how to behave (Damasio, 1994, 1999).

Further support for this hypothesis has come from various sources. Critchley et al. (2000) found using functional magnetic resonance imagery that changes in activity of the prefrontal cortex were related to spontaneous fluctuations in Skin Conductivity Responses (SCR, measuring emotional responses). Since then similar effects have been found using positron emission tomography (Ernst et al., 2002). Then in 2004 research was undertaken with healthy volunteers to examine whether a stronger autonomic response accompanies better learning essentially testing out Damasio's somatic marker hypothesis (Carter & Smith Pasqualini, 2004). This research found that positive emotions enable effective learning and behaviour change.

It would appear that from the literature considered here so far interacting and learning with horses is an emotional experience for us as humans; however the overall impacts seem to be behavioural (see Figure 20.1). Is this mechanism what enables us as human mammals to pass from emotional embodied learning to behaviour change through undertaking EAI?

Emerging ideas from the literature review (Figure 20.1)

In order to explore this relationship between emotions and learning in the context of EAI and to develop research methodologies to describe this process further a team of researchers in the UK have undertaken a small experimental pilot study to attempt to understand whether interventions which include horses may be tapping into this mechanism. In order to do this we have used psychophysiological measurement and qualitative interviews to help us understand the learning taking place on The Horse Course. The aim of the study was to explore the psychophysiological mechanism of action of this equine assisted intervention. The participants were volunteer sports science students in the second year of their degree in a university in the South of England. The following methods of data collection were used to inform this study:

- Analysis of psychophysiology data specifically measuring heart rate, heart rate variability, breathing, galvanic skin response and neurological/emotional measurements (facial EMG) were recorded to establish baseline measures then while the students watched and listened to themselves undertake elements of an EAI within 24 hours of practically undertaking the course.
- Qualitative interviews undertaken with the participants while they watched themselves on video undertaken within five days of undertaking the course. Used in order to explore how they felt (the emotions they experienced) while undertaking the learning experience.

Students were filmed as they learned natural horsemanship skills in the 'field' (indoor equine sand school) for approximately 30 minutes, and then measurements and interviews (in two separate sessions) were carried out within a quiet calm setting (university lab) while students watched and listened to themselves on video to study in detail responses and learning. Students were also asked about their feelings at certain points during the data collection in the laboratory in order to gain further phenomenological insights into their emotions while undertaking the course.

This pilot project with volunteer university sports science students (n=5) as subjects in early 2015 has shown interesting insights into the emotional journey of undertaking elements of The Horse Course. This has been done in order to test and refine this research methodology which was found in this pilot to be effective and engaging for the student participants. Interestingly for these participants the emotional changes shown below were described by them after watching themselves complete a 30-minute period of being taught elements of the course, and being able to rehearse them with the horses. These emotional changes are congruent with previous studies and the evaluation of The Horse Course to date.

Emotional changes described by the pilot study participants (Figure 20.2)

The early psychophysiology results would suggest that the student's skin conductance response (SCR) was activated by asking the horse to do something and the SCR declined immediately if the horse responded appropriately. This response, also known as the electrodermal response (and in older terminology as 'galvanic skin response'), is the phenomenon that the skin momentarily becomes a better conductor of electricity when either external or internal stimuli occur that are physiologically arousing. Arousal is a broad term referring to overall activation, and is widely considered to be one of the two main dimensions of an emotional response. Measuring arousal is therefore not the same as measuring emotion, but is an important component of it. Arousal has been found to be a strong predictor of attention and memory. The stimuli to which skin conductance is sensitive are manifold, including in novel, significant or intense situations or experiences. Many different kinds of events can elevate your response including strong emotion, a startling event or a demanding task. It is unclear at this point whether the participants in this pilot responded to the demands of the course or the emotion of interacting with horses or both.

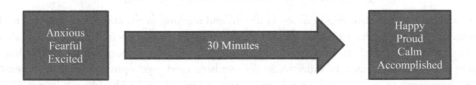

In addition, in the students this SCR response seemed to lower as the horse visibly relaxed (head lowering, blowing out through their nostrils) and vice versa indicating that there may be some kind of reciprocal drop in arousal occurring although this study is obviously limited and all findings require further research. Interestingly in the interviews the participants were not aware of these psychophysiological changes until later . . . around ten minutes later when they started to express feelings of calmness and happiness. This concurs with Damasio's SMH which suggests that this learning is occurring through our emotions and our bodies rather than cognitively; our cognitive recognition of changes in mood or emotion seem to happen later.

The relevance for equine assisted interventions

In relation to the study of equine facilitated interventions, this study offers a small step forward as little has been published to date on the potential mechanism of action for these interventions. It may be possible that this pilot has started to shed light on the possible route to impact of embodied inter species learning and its hypothetical ability to impact our emotions and our learning, therefore potentially influencing our behaviour (the next stage of the study).

The Horse Course intervention does not use cognitive (talking or classroom-based) approaches as is generally the default within interventions for this group currently; indeed students are responded to in the same way as horses by the facilitator, in response to their body language primarily rather than the spoken word. It is particularly important when evaluating an intervention to consider the qualities of the intervention that render it effective. From evaluation of The Horse Course undertaken by the author in a young offenders' institute the immediate feedback 'in the moment' from the horses and the facilitator was an essential quality of the intervention rather than, 'just talking about it' in a classroom. In addition, the researcher observed the participants learning to learn and learning to empathise. They had to try to understand the point of view of the horse as a prey animal in order to be effective when communicating with them through their bodies, the very qualities which Prior and Mason (2010) highlighted when considering the evidence so far on what works to engage young people. As a result of this course, participants learned to 'listen' to another 'being' through their body language and rehearsal and then reflected extensively on the positive impact that had made on their relationships with others which they and the prison staff reported impacted positively on their overall behaviour in prison (Hemingway et al., 2015). Another key element of this intervention is that the facilitator and the student in this intervention are guided by the same principles used for teaching horses, which focus on reading body language and responding appropriately. The course teaches through simulation rather than explanation and uses non-verbal methods (through rehearsal) to positively impact on the thoughts and emotions of the students. In this intervention neither the 'student or the horse' can ever be wrong; each is responding to the other in the moment using body language. Crucially the students are able to try and . . . succeed when learning, possibly the first time for many of these youngsters that they have experienced success in this way.

Conclusion – horses and well-being

Natural horsemanship has a comparatively small but growing following across the world. As the particular version used here has a system and clear games to learn and play it lends itself to evaluative research due to this structure. The communication system allows for detailed observation of the horse and human interaction in a way which has not arguably been possible before and has great potential to further our understanding of this unique cross species 'symphisical' relationship phenomena (vulnerability and togetherness; Acampora, 2006). In addition this pilot study has been the first of its type to focus on evaluating emotional responses and learning in the evaluation of EAI.

Starting to think about how to help our young people develop or learn the path to well-being is a new way of thinking about this area. I would argue that the experience of 'being' with horses offers us as human animals the ultimate in well-being using the 'dwelling, mobility' theory outlined by Todres and Galvin (2010; see also Chapter 8, this volume).

As being together peacefully with a horse has the ability to calm and relax us yet the potential for movement, play and sensory embodied experience and learning in the moment is immense (see Figure 20.3). It is clear that for those youngsters for whom current 'cognitive talking or classroom based' options are not effective or not engaging or both we need to think about innovate routes to well-being. To finish this chapter I would like to share a quote from Martin Seligman whose work on positive psychology has helped to inspire some of the complexity of ideas considered here:

> Question 1 asked of parents: What do you want for your children? If you are like thousands of parents polled you responded, happiness, confidence, contentment, fulfilment, balance, good stuff, kindness, health, satisfaction, love, being civilised, meaning – well-being. Question 2: What do schools teach? Achievement, thinking skills, success, conformity, literacy, maths, work test taking, discipline.
>
> (Seligman, 2011, p. 78)

I believe that we should consider how nature, of which both ourselves and animals are part can help us towards well-being. Indeed I would argue that our 'nature' enables us to engage in an embodied way

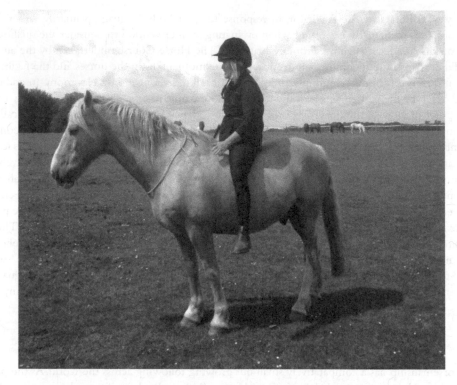

Figure 20.3   Ann Hemingway with Arn, their variation of embodiment of the dwelling mobility theory of wellbeing

with learning or recognising what it is to be well. I would suggest that along with exposure to nature of all kinds in the school curriculum that embodied routes to well-being should be considered as the answer to some of the public health issues we face today and that our obsession with waiting until young people are struggling and then relying on cognitive (talking) and pharmacological remedies as the only options for investment in terms of research and development should urgently be questioned by researchers, funders and practitioners alike.

Acknowledgements

Heartfelt thanks for the support and inspiration to Nigel, Mac, Arni, Coco, Harriet Laurie, Dr Sid Carter, Dr Emma Kavanagh, Dr Andy Callaway, Shelley Broomfield, Prof Kate Galvin, Prof Les Todres, Dr Caroline Ellis Hill and Dr Liz Norton.

References

Acampora, R. 2006. *Corporal Compassion*. Pittsburgh: University of Pittsburgh Press.
Alfonso, S.V., Alfonso, L.A., Llabre, M.M., & Fernandez, M.I. 2015. Project Stride: An equine assisted intervention to reduce symptoms of social anxiety in young women. *Explore*, Nov/Dec, 11(6), 461–467.
All, A.C., Loving, G.L., & Crane, L.L. 1999. Animals, horseback riding, and implications for rehabilitation therapy. *Journal of Rehabilitation*, Jul/Aug 65(3).
All Party Parliamentary Health Group & The Health Foundation. 2016. *A Healthier Life for All: The Case for Cross Government Action*. London: APPHG & THF.
Anderson, R., Mikulic, B., & Sandor, E. 2010. *Quality of Life in the EU: Trends in Key Dimensions 2003–2009*. Paper presented at the 96th Directors General of the National Statistical Institutes (DGINS) conference, Sophia (Bulgaria), 30

September 2010. Retrieved December 19, 2011, from www.dgins-sofia2010.eu/pdocs/Eurofound%20Quality%20 of%20life%20in%20the%20EU%20Trends%20in%20key%20dimensions.pdf.

Araujo, T.B., Silva, N.A., Costa, J.N., Pereira, M.M. & Safons, M.P. 2011. Effect of equine-assisted therapy on the postural balance of the elderly. *Revista Brasileria De Fisioterapia*, 15(5), 414–419.

Bateson, G. 1972. *Steps to an Ecology of Mind*. New York: Ballantine.

Benda, W., McGibbon, N., & Grant, K.L. 2003. Improvements in muscle symmetry in children with cerebral palsy after equine-assisted therapy (hippotherapy). *The Journal of Alternative and Complementary Medicine*, 9(6), 817–825.

Birch, M. 2005. Cultivating wildness: Three conservation volunteers' experiences of participation in the Green Gym scheme. *British Journal of Occupational Therapy*, 68(6), 244–252. doi:10.1177/030802260506800602

Bohnke, P. 2008. Does society matter? Life satisfaction in the enlarged Europe. *Social Indicators Research*, 87(2), 189–210.

Brogen, E., Hadders-Algra, M., & Forssberg, H. 1996. Postural control in children with spastic diplegia: Muscle activity during perturbations in sitting. *Developmental Medicine & Child Neurology*, 38, 379–388.

Burgon, H.L. 2011. 'Queen of the world': the experiences of at risk young people participating in equine assisted learning. *Journal of Social Work Practice*, June, 25(2), 165–183.

Camfield, L. & Skevington, S.M. 2008. On subjective well-being and quality of life. *Journal of Health Psychology*, 13(6), 764–775.

Carter, S. & Smith Pasqualini, M.C. 2004. Stronger autonomic response accompanies better learning: A test of Damasio's somatic marker hypothesis. *Cognition & Emotion*, 18, 901–911.

Cerino, S., Cirulli, F., Chiarotti, F., & Seripa, S. 2011. Non conventional psychiatric rehab in schizophrenia using therapeutic riding: The FISE multicentre Pindar Project. *Annali dell'Istituto Superiore di Sanita*, 47, 409–414.

Christian, J.E. 2005. All creatures great and small: utilising equine-assisted therapy to treat eating disorders. *Journal of Psychology and Christianity*, 24(1), Spr, 65–67.

Cresswell, J. 2010. Using the Blue Gym. *SportEX Health*, 24, 14–15.

Critchley, H.D., Elliott, R., Mathias, C.J., & Dolan, R.J. 2000. Neural activity relating to generation and representation of galvanic skin conductance responses: A functional magnetic resonance imaging study. *The Journal of Neuroscience*, 20(8), 3033–3040.

Csikszentmihalyi, M. 2004. What we must accomplish in the coming decades. Zygon, 39(2), 359–366.

Dabelko-Schoeny, H., Phillips, G., Darrough, E., DeAnna, S., Jarden, M., Johnson, D., & Lorch, G. 2014. Equine assisted intervention for people with dementia. *Anthrozoos*, 27(1), 141–155.

Damasio, A.R. 1994. Descartes' *Error: Emotion, Reason, and the Human* Brain. New York: G.P. Putnam.

Damasio, A.R. 1999. The *Feeling of What Happens: Body and Emotion in the Making of* Consciousness. San Diego, CA: Harcourt.

Damasio, A.R. 2010. *Self Comes to Mind: Constructing the Conscious Brain*. New York: Pantheon Books.

Dell, C.A., Chalmers, D., Bresette, N., Swain, S., Rankin, D., & Hopkins, C. 2011. A healing space: The experiences of First Nations and Inuit youth with equine-assisted learning (EAL). *Child Youth Care Forum*, 40, 319–336.

Del Rosario-Montejo, O., Molina-Reuda, F., Munoz-Lasa, S., & Alguacil-Diego, I.M. 2013. Effectiveness of equine therapy in children with psychomotor impairment. *Neurologia*, 30, 425–432.

De Villers, B., Ansorge, J., & Boissin, T. (2013). Camargue horses meeting with inmates: A psychoanthropological study on equine mediation's therapeutic aspects in a prison setting. In *International Conference on Human Animal Interactions, Chicago*. www.iahaio.org/files/conferences2013chicagopdf Accessed 29 January 2018.

Dodge, K.A. & Somberg, D.R. 1987. Hostile attributional biases among aggressive boys are exacerbated under conditions of threats to the self. *Child Development*, 58, 213–224.

Eckersley, R. 2004. *Well & Good: How We Feel and Why It Matters*. Melbourne, Australia: Text Publishing.

Ernst, M., Bolla, K., Mouratidis, M., Contoreggi, C., Matochik, J.A., Kurian, V., Cadet, J., Kimes, A.S., & London, E.D. 2002. Decision-making in a risk-taking task: A PET study. *Neuropsychopharmacology*, 26(5), 682.

Ferriss, A.L. 2010. *Approaches to Improving the Quality of Life: How to Enhance the Quality of Life*. Berlin: Springer.

Gabriels, R.L., Pan, Z., Dechant, B., Agnew, J.A., Brim, N., & Mesibov, G. 2015. Randomised controlled trial of therapeutic horseback riding in children and adults with autism spectrum disorder. *Journal of the American Academy of Child & Adolescent Psychiatry*, Jul, 54(7), 541–549.

Gibbons, J.L., Cunningham, C.A., Paiz, L., Poelker, K.E., & Cardenas, M.A.M. 2015. "Before he fought every day with the horse and me": Reducing violence in a Guatemalan community through a horse handling program. *Human Animal Interaction Bulletin*, 3(2), 37–55.

Griffin, K.W., Epstein, J.A., Botvin, G.J., & Spoth, R.L. 2001. Social competence and substance use among rural young: Mediating role of social benefit expectancies of use. *Journal of Youth and Adolescence*, 30, 485–498.

Haehl, V. 1996. The influence of hippotherapy on the kinematics and functional performance of two children with cerebral palsy. *Pediatric Physical Therapy*, 11, 89–101.

Hakanson, M., Moller, M., Lindstrom, I., & Mattsson, B. 2009. The horse as the healer – a study of riding in patients with back pain. *Journal of Bodywork and Movement Therapies*, 13(1), 43–52.

Hanlon, P., Carlisle, S., Hannah, M., Reilly, D., & Lyon, A. 2011. Making the case for a 'fifth wave' in public health. *Public Health*, 125(1), 30–36.

Haumery, L., Delavous, P., Teste, B., Leroy, C., Gaboriau, J.C., & Berthier, A. 2010. Equine assisted therapy and autism. *Annales Medico Psychologiques*, Nov, 168(9), 655–659.

Hemingway, A. 2011. Lifeworld led care wellbeing, and the 5th wave of public health. *International Journal of Qualitative Studies on Health and Well-Being*, 6(4).

Hemingway, A., Meek, R., & Ellis Hill, C. 2015. An exploration of an equine facilitated learning intervention with young offenders. *Society and Animals*. 1–25.

Kamioka, H., Okadah, H., Tsutan, K., Park, H., Okuizumi, H., Handa, S., Oshio, T., Park, S., Kitayuguchi, J., Abe, T., Honda, T., & Mutoh, Y. 2014. Effectiveness of animal-assisted therapy: A systematic review of randomized controlled trials. *Complementary Therapies in Medicine*, 22(2), 371–390.

Kendall, E., Maujean, A., Pepping, C.A., Downes, M., Lakhani, A., Byrne, J., & Macfarlane, K. 2015. A systematic review of the efficacy of equine-assisted interventions on psychological outcomes. *European Journal of Psychotherapy & Counselling*, 17(1), 57–59.

Klontz, B.T., Bivens, A., Leinart, D., & Klontz, T. 2007. The effectiveness of equine assisted experiential therapy: results of an open clinical trial. *Society and Animals*, 15, 257–267.

Lane, R. E. 2000. *The Loss of Happiness in Market Democracies*. London: Yale University Press.

Lasa, S.M., Bocanegra, N.M., Alcaide, V.R., Arratibel, M.A.A., Donoso, E.V., & Ferriero, G. 2013. Animal assisted interventions in neurorehabilitation: A review of the most recent literature. *Neurologia*, 30(1), 1–7.

Le Masurier, G.C., Corbin, C.B., Greiner, M., & Lambdin, D.D. 2010. *Fitness for Life: Elementary School Physical Education Lesson Plans*. Champaign, IL: Human Kinetics.

Lessick, M., Shinaver, R., Post, K., Rivera, J.E., & Lemon, B. 2004. Therapeutic horseback riding. *AWHONN (Association of Women's Health, Obstetric and Neonatal Nurses) Lifelines*, February 2004 8(1), 46–53.

Lo, A.W. & Repin, D.V. 2002. The psychophysiology of real-time financial risk processing. *Journal of Cognitive Neuroscience*, 14(3), 323–339.

Local Government Improvement and Development. 2010. *The Role of Local Government in Promoting Wellbeing: Healthy Communities Programme*. National Mental Health Development Unit. January 19, 2012. www.idea.gov.uk/idk/aio/23693073.

MacPhail, H.E.A., Edwards, J., Golding, J., Miller, K., Mosier, C., & Zwiers, T. 1998. Trunk postural reactions in children with and without cerebral palsy during therapeutic horseback riding. *Pediatric Physical Therapy*, 10, 143–147.

May, D.K., Nicholas, P., Seivert, A.C., Casey, R.J., & Johnson, A. 2016. Animal assisted therapy for youth: A systematic methodological critique. *Human-Animal Interaction Bulletin*, 4(1), 1–18.

McGibbon, N.H., Andrade, C.K., Widener, G., & Cintas, H.L. 1998. Effect of an equine movement therapy program on gait, energy expenditure, and motor function in children with spastic cerebral palsy: A pilot study. *Developmental Medicine & Child Neurology*, 40, 754–762.

McGlaskin, T.H. & Fenton, W.S. 1992. The positive negative distinction in schizophrenia: Review of natural history validators. *Archives of General Psychiatry*, 49, 381–395.

McMahan, E. & Estes, D. 2010. Measuring lay conceptions of well-being: The beliefs about well-being scale. *Journal of Happiness Studies*, 12(2), 267–287.

Nawijn, J. 2010. The holiday happiness curve: a preliminary investigation into mood during a holiday abroad. *International Journal of Tourism Research*, 12, 281–290.

Nussbaum, M.C. 1988. *Nature Function and Capability: Aristotle on Political Distribution*, Oxford studies in ancient philosophy (supplementary volume); Potvin, L., Gendron, S., Bilodeau, A., & Chabot, P. (eds.). Oxford: Oxford Press

Parelli. 2011. www.parellinaturalhorsetraining.com/natural-horsemanship/ Accessed 21 July 2011.

Pendry, P. & Roeter, S. 2013. Experimental trial demonstrates positive effects of equine facilitated learning on child social competence. *Human-Animal Interaction Bulletin*, 1(1), 1–19. Princes Trust (2005)

Prior, D. & Mason, P. 2010. A different kind of evidence? Looking for what works in engaging young offenders. *Youth Justice*, Dec, 10(3), 211–226.

Rockhill, C.M., Vander Stoep, A., McCauley, E., & Katon, W.J. 2009. Social competence and social support as mediators between comorbid depressive and conduct problems and functional outcomes in middle school children. *Journal of Adolescence*, 32, 535–553.

Rothe, E.Q., Vega, B.J., Torres, R.M., Soler, S.M.C., & Pazos, R.M.M. 2007. From kids and horses: Equine facilitated psychotherapy for children. *International Journal of Clinical and Health Psychology*, 5(2), 373–383.

Schultz, P.N., Remick-Barlow, A., & Robbins, L. 2007. Equine-assisted psychotherapy: a mental health promotion/intervention modality for children who have experienced intra-family violence. *Health and Social Care in the Community*, 15(3), 265–271.

Selby, A. & Smith-Osborne, A. 2012. A systematic review of effectiveness of complementary and adjunct therapies and interventions involving equines. *Health Psychology*, 32, 418–432.

Seligman, M. 2011. *Flourish: A New Understanding of Happiness and Wellbeing*. New York: Nicholas Brealey Publishing.

Sen, A. 2002. Why health equity? *Health Economics*, 11, 659–666.

Shambo, L. 2008. Equine facilitated psychotherapy for trauma related disorders: Pilot study. *Human Equine Alliances for Learning*. http://humanequinealliance.org/wp- content/uploads/2010/HEAL-PTSD-Research-Summary.pdf Accessed 29 January 2018.

Shonkoff, J. & Phillips, D. 2000. *From Neurons to Neighborhoods: The Science of Early Childhood Development*. Washington, DC: National Academy Press.

Sorlie, M., Hagen, K.A., & Ogden, T. 2008. Social competence and anti social behaviour: Continuity and distinctiveness across early adolescence. *Journal of Research on Adolescence*, 18, 121–144.

Sorlie, M.A. & Nordahl, T. 1998. *Problem Behaviour in Schools: Main Findings, Explanations and Educational Implications. School and Difficult Social Interactions*. Oslo: NOVA.

The Horse Course (THC). 2015. *Evidence Summary THC*. www.thehorsecourse.org/docs/THC_Youth_Sum mary_2015.pdf Accessed 29 January 2018.

Todres, L. & Galvin, K. 2010. "Dwelling-mobility": An existential theory of well-being. *International Journal of Qualitative Studies on Health and Well-Being*, 5, 5444. doi:10.3402/qhw.v5i3.5444.

Trotter, K.S., Chandler, C.K., Goodwin-Bond, D., & Casey, J. 2008. A comparative study of the efficacy of group equine assisted counseling with at-risk children and adolescents. *Journal of Creativity in Mental Health*, 3(3), 254–284.

Wentzel, K.R. 1991. Relations between social competence and academic achievement in early adolescence. *Child Development*, 62, 1066–1078.

Wu, C-H., Chen, L., & Tsai, Y-M. 2009. Investigating importance weighting of satisfaction scores from a formative model with partial least squares analysis. *Social Indicators Research*, 90(3), 351–363. doi:10.1007/s11205-008-9264-1.

Yorke, J., Nugent, W., Strand, E., Bolen, R., New, J., & Davis, C. 2013. Equine assisted therapy and its impact on cortisol levels of children and horses: A pilot study and meta-analysis. *Early Childhood Development and Care*, 183(7), 874–894.

21

WELL-BEING AND QUALITY OF LIFE IN A MATERNAL HEALTH CONTEXT

Julie Jomeen and Colin R. Martin

Introduction

The optimum state of health in postpartum women is articulated in the World Health Organization's (WHO) definition of general health as the physical, mental and social well-being of a person (WHO and UNICEF 1978). The term well-being is further defined by several other authors as 'being equivalent to the state of set conditions which fulfil or enable a person to work or fulfil her realistic chosen and biological potentials' (Lucey 2007, p. 103) and 'creatively build strong and positive relationships with others and contribute the [*sic*] their chosen community' (Beddington et al. 2008)

Well-being is currently a prevailing theme in the health care arena and suggests a concentration of capabilities and positive emotions rather than negative emotions, illness or disability (Kinderman, Schwannauer and Tai 2011). Well-being aims to encompass multiple domains which can be experienced spatially, temporally, inter-personally, bodily, as well as in mood and personal identity (Galvin and Les Todres 2011; see also Chapter 30, this volume). Each aspect of well-being inter-relates with perceived importance differing between individuals; this in turn can alter behaviour and consequently well-being is ever changing (Allen, Carrick-Sen and Martin 2013). It is undoubtedly a complex construct, which lacks universal definition and there is clear recognition of the overlap with other related concepts (Kinderman et al. 2011), which would seemingly reflect common characteristics between these constructs.

Conceptualising perinatal well-being

In a perinatal context, well-being is a well-used idiom but as in other areas it is used interchangeably with other terms such as quality of life and general health. Quality of life has increasingly been shown to play a significant role in the psychological well-being of pregnant and postnatal women (Morrell et al. 2013) and it is argued that the concept of well-being is of particular import in the perinatal period. Pregnancy, labour and the postnatal period are recognised as a period of physiological and psychological transition (Darvill, Skirton and Farrand 2010). The physiological, such as changing body shape, nausea and fatigue, are obvious, but are coupled with intense emotional involvement which may not be as transparent. The perinatal period is acknowledged as a transition phase in women's lives and emotions are ever changing across this time (Matthey et al. 2000). Though pregnancy and childbirth are universally biological events they also occur within a socio-cultural context that is individual to the women and contingent on her values, attitudes and beliefs, which is turn are influenced by culture, race, religion, social norms (Ottani 2002) and the personal and social context within which the woman lives, including her economic circumstance (Bennett 2005) and support network (Darvill et al. 2010).

As a consequence of the multifactorial nature of women's perinatal experience and the associated intensity of adaptation required there is a tendency to explore associations with negative psychological consequences and sequelae and conceptualise well-being in relation to maternal mental health (Alderdice, McNeill and Lynn 2013). Allen and colleagues (2013) highlight 'the magnitude of literature examining psychological problems in the perinatal period which dwarfs the literature on positive psychological functioning' (p. 387). For a smaller albeit significant proportion of women, perinatal adaptation will result in pathological changes (Raynor and England 2010) leading to mental health problems and evidence clearly supports the criticality of accurate identification of women at risk to prevent long-term consequences for mothers, babies and families (NICE 2014) as well as societal economic burden (Bauer et al. 2014). It carries with it however a concomitant a risk of over-pathologisation of emotional lability and life appraisal and risks potential stigmatisation of women in a period of normative adaptation to a major life event. The well-being perspective, therefore, offers a potent framework to encompass and exemplify the holistic nature of new motherhood, one which can involve a multi-faceted and evolving continuum ranging from a positive to a negative sense of well-being. There is an urgency to consider how we can best support women in pregnancy to maximise well-being (Alderdice, McNeill and Lynn 2013).

Critical to the construct seems to be individual perception and self-evaluation (Allen et al. 2013) of the physical, emotional and life changes that occur to women in a perinatal context. In considering well-being as not merely the absence of psychological symptomology or illness (Ryff 1995) and positive affect as not merely the opposite of negative affect, it is evident that socio-cultural factors will inevitably impact on how a woman adjusts to perinatal changes and as a result their self-evaluation of their life at that time. Indicators of perinatal well-being can focus on physical characteristics relating to perceived perinatal health, pain, pregnancy symptomology, bodily changes and are factors related to a low sense of subjective well-being (Bennett 2005), but assessment of well-being is not reducible to physical attributes only, as it can be derived from the realisation of goals or valued outcomes (Tinkler and Hicks 2011). Hence, can include emotional assessments relating to happiness, mood, sense of the future, self-esteem, quality of life, satisfaction with life, family functioning and independence (Allen et al. 2013) as well as self-compassion (Felder et al. 2016). Such a model explains why many pregnant women experience pregnancy as a pleasurable experience, birth as satisfying and experience enhanced self-esteem and a sense of optimism (DiPietro et al. 2004), reporting motherhood as a positive experience (Green and Kafetsios 1997). It is important to acknowledge that women's perception of well-being is biologically as well as socially and psychologically mediated. Postpartum physical status and maternal emotional well-being are correlated, with physical recovery positively associated with improving psychological profiles (Jomeen and Martin 2008). In turn this physical recovery facilitates the process of attaining a maternal identity that consists of developing an attachment with their baby, competence in mothering behaviours and experiencing pleasure when interacting with their baby (Olsson et al. 2005). This process of personal growth in becoming a mother is described as a process of appreciation, discovery, learning and acceptance of the woman's new role which results in a positive and worthwhile experience (Martell 2001). This fits with the notion of well-being as encapsulating the presence of positive capabilities and emotions (Kinderman 2011) but seemingly in the ability of women to self-appraise the domains of the experience. Hence, the complexity is not merely in defining the components and overall construct of perinatal well-being but recognising them as inherently implicated and rooted in the intrinsic abilities of women themselves as well as the proposed fluidity of the construct across a puerperium that is distinctively dynamic for women (Spiteri, Jomeen and Martin 2013).

Identifying and considering the dimensions relevant to perinatal well-being are essential in moving toward a better understanding of the concept. Conceptual understanding and clarity is critical to counterbalance the attention given in the international literature and policy on identifying perinatal morbidity (CEMACE 2011).

Defining perinatal well-being

Allen et al. (2013) who to date have provided, via a concept analysis, the only empirically derived definition of perinatal well-being ultimately describes perinatal well-being as

> the cognitive and/or affective self-evaluation of the individuals life specific to the period before and/or after childbirth, which encompasses a multitude of elements; physical, psychological, social, spiritual, economical and ecological.
>
> (p. 390)

It is their assertion that it is the inter-relating dimensions that separate perinatal from the concept of well-being more broadly, suggesting that acknowledgment of the socio-cultural environment and the fluctuating nature of emotions during the transition from pregnancy to motherhood influences a woman's perception and self-evaluation of life during this time.

Assessing perinatal well-being

If current assessment seeks to identify 'deviation from the norm', in particular poor psychological health, rather than focus on identifying positive adjustment, it raises the question of how perinatal 'health' can be assessed within a positive normative frame rather than from negative focus. This could facilitate a normalising context and help practitioners to promote a positively oriented model of perinatal health and/or recovery. There are currently many validated tools developed to measure well-being – taking different conceptualisations of the term as their starting point – and many to measure concepts that relate to well-being. Existing instruments focus on quality of life, happiness, satisfaction or aim to assess depression, anxiety and stress. As previously described, the constructs of health, quality of life (QoL) and well-being are often used interchangeably, with QoL often used as a proxy measure of well-being. Both concepts are difficult to define, measure and interpret but QoL can be described as a multi-dimensional concept that includes domains of emotional, physical and social functioning, which can improve or worsen over time, while well-being relates to positive self-evaluation of life, such as positive emotions, happiness and life satisfaction (Allen et al. 2013; Alderdice et al. 2017). Hence the evident synergy and interrelationship between health, well-being and QoL (Morrell et al. 2013) might explain why QoL measures are often accepted and utilised as measures of well-being.

Quality of life assessment

The most commonly used measure of health-related QoL internationally is the Medical Outcomes Survey Short-Form 36 (SF-36) (Ware and Sherbourne 1992), originally developed to monitor patient outcomes in medical practice, to survey health status in general populations and to conduct health policy evaluations, research and clinical practice. The instrument was developed to measure a range of health concepts and detect clinically and socially relevant differences in health status and changes over time. The questionnaire consists of eight health domains and reports two summary measures: emotional and physical role limitation and demonstrates good psychometric performance. The SF-12 is a short version and also performs well psychometrically.

The SF-36 has been validated for use in early pregnancy (Jomeen and Martin, 2005), and has been used in several studies. Studies using the SF-36 and SF-12 have demonstrated a general negative impact of pregnancy on vitality with decreased physical functioning and increased bodily pain as pregnancy progresses (Hueston and Kasik-Miller 1998); others have identified the specific role of early pregnancy, nausea and vomiting on physical and mental QoL, with physical role and vitality more negatively affected than other

SF-36 domains (Chan et al. 2010; Gartland et al. 2010; Lacasse et al. 2008). Setse et al. (2009) highlighted a substantial impact of depressive symptoms on functioning during pregnancy. Comparisons with normative population values demonstrated role limitation due to physical health, vitality and physical function in the third trimester of pregnancy (Da Costa et al. 2010), with poorer physical and mental QoL associated with sleep problems (Jomeen and Martin 2007). These findings illustrate the value of measuring QoL in the perinatal period but whether this can be considered an assessment of perinatal well-being is another question

Measurement of emotional well-being

A recent review by Morrell and colleagues (2013) sought to identify pregnancy-focused measures of psychological well-being. A range of instruments were reviewed, which in some way purported to measure psychological well-being in pregnancy. The main focus of the measures reviewed appears to be the nature and extent of worries in pregnancy, fear, distress and social support, measured as distinct aspects of health and well-being. Very few of the instruments reviewed focused on positive emotions and so would fail to be measuring the construct of well-being as described by Allen et al. (2013)

General Health Questionnaire

One instrument that has been specifically adapted and subsequently psychometrically evaluated to assess well-being in a perinatal population is the General Health Questionnaire-12 (GHQ-12). In the absence of a measure of well-being designed for or validated in a postpartum population at the time of the study and the potential congruence of the concepts of general health and well-being – acknowledged by other authors (Tennant et al. 2007; Kinderman et al. 2011) – the GHQ-12 was considered as a potentially useful instrument to assess well-being (for full description of the development of the measure see Spiteri et al. 2013). The aim was to facilitate the use of the measure as one of well-being rather than a case detector for psychological morbidity; this was achieved using an alternative approach to scoring. One approach which facilitates a scaling of the intensity of the mother's feelings associated with their emotional health is the use of the visual analogue scales (VAS). This facilitates an element of self-evaluation which has been highlighted as particularly pertinent to the dynamic perinatal context and the construct of perinatal well-being. The advantage of VAS, therefore, over a categorical scale is that they do not limit subjects to a number of possible responses but offer a continuum, which offers both greater sensitivity and enables potentially finer distinctions to be made (Waltz, Strickland and Lenz 2005). In line with the conceptualisation of well-being, these scales were on a positive trend and were scored by measuring the distance from the low end (zero point) to the specified place on the mother's mark.

The psychometric properties of the GHQ-12(WB) were explored using confirmatory factor analysis, discriminant and divergent validity and reliability analysis. The GHQ-12(WB) demonstrated good divergent and known-groups validity and internal consistency. However, overall consistent best-fit to the data was an eight-item, two-factor model (GHQ-8). Findings generally support the reliability and validity of the GHQ-12(WB) and model fit changes demonstrated over time reflect and confirm the dynamic nature of postpartum recovery. There seems to be a case for further work evaluating this instrument as a measure of emotional well-being. Despite its potential utility, the adapted GHQ is only addressing one domain of well-being of the construct as defined by Allen and colleagues (2013).

Well-being in Pregnancy (WiP) Questionnaire

Recent work by Alderdice et al. (2017) has sought to develop a measure that recognises the concept of well-being as multi-faceted and encompassing both positive and negative emotions as well as satisfaction with life. They have developed the WiP in an attempt to measure both positive and negative thoughts and emotions and the positive aspects of health and well-being. In preliminary testing, the psychometric properties of the questionnaire were explored using exploratory factor analysis and correlations to explore the relationship between the WiP questionnaire and other validated generic well-being measures. The WiP identified two factors, the first reflecting positive effect and satisfaction and the second concerns. This preliminary testing indicated that the scale demonstrates good reliability and correlates well with the other well-being scales. The ability to measure positive as well as negative emotions is a significant step forward in the assessment of perinatal well-being that could be of value in practice as well as research-based settings.

Discussion

The appraisal of the literature of quality of life and well-being summarised in the current chapter presents fundamental challenges in the application of these concepts to maternal and perinatal health. The literature reveals that quality of life can be reliably assessed by questionnaire measures and indeed, many generic quality of life measures have been applied to the maternal and perinatal health arena. The notion of maternal and perinatal well-being, however, represents a more diffuse concept than quality of life and this is seen in the literature, both in terms of the maturity of conceptual exposition, and the general lack of robust and conceptually congruent measures of the concept of well-being.

This tension is likely to be, at least in part, consequential of a distinction between the research themes of concept analysis within the perinatal field, and the development of maternal and perinatal health-specific measures of well-being based on robust and replicable psychometric principles. This issue is compounded by proxy measures of well-being. First, the use of quality of life measures as proxies for well-being represents a conceptual misspecification. Given that any assessment by a questionnaire measure represents the assessment of concept itself *and* associated error, a conceptual misspecification in the use of a proxy measure for a concept represents an additional source of error. Importantly, this additional source of error cannot be estimated in terms of magnitude and effect since the critical level of error is not one of measurement, but conceptual congruence. Contemporary research work on concept analysis of well-being has focused on the perinatal period, yet, to generalise such a framework to the broader arena of maternal health in general requires further work and indeed, the evidence may suggest distinct and time-differentiated characteristics at the conceptual level. Researchers and practitioners may be readily seduced into using quality of life measures as proxies for well-being because of both the availability of the former, and the ready availability of the measures themselves, normative data, known psychometric properties and so forth. The use of these measures undoubtedly has utility when used contextually but offers a limited ability to assess and measure the well-being of pregnant women and capture positive psychological pregnancy outcomes (Morrell et al. 2013). It needs to be acknowledged that well-being is not quality of life (in terms of quality of life measurement tools) and to use measures as such, and uncritically, perpetuates a conceptual error which in turn contributes to a lack of innovation in evidence-based and conceptually adherent measures of maternal and perinatal well-being.

An important pursuit then, is the development and application of conceptually valid and psychometrically robust measures of maternal and perinatal well-being. This work has commenced, as evidenced by the WiP (Alderdice et al. 2017). An important caveat to this important future work is an integral consideration of the important and profound physiological challenges that accompany, for example, the course of pregnancy and how this may be accommodated within both a coherent conceptual framework and a robust and psychometrically reproducible measurement structure. The key philosophical and pragmatic consideration in achieving this goal, essentially, a robust measure of maternal and perinatal well-being, must be a considered and reflective discussion on the merits and appropriateness of specific methodological paradigms. The methodological framework to support such an enterprise must incorporate both the conceptual and measurement aspects and bring them together as gestalt. This must acknowledge the dynamic and complex interplay inherent in the emotional and physiological change that defines maternal and perinatal well-being as well as acknowledge the social, spiritual, economical and ecological domains within a framework of self-evaluation and consider how that can be brought to the measurement context.

A mixed-method approach (Creswell and Plano-Clark 2011) to instrument design could be considered the most suitable approach, capturing the relevant qualitative and quantitative threads implicit to the successful development of a 'condition-specific' and psychometrically robust measurement tool. Importantly, an appropriate mixed-method design is available and suitable for this endeavour, two-stage qualitative-quantitative instrument development design. This design, though eminently suitable for such a task, would need to be considered in great detail to accommodate in a meaningful way the dynamic change states associated with maternal and perinatal health. Consistent with this, both in terms of the qualitative and quantitative components of the study would be the distinct timelines in sampling. Given that many quality of life and well-being tools are developed using a cross-sectional design, with perhaps a small (percentage-wise) follow group being used to evaluate test-retest reliability of the developed measure, this approach, even within the context of a mixed-methods design, would be clearly insufficient to capture the cognitive, conative and physiological dynamism exemplified by maternal and perinatal life course. Incorporating within the design a structure that can capture the essence of these domains across timelines circumscribed by the maternal and perinatal health constructs is critical to success in the development of a valid and reliable well-being measure.

It is noteworthy that the current 'crisis' in psychology, essentially, the difficulties faced in replicating findings of studies, would be a very important consideration in the context of the development of a maternal and perinatal well-being assessment tool. It is unlikely that an approach which does not incorporate timeline considerations within the fabric of the instrument would be successful either conceptually, or in terms of exemplary measurement characteristics. Recognising that incorporation of inherent timelines into the development of such a well-being measure highlights a salient prima facie consideration, that is that the tool itself is likely to be multi-dimensional and that such multi-dimensionality may be specific to defined time periods over the maternal and perinatal health timeline.

Conclusion

This chapter has sought to provide a valuable summary of the current evidence and gaps in evidence related to the state of knowledge in the arena of perinatal well-being. It also provides the opportunity to reflect on what needs to be considered by practitioners and researchers on their potential role in the field going forward. There is clearly a lack of evidence at this time on which to base well-being interventions. New interventions would also need evaluation in terms of outcomes and whilst we see the emergence of measures which focus on a construct of well-being this is early work and it would be premature to consider we had fully defined the construct or determined a robust way of assessing and measuring it. There is much future work to be done that could add value to this area.

References

Alderdice, F., McNeill, J., Gargan, P., & Perra, O. (2017) Preliminary evaluation of the Well-being in Pregnancy (WiP) questionnaire. *Journal of Psychosomatic Obstetrics and Gynecology*. Available from www.tandfonline.com/doi/full/10.1 080/0167482X.2017.1285898

Alderdice, F., McNeill, J., & Lynn, F. (2013) A systematic review of systematic reviews of interventions to improve maternal mental health and well-being. *Midwifery*, 29(4), 389–399.

Allen, C., Carrick-Sen, D., & Martin, C.R. (2013) What is perinatal wellbeing? A concept analysis and review of the literature. *Journal of Reproductive and Infant Psychology*, 31(4), 381–398.

Bauer, A., Parsonage, M., Knapp, M., Lemmi, V., & Adelaja, B. (2014) *Costs of Perinatal Mental Problems*. London: London School of Economics and Political Science.

Beddington, J., Cooper, C.L., Field, J., Goswami, U., Huppert, F.A., Jenkins, J., et al. (2008). The mental wealth of nations. *Nature*, 455(23), 1057–1060.

Bennett, K.M. (2005) Psychological wellbeing in later life: the longitudinal effects of marriage, widowhood, and marital status change. *International Journal of Geriatric Psychiatry*, 20, 280–284.

Centre for Maternal and Child Enquiries (CEMACE). (2011) Saving mothers' lives: reviewing maternal deaths 2006–2008. *British Journal of Obstetrics and Gynaecology*, 118(Suppl. 1), 1–203.

Chan, O.K., Sahota, D.S., Leung, T.Y., Chan, L.W., Fung, T.Y., & Lau, T.K. (2010) Nausea and vomiting in health-related quality of life among Chinese pregnant women. *Australian and New Zealand Journal of Obstetrics and Gynaecology*, 50, 512–518.

Creswell, J.W. & Plano Clark, V.L. (2011) *Designing and Conducting Mixed Methods Research*. Los Angeles: Sage.

Da Costa, D., Dritsa, M., Verreault, N., Balaa, C., Kudzman, J., & Khalife, S. (2010) Sleep problems and depressed mood negatively impact health-related quality of life during pregnancy. *Archives of Women's Mental Health*, 13, 249–257. doi:10.1007/s00737-009-0104-3

Darvill, T., Skirton, H., & Farrand, P. (2010) Psychological factors that impact on women's experiences of first-time motherhood: A qualitative study of the transition. *Midwifery*, 26, 357–366.

DiPietro, J.A., Ghera, M., Costigan K., Hawkins, M. (2004) Measuring the ups and downs of pregnancy stress. *Journal of Psychosomatic Obstetrics and Gynecology*, 25, 189–201.

Felder, J.N., Lemon, E., Shea, K., Kripe, K., & Dimidjian, S. (2016) Role of self-compassion in psychological wellbeing among perinatal women. *Archives of Women's Mental Health*, 19, 687–690.

Galvin, K.T. & Les Todres, L. (2011) Kinds of well-being: a conceptual framework that provides direction for caring. *International Journal of Qualitative Studies in Health and Well-Being*, 6, 1–13.

Gartland, D., Brown, S., Donat, S., & Perlen, S. (2010) Women's health in early pregnancy: findings from an Australian nulliparous study. *Australian and New Zealand Journal of Obstetrics and Gynaecology*, 50, 413–418.

Green, J. & Kafetsios, K. (1997) Positive experiences of early motherhood: predictive variables from a longitudinal study. *Journal of Reproductive and Infant Psychology*, 15(2), 141–157.

Heuston, W. & Kasik-Miller, S. (1998) Changes in functional health status in normal pregnancy. *Journal of Family Practice*, 47, 209–212.

Jomeen, J. & Martin, C.R. (2005) The factor structure of the SF-36 in early pregnancy. *Journal of Psychosomatic Research*, 59, 131–138.

Jomeen, J. & Martin, C.R. (2007) Assessment and relationship of sleep quality to depression in early pregnancy. *Journal of Reproductive and Infant Psychology*, 25, 87–99.

Jomeen, J. & Martin, C.R. (2008) The impact of choice of care on psychological health outcomes for women during pregnancy and the postnatal period. *Journal of Evaluation in Clinical Practice*, 14(3), 645–648.

Kinderman, P., Schwannauer, M., & Tai, S. (2011) The development and validation of a general measure of well-being: the BBC well-being scale. *Quality of Life Research*, 20, 1035–1042.

Lacasse, A., Rey, E., Ferreria, E., Morin, C., & Bérard, A. (2008) Nausea and vomiting in pregnancy: What about quality of life? *British Journal of Obstetrics and Gynaecology*, 115, 1484–1493.

Lucey, P. (2007) Social determinates of health. *Nursing Economics*, 25(2), 103–109.

Martell, L.K. (2001) Heading towards the new normal: a contemporary postpartum experience. *Journal of Obstetric, Gynecological and Neonatal Nursing*, 30, 496–506.

Matthey, S., Barnett, B., Ungerer, J., & Waters, B. (2000) Paternal and maternal depressed mood during the transition to parenthood. *Journal of Affective Disorders*, 60, 75–85.

Morrell, C.J., Cantrell, A., Evans, K., & Carrick-Sen, M. (2013) A review of instruments to measure health-related quality of life and well-being among pregnant women. *Journal of Reproductive and Infant Psychology*, 31(5), 512–530.

National Institute for Health and Clinical Excellence (NICE). (2014) *Antenatal and Postnatal Mental Health: Clinical Management and Service Guidance*. London: NICE.

Olsson, A., Lundqvist, M., Faxelid, E., & Nissen, E. (2005) Women's thoughts about sexual life after childbirth: focus group discussions with women after childbirth. *Scandinavian Journal of Caring Science*, 19, 381–387.

Ottani, P.A. (2002) When childbirth preparation isn't a cultural norm. *International Journal of Childbirth Education*, 17, 12–16.

Raynor, M. & England, C. (2010) *Psychology for Midwives: Pregnancy, Childbirth and Puerperium*. Maidenhead: Open University Press.

Ryff, C.D. (1995) Psychological wellbeing in adult life. *Current Directions in Psychological Science*, 4, 99–104.

Setse, R., Grogan, R., Pham, L., Cooper, L.A., Strobino, D., Powe, N.R., et al. (2009). Longitudinal study of depressive symptoms and health-related quality of life during pregnancy and after delivery: the Health Status in Pregnancy (HIP) study. *Maternal & Child Health Journal*, 13, 577–587. doi:10.1007/s10995-008-0392-7.

Spiteri, C.M., Jomeen, J., & Martin, C.R. (2013) Reimagining the general health questionnaire as a measure of emotional wellbeing: a study of postpartum women in Malta. *Women and Birth*, 26(4), e105-e111.

Tennant, R., Hiller, L., Fishwick, R., Platt, S., Joseph, S., Weich, S., et al. (2007). The Warwick– Edinburgh Mental Well-being Scale (WEMWBS): development and UK validation. *Health and Quality of Life Outcomes*, 5(63). Available at www.hqlo.com/content/5/1/63.

Tinkler, L. & Hicks, S. (2011) *Subjective Wellbeing*. London. Office for National Statistics.

Waltz, C.F., Strickland, O.L., & Lenz, E.R. (2005) *Measurement in Nursing and Health Research*. (3rd ed.). New York: Springer Publishing Company.

Ware, J.E., & Sherbourne, C.D. (1992) The MOS 36-item short-form health survey (SF-36). Conceptual framework and item selection. *Medical Care*, 30, 473–483.

World Health Organization (WHO) & UNICEF. (1978) *Declaration of Alma-Alta*. International Conference on Primary Health Care, Alma-Ata, USSR, 6–12 September. WHO.

22
WELL-BEING AND SELF-INTEREST
Personal identity, Parfit, and conflicting attitudes to time in liberal theory and social policy

Steven R. Smith

Introduction

Classical liberal accounts of well-being and its enhancement depend on particular views of self-interest, attitudes to time, and personal identity. For example, Adam Smith (2011, p. 216), Henry Sidgwick (1981, p. 381), and John Rawls (1973, p. 420), variously argue that someone acting in her self-interest has a neutral attitude to time. Her future self has the same importance to her as her present self, and she acts accordingly. This enables her to plan for her future – sometimes enduring short-term present pain for long-term future well-being – knowing that overall her life will go better. These prudent choices are therefore informed by her taking stock of her life led *as a whole*, having no bias to specific time periods (also see Brink, 2003, 1997).

However, there are problems viewing the experience of time neutrally which Derek Parfit explores in his seminal book *Reasons and Persons* (1987). Promoting temporal neutrality, which may explain our attitudes and preferences regarding many of our future plans, does not accommodate other emotional biases we have toward the present and near future, over the past and distant future (Parfit, 1987, pp. 149–186). Typically, a person is emotionally relieved when her past pain is over but dreads her near-future anticipated pain. These highly contrasting affective responses to personal pain are understandable, given our experiences across time, but are straining the temporal neutrality promoted by classical liberals.

The argument here, though, is that despite Parfit's insights, his conclusions about personal identity oppose key aspects of many contemporary conceptions of well-being. Parfit's reductionist understanding of personal identity argues that identity is reducible to the physical and especially the psychological characteristics of 'continuity and connectedness' which are often fragile over time (Parfit, 1987, pp. 261–275, 312–315). Consequently, personal identity is not indivisible and definitively singular, but plural and ambiguous, which explains why we are not temporally neutral when we protect our self-interest and enhance our well-being over time. Consider who we are now as, say, middle-aged adults, compared with who we were in our twenties, and then as young children. Our desires, preferences, goals, ambitions, and psychological make-up, are/were very different in each time period reflecting the very different identities we possess over our lifetimes (Parfit, 1987, pp. 313–314). However, a non-reductionist view of identity ignores the inevitable and reasonable bias we have to the different person we are now over the different person we might be in the medium- to long-term future (Parfit, 1987, pp. 277–278, 317–320).[1] Instead, temporal neutrality assumes we have the same identity and so are the same beneficiary over time, and that this identity therefore exists separately to our changing psychological and physical experiences (Parfit, 1987, p. 275).

Nevertheless, Parfit's reductionist view, notwithstanding its insights, complicates any evaluation of a person's life concerning her well-being, as evaluating how well a life is going *overall* is made more difficult than the non-reductionist view. Interpersonal comparisons of welfare are notoriously problematic as the levels and quality of well-being is hard to meaningfully measure between different persons. But these problems also become salient with intrapersonal comparisons if plural identities occur over time for one person, as Parfit's reductionism has it (and see Braddon-Mitchell and West, 2001). Nevertheless, the main recommendation here is to offer a 'hybrid' account of personal identity, combining both reductionist and non-reductionist views which, it is claimed, makes better sense of contemporary social policy debates about well-being enhancement, even though these views pull in opposite directions. Old-age pensions and disability policy are examined to address these issues and the above complexities and difficulties.

Liberal self-interest and rationality

Parfit's insights, just outlined, raises serious difficulties for classical liberals, such as Henry Sidgwick, Adam Smith, and John Rawls, as he is fundamentally challenging their accounts of rationality, individual self-interest, and, by implication, well-being promotion. The logical scheme of these classical liberals regarding their view of individual self-interest and rationality runs roughly as follows:

> *Premise 1:* A person acting rationally and in her self-interest will impartially reflect on her life overall, and will realise:
> *Premise 2:* Her future self has the same importance to her as her present self, as both are equally connected to her as one indivisible person.
> *Therefore:* Insofar as she can be sure of what will happen in the future, she should give as much consideration to her future self as her present self so exercising 'temporally neutrality', given she is the same beneficiary in each time period.

Following the above, rational long-term plans are implemented contributing to a person's life going well overall, enhancing her well-being. So, there are good reasons for accepting some pain and hardship now, if this furthers her long-term future interests. She studies hard now, sacrificing present pleasures, enabling her to pass exams and get a good job in the future; she undergoes painful and uncomfortable exercise now to become, in the future, fit and healthy, and so on. Consequently, this person views time neutrally, enduring present pain and hardship to further her future self-interest, but thereby enhancing her well-being over the whole of her life. This is seen as rational because she sees herself as the same beneficiary, both now and in the future, and therefore rationally can give equal weighting to her interests over time.

The problem though, identified by Derek Parfit, is that temporal neutrality seems irrational when we reflect on our emotional responses to experiences in the past, the present, the near and long-term future. For example, past pain matters much less to us now than pain in the near future. We fearfully dread pain when we know we will experience pain soon, but we are relieved when our pain is over. For Parfit, this affective bias we have toward near-future pain over past pain is straightforwardly explained: "We are concerned about these future pains simply because they are not yet in the past" (Parfit, 1987, p. 168). However, if this is the case, then we cannot always associate temporal neutrality with rationality.

> If [the person who is temporally neutral] condemns the bias towards the near because it cannot have rational significance *when* some pain is felt, he must condemn the bias towards the future. He must claim that it is irrational to be relieved when some pain is in the past. Most of us would find this hard to believe ... most of us would disagree.
>
> (Parfit, 1987, p. 170 – his emphasis)

This chapter now examines Parfit's position more closely, exploring how his argument also depends on a reductionist view of personal identity. This view, though, also raises difficult problems for contemporary understandings of well-being and how these understandings are, in turn, applied to social policy and welfare practice.

Parfit and the problems of reductionism

Underpinning Parfit's objections to temporal neutrality, and the classical liberal view of rationality and self-interest, is his reductionist view of personal identity which radically contrasts with the non-reductionist view underpinning these classical liberal accounts (for example, see Parfit, 1987, pp. 313–315). Returning to premises 1 and 2 outlined above, part of the classical liberal case for temporal neutrality depends on the further assumption that we have one irreducible identity which is the same across time, and to which we self-reflectively refer when making plans. Consequently, a person impartially reflects on her life overall (premise 1), and, in the process, different periods of her life are given equal consideration (premise 2), only by further assuming that the person who experiences the future is irreducibly identical with the person she is now, or the person she once was when considered from this future perspective. If we assume this non-reducible "further fact" concerning personal identity – that a person's identity is exactly the same over time, and so occurring separately to her physical and psychological characteristics which change over time (Parfit, 1987, p. 210) – then we can understand why a person endures pain now, anticipating her future long-term interests will be enhanced. She enhances her future self-interest, even if this involves experiencing pain now, because she knows now that she will be exactly the same person in the future. Indeed, without the assumption of this "further fact", occurring separately to her physical and psychological characteristics, we cannot make sense of temporal neutrality. Briefly put, there would be much less reason for her to act in support of her future long-term interests, as the 'her' may be a different person and so not therefore irreducibly identical in each time period (and see Stocker, 1997; Braddon-Mitchell and West, 2001; Brink, 2003, p. 223).

However, according to Parfit, despite its intuitive attractions we cannot just assume this further fact, as personal identity over time, contra the classical liberal account, is indeterminate and ambiguous (for example, Parfit, 1987, pp. 213–215). Rather, what matters in questions of 'identity' is psychological continuity and connectedness (memory, personality, opinions, ambitions, desires, values, and so on) which may relate, to lesser or greater *degrees*, to a person's past, present, and future selves. Therefore, Parfit views 'identity' as potentially dissipated and plural over time. What we value and pursue now, for example, may be very different to what we valued and pursued in our distant past, and what we will value in the future, especially the long-term future (and see Stocker, 1997).

However, even if we give some credence to Parfit's account, measurements and evaluations concerning a person's well-being and how well 'her' life is going overall is much more difficult to assess as a result. So, many philosophical conceptions of well-being rely on the exercise of individual agency, where a person who is able to devise plans for herself and implement them is likely to increase her well-being (for example, see Griffin, 1988; Raz, 1988; Sumner, 1999; Haybron, 2008; Tiberius, 2008; and my arguments in Smith, 2013). Individual agency, for many though, necessarily involves a capacity to devise and execute plans *across* a whole life. Here, the 'further fact' of a singular identity provides the coherency and continuity to one person's narrative, where she views herself as '*the* author' of her life, despite her changing psychological and experiential landscapes across time. Whereas, following Parfit's reductionism, not assuming this 'further fact' risks undermining this person's ability to act as 'an author' of her life, given that her personal identity is not constant but multiple and ambiguous (and see Korsgaard's criticism of Parfit, 1989; Blackburn, 1997). This inability, in turn, risks diminishing her overall well-being, if enhancing a person's well-being is conceptualised as including the capacity to successfully implement long-term plans that this person considers valuable to pursue over time and across the whole of her life.

Moreover, if personhood is identified as a singular irreducible entity occurring separately to her changing psychological and experiential make-up, then a person's life can be more straightforwardly evaluated as a whole concerning her *overall* well-being. Evaluations and comparisons are easier to make when there is only one 'identity target' and one neutral 'temporal weighting' taking place across time. For example, long-term strategies for policy can be implemented more readily if it is assumed that persons are the same beneficiaries over time, thus providing a more coherent justification for policies which may require some pain now, anticipating that the present generation's future long-term interests will be enhanced.

To summarise so far, then, we seem to be facing an uncomfortable choice or dilemma. We either accept the non-reductionist classical liberal account of temporal neutrality and the pursuit of rational self-interest, ignoring the problems Parfit highlights concerning our bias attitudes toward time which seem highly plausible. Or, we accept Parfit's objection and abandon key aspects of the more straightforwardly applicable non-reductionist accounts of well-being just outlined, which also seems plausible. There is, though, another response – namely, to resist choosing between an either/or understanding of identity and well-being, and instead offer a more hybrid view, combining both perspectives but recognising these also conflict philosophically, and when applied to social policy and welfare practice.

The 'hybrid response' and social policy

The main claim is that the hybrid view is consistent with our common intuitions about living a life well, and many contemporary philosophical accounts of well-being. On the reductionist side, a person who is unreflectively absorbed in a presently lived satisfying activity, often experiences well-being enhancement. For example, Valerie Tiberius (2008, pp. 74–75) and Daniel Haybron (2008, pp. 115–117) argue that living in 'the present' can enhance a person's well-being and happiness. So, according to Tiberius:

> if the values that constitute a good life are many, we must be able to take different practical perspectives at different times. Sometimes we should be focused on friendship, sometimes absorbed by our careers, and sometimes overwhelmed by the beauty of nature. . . . 'Being in the moment', although now a cliché, has much to recommend it.
>
> (Tiberius, 2008, p. 75)

More abstractly, Gereon Kopf (2002, pp. 224–245) explores how 'the present' can be experienced as 'eternal' with no temporal dimension if a person is unreflectively absorbed in her present activities. The point here is that a person's identity, occurring separately to her subjective experiences as a further irreducible fact (underpinning the non-reductionist view), does not fit so readily with this account. For example, if she is utterly absorbed in her presently orientated experiences, then she is less able to be temporally neutral, reflecting Parfit's reductionism. This is because her identity is so embedded in the subjectively experienced present that she will have little or no objective regard for her future or her past.

However, at other times, she may break away from her subjectively absorbed world, to gain a wider more objective perspective, enabling her to have 'attentional flexibility' as Tiberious calls it – where she can consider the possibility of having new experiences via the judgements she makes about her life overall (Tiberius, 2008, pp. 65–88). For Tiberius:

> To have attentional flexibility, then, is to be open to considerations that are not the focus of our current practical perspective . . . and to be able to make judgments on the basis of these considerations about our current perspective.
>
> (Tiberius, 2008, p. 83)

The point here is that when this attentional flexibility occurs a person can view herself more objectively or impartially, in effect assuming the non-reducible identity of a singular agent, functioning as 'the author' of her overall life-plans. Christine Korsgaard objects to Parfit's reductionism on precisely these grounds, arguing, from a Kantian viewpoint, that it is important for our identities (and by implication our well-being) that we consider ourselves as authors of our lives (Korsgaard, 1989; and see Blackburn, 1997; for a Parfitian counter-argument to Korsgaard, see Shoemaker, 1996).

In summary, then, promoting the hybrid view resists an oversimplified choice – between the non-reductionist view of agency, self-interest, and temporal neutrality; or the reductionist view, having a bias towards the present and near future, over the past and distant future. So, how can this hybrid view be applied to social policy – particularly to pensions and disability policy?

Policy debate over pensions typically focuses on the problems governments have persuading younger workers to invest in their futures, given their present preferences which do not regard this investment as important (Foster, 2010; Evandrou and Falkingham, 2009; Pettigrew et al., 2007). Following the arguments here, there is a conflict, therefore, between policy-makers who are trying to promote long-term self-interest and temporal neutrality amongst younger workers – and the non-neutral temporal attitudes of these younger people who are absorbed in the present. Policy-makers argue, subsequently, that young people acting in their self-interest should have a neutral attitude to time, and so view their future selves as having the same importance as their present selves, and act prudently – thereby furthering their long-term self-interest and well-being for their lives overall.

However, the hybrid view would regard temporal neutrality as only part of the story. So, acknowledging Parfit's criticisms, policy-makers from this viewpoint should not regard the inability of young people to save for their pensions as *merely* reflecting an irrational disregard for their future selves and well-being. Rather, it also reflects an appropriate bias toward the present, consistent with the kinds of creatures we all are, young or old. Therefore, the pursuit of rationality and self-interest are rightly made relevant to our lives as these are lived now, recognising that this absorbed focus on the present can enhance our well-being. If a young person, subsequently, becomes absorbed in her present experiences, she will often enhance her well-being and, *rationally*, will, as a result, refuse to become preoccupied with her long-term future interests (Shoemaker, 1996; Tiberius, 2008, p. 75; Haybron, 2008, pp. 115–117; Parfit, 1987, pp. 313–314).

Moreover, having this presently orientated bias also reveals, more abstractly, how we are profoundly limited by beginnings and ends, or our finiteness (and see my arguments in Steven Smith, 2011, 2013). For example, we are constrained by our social and physical environments, our inability to be in two places simultaneously, to be more than one person at a time, as well as our inability to imagine with complete accuracy what our personal identities will be like in the long-term future. These limitations are universal, applying to us all whether young or old, where we often are not in full control of our circumstances, and will have incomplete information when making decisions about our futures. Regarding pension policy, it is important to acknowledge that these limitations also make us vulnerable to harm, disappointment, failure, conflicting choices, and error, when calculating what is in our best interest to pursue, and especially concerning our long-term futures (and see Sobel, 1994). The broad recommendation here, then, is that this vulnerability should be accommodated for in pension policy, where mechanisms should be implemented to ensure that the long-term future well-being of vulnerable populations are protected (Foster, 2010; Goodin, 1985, 1988). This protection will also allow a young person to rationally pursue her interests now without being overly concerned about her future (reflecting the reductionist view), but still also be secure knowing that her long-term future interests are not being neglected (reflecting the non-reductionist view). Of course, the hybrid response recognises that these views conflict. However, by placing the onus of responsibility on governments through collective provision to meet the legitimate temporally neutral demands of non-reductionism, it allows all younger individual workers, and especially including those who will be most vulnerable as pensioners, to be biased toward their present lives, consistent with reductionism.

Turning to disability policy, I have argued elsewhere the important role that the value of individual agency plays, not only in contemporary accounts of well-being, but also within the disability rights movement and its promotion of the social model of disability (Steven Smith, 2011, pp. 131–152, 2013). So again reflecting the non-reductionist view of identity, a disabled person may see herself as possessing a singular and determinate identity, existing as an objective 'further fact' behind presently experienced physical and/ or psychological circumstances and relations. The point here is that her identity as a person *first*, that is, as an objective further fact occurring separately to her experiences of impairment, then allows for a critique of the medical model – which is a model that is seen as mistakenly reducing 'the disabled person' to a set of characteristics associated with medical 'dysfunction' and 'abnormality'. This radical process of 'objectification' (as it can now be called), renders classical liberal accounts of self-interest more plausible, despite Parfit's criticisms. Temporally neutral self-reflective judgements are made by a disabled person concerning her life-plans over time, and contribute to her well-being enhancement, because she is now viewed as 'the author' of her life in exactly the same way as a non-disabled person; her physical and psychological characteristics having no bearing at all on this 'further fact' of authorship (also see my arguments about these Kantian implications of *some* aspects of the disability movement's position in Smith, 2005b).

Moreover, for the disability movement, social expectations, reflecting the medical model, often mistakenly single out only disabled people as 'limited' and so leading lives of 'lesser' value than non-disabled people. Whereas, the social model views impairment as signifying restrictions in certain respects, but also as life enhancing in others (Morris, 1991; Swain, French, and Cameron, 2003; and Smith, 2001, 2009, 2011). The point here is that social policy and welfare practice should ensure the full expression of the latter view, where the training of welfare practitioners, for example, would assume that value is brought to a person's life often *because* and not despite of her impairment. Therefore, instead of a practitioner administering 'care' to the 'unfortunate victim' or 'tragically disabled', she would be open to learning from the personal experience of the disabled person she is caring for. That is, assuming the life led by an impaired service-user can be a positive one which contributes to her well-being and the life of others (Morris, 1991; Kittay, 2005, 1999).

However, difficult questions concerning how we understand and promote well-being within disability care are thrown into sharp relief as a result, and have a profound bearing on how the hybrid view is understood and promoted. For example, to what degree should a welfare practitioner accommodate for the present cognitive perspective of a disabled person in her care, given it is held by the service-user now? Or, to what degree should a welfare practitioner assume an impartial or temporary neutral perspective, which may go against the present perspective of the service-user? The point here is that recognising the presently orientated bias of the service-user, which may enhance presently occurring subjective well-being reflecting the reductionist view (and see Eid and Larson, 2008), may nevertheless conflict with the need for change and the possession of enhanced objective capacities for the service-user in the future – that, if implemented, would also enhance a person's long-term well-being (and see Nussbaum, 2011, 2006). The broader recommendation from the arguments presented in this chapter is that *holding* these conflicts as necessary tensions, is integral to how well-being, disability, and effective welfare practice is understood, across the various trajectories – actual *and* potential – of a disabled person's life. The practitioner must therefore manage the difficult balance of taking seriously the proposition that a life presently lived by a disabled person is worthwhile and valuable, not despite, but often because of their impairment, but also implement a future set of possibilities for the disabled person which expands this person's choices, opportunities, and agency, so enhancing their long-term future well-being.

Conclusion

As finite creatures we are all subjectively limited. But this gives shape to our lives, and, paradoxically, enables us to enjoy our lives as we become positively immersed 'in the moment' and 'who we are now'. For contemporary commentators on well-being, and consistent with Parfit's reductionism, we can also become better "engaged" with our lives (Haybron, 2008, pp. 114–115) – whole-heartedly committing to what we presently aim for and seek to accomplish, so enhancing our well-being. This enhancement occurs because we can be satisfied with our achievements now, but with these achievements reflecting our present temporally bounded identities and biases.

However, on other occasions we are more objectively reflective and so will maintain a more temporally neutral or impartial view of our lives. For example, when ensuring our long-term interests are protected we implement plans now to enhance our long-term future capabilities for well-being enhancement. This future-orientated implementation strategy readily reflects a non-reductionist view of identity, which assumes a "further fact" of a constant and unchanging identity occurring separately to changing circumstances, experiences, and psychological relations, and so existing as a singular determinate entity across time. The point here is that maintaining this temporal neutrality and impartiality can lead to conflicts within a person, between fulfilling present aims, so remaining 'authentic' and 'true to herself' now (reflecting the reductionist view) – but also, simultaneously, imagining new possibilities for her future which could be undermined if all these present aims are now met (reflecting the non-reductionist view; and see Sumner, 1999; Brink, 2003). Recognising this conflict and the resulting dilemmas underpins the hybrid view which combines reductionism and non-reductionism, and, it is argued here, is essential for understanding how best to develop social policies and welfare practices. The main conclusion is that when this conflict *within* persons is extended to populations and groups, social policy and welfare practice dilemmas are also produced concerning, not only how individual agency is exercised presently, but also how well-being is enhanced over generations and across communities. In short, the problem is how to manage these conflicts and tensions while resisting the temptation to 'dissolve' them.

Finally, following from the above, we can see that all our lives, whatever our social and other circumstances, are often led in complex and multi-layered ways, where many aspects of our well-being are not merely subjectively experiential, so occurring in the here-and-now, but also contain objective or impartial elements which then may facilitate appropriate attitudes of temporal neutrality. However, this pull toward temporal neutrality, despite our present-orientated bias, refers not only to one person's life where, contra Parfit, she treats her identity as a 'further fact' making herself the sole beneficiary of decisions made as the author of her life. It also can facilitate a neutral attitude *between* persons where a person considers her own interests as being equally weighted to others within any given community. This then leads to other questions concerning the interplay between these subjective and objective viewpoints or perspectives. For example, I have argued elsewhere (for example, see Smith, 2005a, 2011, pp. 83–106), that we often subjectively experience 'other regarding' emotions such as compassion for another's suffering, but which prompt us, more objectively and impartially, to imagine the life of others as being equally important to our own (and see Nagel, 1989). Given these latter demands of impartiality and objectivity within these wider social contexts, good reasons are often provided for policies that redistribute resources from the better-off to the worst-off, to rectify inequalities and enhance well-being for everyone.

Note

1 Indeed, for Parfit, in certain ways it might be better for us if we were more like 'Timeless' – a creature who has no bias toward the present and the near future over the past and distance future (see Parfit, 1987, pp. 176–177). The problem though, for Parfit, is that we are not like Timeless.

References

Blackburn, Simon. (1997) "Has Kant Refuted Parfit?" in Jonathan Dancy (ed), *Reading Parfit*, (Oxford: Blackwells), 180–201.

Braddon-Mitchell, David and Caroline West. (2001) "Temporal Phase Pluralism," *Philosophy and Phenomenological Research*, 62, 59–83.

Brink, David O. (2003) "Prudence and Authenticity: Intrapersonal Conflicts and Values," *The Philosophical Review*, 112, 215–245.

———. (1997) "Rational Egoism and the Separateness of Persons," in Jonathan Dancy (ed), *Reading Parfit* (Oxford: Blackwells), 96–134.

Eid, Michael and Randy Larsen. (eds.) (2008) *The Science of Subjective Well-Being* (New York: The Guilford Press).

Evandrou, Maria and Jane Falkingham. (2009) "Pensions and Income Security in Later Life," in J. Hills, T. Sefton and K. Stewart (eds), *Towards a More Equal Society? Poverty, Inequality and Policy Since 1997* (Bristol: Policy Press).

Foster, Liam. (2010) "Towards a New Political Economy of Pensions? The Implications for Women," *Critical Social Policy*, 30(1), 27–47.

Goodin, Robert. (1985) *Protecting the Vulnerable: A Re-Analysis of Our Social Responsibilities* (Chicago: University of Chicago Press).

———. (1988) *Reasons for Welfare: The Political Theory of the Welfare State* (Princeton, NJ: Princeton University Press).

Griffin, James. (1988) *Well-Being: It's Meaning, Measurement and Moral Importance* (Oxford: Clarendon Press).

Haybron, Daniel. (2008) *The Pursuit of Unhappiness: The Elusive Psychology of Well-Being* (Oxford: Oxford University Press).

Kittay, Eva. (2005) "At the Margins of Moral Personhood," *Ethics*, 116(October), 100–131.

———. (1999) *Love's Labor: Essays on Women, Equality and Dependency* (New York: Routledge).

Kopf, Gereon. (2002) "Temporality and Personal Identity," *Philosophy East and West*, 52, 224–245.

Korsgaard, Christine. (1989) "Personal Identity and the Unity of Agency: A Kantian Response to Parfit," *Philosophy and Public Affairs*, 18.

Morris, Jenny. (1991) *Pride Against Prejudice* (London: Women's Press).

Nagel, Thomas. (1989) *The View from Nowhere* (New York: Oxford University Press).

Nussbaum, Martha. (2011) *Creating Capabilities: The Human Development Approach* (Cambridge, MA: Harvard University Press).

———. (2006) *Frontiers of Justice: Disability, Nationality, Species Membership* (Cambridge: MA: Harvard University Press).

Parfit, Derek. (1987) *Reasons and Persons* (Oxford: Oxford University Press, 1987 – first published in 1984).

Pettigrew, Nick, Jayne Taylor, Caroline Simpson, Joe Lancaster and Richard Madden. (2007) *Department for Work and Pensions Research Report No 438: Live now, save later? Young people, saving and pensions* (Norwich: HMSO).

Rawls, John. (1973) *A Theory of Justice* (Oxford: Oxford University Press, 1973 – first published in 1972).

Raz, Joseph. (1988) *The Morality of Freedom* (Oxford: Oxford University Press).

Shoemaker, David W. (1996) "Theoretical Persons and Practical Agents," *Philosophy and Public Affairs*, 25(3), 18–32.

Sidgwick, Henry. (1981) *The Methods of Ethics* (Indianapolis: Hacket Publishing Company – first published in 1874).

Smith, Adam. (2011) *Theory of Moral Sentiments* (London: Penguin Classics – first published in 1759).

Smith, Steven R. (2011) *Equality and Diversity: Value Incommensurability and the Politics of Recognition* (Bristol: Policy Press).

———. (2005a) "Equality, Identity and the Disability Rights Movement: From Policy to Practice and From Kant to Nietzsche in More Than One Uneasy Move," *Critical Social Policy*, 25(4), 554–576.

———. (2005b) "Keeping Our Distance in Compassion-Based Social Relations," *Journal of Moral Philosophy*, 2(1), 69–88.

———. (2013) "Liberal Ethics and Well-Being Promotion in the Disability Rights Movement, Disability Policy, and Welfare Practice," *Ethics and Social Welfare*, 7(1), 20–35.

———. (2001) "The Social Construction of Talent: A Defence of Justice as Reciprocity," *Journal of Political Philosophy*, 9, 19–37.

———. (2009) "Social Justice and Disability: Competing Interpretations of the Medical and Social Models," in Kristjana Kristiansen, Simo Vehmas and Tom Shakespeare (ed), *Arguing About Disability: Philosophical Perspectives* (Abingdon: Routledge).

Sobel, David. (1994) "Full Information Accounts of Well-Being," *Ethics*, 104, 784–810.

Stocker, Michael. (1997) "Parfit and the Time of Value" in Jonathan Dancy (ed), *Reading Parfit*, (Oxford: Blackwells), 54–71.

Sumner, Leonard W. (1999) *Welfare, Happiness and Ethics* (Oxford: Clarendon Press).

Swain, John, Sally French and Colin Cameron. (2003) *Controversial Issues in a Disabling Society* (Buckingham: Open University Press).

Tiberius, Valerie. (2008) *The Reflective Life: Living Wisely with Our Limits* (New York: Oxford University Press).

23

VALUES-BASED PRACTICE

At home with our values

K.W.M. (Bill) Fulford and Kathleen T. Galvin

What is well-being without values? Several chapters in this book attest to the role of values in well-being in areas ranging from health (see for example Burwood, Chapter 13; illness, for example Eatough, Chapter 17; in psychosomatic conditions, Bullington, Chapter 5 and in a maternal context, Jomeen and Martin, Chapter 21), through work modern and professional life (Prendergast and Leggo, Chapter 27), caring practices (Dahlberg and Ranheim, Chapter 14) to relationships (for example, Knowles, Chapter 6; Hemingway, Chapter 20; Calder, Chapter 9). The very word *well*-being is explicitly value-laden. Small wonder then that well-being is challenging. For values themselves are challenging. They are challenging theoretically: values have been a focus of philosophical enquiry for over two millennia. They are also in various respects challenging practically.

This chapter outlines the potential contribution of values-based practice to well-being. Values-based practice has been developed thus far mainly in healthcare. In this context as the chapter will indicate it has proved effective in supporting balanced clinical decision-making where challenging values issues are in play. This is why it has potential for well-being. To the extent that the challenges of well-being are or reflect values challenges they should be susceptible to similar values-based approaches. One way to understand the impact of values-based practice in healthcare is indeed, as the chapter will show, that it shifts the aims of care from curing disease to enhancing well-being.

The chapter starts with a short interactive exercise exhibiting three features of values that are important for understanding the challenges they present for practice. This is followed by an overview of values-based practice indicating how it supports stakeholders in responding to the values challenges of practice. Examples are then given of how values-based practice has been applied in two contrasting areas of healthcare, surgery and mental health. The chapter concludes with a brief review of continuities and discontinuities between values-based practice in healthcare and work on well-being.

Values

The features of values of particular relevance to values-based practice are best appreciated from personal experience. Hence rather than just reading straight on you may like to try the following brief exercise for yourself.

The exercise explores the deceptively simple question of what you understand by values. It has two distinct steps:

- Step 1 – write down three words that mean 'values' to you.
- Step 2 – then (and only when you have written down your own three words) compare what you have written with the responses of others given in the Figure 23.1 over-page.

Note: it is important to actually write down your own three words – don't just think of them 'in your head'. It is also important to write down your own three words before looking at what others have come up with. This is why Figure 23.1 is given over-page. The temptation is to check what others have written before committing yourself. It is natural to seek the reassurance of conformity. But remember that the exercise aims to explore your own individual understanding of values. And as Figure 23.1 shows, when it comes to values everyone is different.

The 'three words' responses shown in Figure 23.1 are taken from an early seminar with a clinical team working on values-based surgical care (more on values-based practice in surgery below). But the responses are typical. The exercise always produces a diverse range of responses similar to those shown in Figure 23.1. It is a good bet that your response is different again. It is possible you came up with a triplet of words that is the same as one of those in Figure 23.1. But the odds are heavily against this. There are different values expressed ('respect' and 'transparency', for example); different categories of values ('principles', 'codes' and 'ethics'); different ideas about the role of values ('What makes me tick') and about their origins ('personal to me', 'cultural').

There are overlaps of course. Words occurring more than once in Figure 23.1 include 'principles' and 'respect'. Such overlaps are important for values-based practice. They are the basis for the frame-works of shared values within which as described further below values-based decision-making takes place. But the first point about values to take from this exercise is, in a word, *diversity*. Figure 23.1 graphically illustrates this diversity in the range of responses to that deceptively simple question about what values mean to you.

A second point to take from the exercise is summed up in the word *surprise*. Most people doing this exercise for the first time are surprised by the diversity of responses it evokes. Even the person sitting next to them and that they may have known for years often has a completely different response to their own. It is natural to be surprised by this. The word 'values', after all, is familiar in everyday use. It is thus natural to assume that 'we' know what it means. In a sense we do. We use 'values' seamlessly and by and large unreflectingly in contrast with for example a technically challenging word like 'metaphysics'. But what this exercise brings home from direct personal experience is that the very meaning each of us attaches to the word 'values' in a given context is not only highly diverse but surprisingly so.

With these two points it can already be seen why values are challenging in practice. If the degree to which values are individually diverse is not self-evident (if they are surprisingly diverse), it is small wonder they cause difficulties in practice. The main barrier to be overcome in values-based training is indeed what might be called the 'assumption of sameness'. This assumption, as will be illustrated with case 1 below, is a particular challenge in clinical decision-making.

Figure 23.1 Example triplets of words in feedback from the 'three words' exercise

Preferences	How we treat people
Needs	Attitudes
Cultural	Principles
Respect	Non-violence
Personal to me	Compassion
Difference . . . diversity	Dialogue
Codes	Responsibility
Right/wrong to me	Respect
What I am	Transparency
Belief	What I *believe*
Principles	What makes me tick
Things held dear	What I won't compromise
Subjective merits	'Objective' core
Meanings	Confidentiality
Person-centred care	Ethics

But there is a further reason why values are challenging: even where values are shared they may be *complex and conflicting*. Again, this is evident from Figure 23.1. The value of respect for example (one of the repeat words in Figure 23.1) is widely shared particularly in healthcare. But exactly what respect means in any given context is highly variable from one person to the next. Respect is in this sense a complex value. It is also to a greater or lesser extent in conflict with other widely shared values. Thus, respect may come into conflict with transparency (another of the repeat words in Figure 23.1). In healthcare contexts, for example, respecting a patient's confidentiality may involve being less than transparent with the patient's relatives.

The three features of values just outlined are summarised in Figure 23.2. They capture between them much that is challenging about working with values in healthcare. This is why raising awareness of these features, using the 'three words' and other exercises, is the foundation for values-based training. So, how does values-based practice help us to respond to the values challenges of healthcare?

Figure 23.2 Three practically challenging features of values

Values are

1) **Individually diverse**: each of us has a unique 'values fingerprint'
2) **Surprisingly diverse**: other people's values are often very different from what we imagine them to be (overcoming the 'assumption of sameness' is thus key to values-based practice)
3) **Complex and conflicting**: even where our values are shared they are likely to be individually complex ('respect' for example means different things to different people) and jointly conflicting ('respect' may be in conflict with 'transparency', for example – see text)

Values-based practice

One way of responding to the values challenges of healthcare is to seek consensus. Ethics for example, in healthcare contexts, seeks consensus on values. Given a contested area of decision-making, ethics seeks consensus on values by which the outcomes of an action may be judged to be right or wrong. Autonomy of patient choice is one such value widely reflected in contemporary codes of medical practice.

Values-based practice takes a different approach. Instead seeking consensus on right outcomes it offers a process that supports stakeholders in finding answers for themselves in the particular circumstances presented by a given situation (Fulford, Peile and Carroll, 2012). Values-based practice is in this respect like evidence-based practice. The two indeed are partners in clinical decision-making. Evidence-based practice offers a process that supports stakeholders where complex and conflicting evidence is in play. Values-based practice offers a process that supports stakeholders where complex and conflicting values are in play.

The processes are different of course. Evidence-based practice employs meta-analyses of high-quality research to come to a consensus on current best evidence informing decision-making in a given area. Values-based practice builds rather on learnable clinical skills and other elements to support balanced decision-making within frameworks of shared values. But the principle of providing support for decision-makers rather than handing down answers is the same.

The process of values-based practice is summarised in Figure 23.3 and brief definitions of its process elements are given in Figure 23.4. Values-based practice as these figures show is premised on respect for differences of values. Within this premise, values-based practice builds on four key areas of learnable clinical skills. Raised awareness as noted above is the starting point. Also important are skills of knowledge acquisition, reasoning and certain aspects of communication skills. As illustrated below, skills for eliciting values are a key communication skill for values-based practice. Good clinical skills however will be ineffective without an appropriate service context. Values-based practice depends on services that are person-centred (focusing on what matters or is important to the person concerned) and multidisciplinary (in values-based practice a range of team values is important as well as of knowledge and skills).

The three principles linking values and evidence capture between them the importance of partnership between evidence-based and values-based approaches. Although often neglected nowadays, the partnership between evidence and values was emphasised by the pioneers of evidence-based practice. David Sackett, for example, writing as the first Director of Oxford's Centre for Evidence-based Medicine defined evidence-medicine as combining best research evidence with experience and with values (Sackett et al., 2000, p. 1). Contemporary evidence-based guidelines from the UK's NICE (National Institute for Health and Care Excellence) reflect this in requiring those using the guidelines to take

Figure 23.3 A diagram of values-based practice

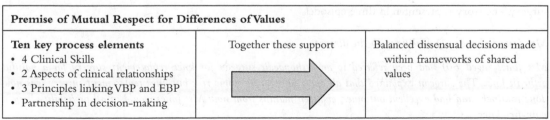

Premise of Mutual Respect for Differences of Values		
Ten key process elements • 4 Clinical Skills • 2 Aspects of clinical relationships • 3 Principles linking VBP and EBP • Partnership in decision-making	Together these support	Balanced dissensual decisions made within frameworks of shared values

Figure 23.4   Brief definitions of the elements of values-based practice

Values-based practice	Brief definition
Premise of mutual respect	Mutual respect for differences of values
Skills – awareness	Awareness of values and of differences of values
Skills – knowledge	Knowledge retrieval and its limitations
Skills – reasoning	Used to explore the values in play rather than to 'solve' dilemmas
Skills – communication	Especially for eliciting values and conflict resolution
Person-values-centred care	Care centred on the actual rather than assumed values of the patient
Extended MDT	MDT role extended to include a range of value perspectives as well as of knowledge and skills for interagency working
Two feet principle	All decisions are based on the two feet of values and evidence
Squeaky wheel principle	We notice values when they cause difficulties (like the squeaky wheel) but (like the wheel that doesn't squeak) they are always there and operative
Science-driven principle	Advances in medical science drive the need for VBP (as well as EBP) because they open up choices and with choices go values
Partnership	Decisions in VBP (although informed by clinical guidelines and other sources) are made by those directly concerned working together in partnership
Frameworks of shared values	Values shared by those in a given decision-making context and within which balanced decisions can be made on individual cases
Balanced dissensual decision-making	Decisions in which the values in question remain in play to be balanced sometimes one way and sometimes in other ways according to the circumstances of a given case

into account 'the individual needs, preferences and values of their patients or service users' (see websites below).

These elements, as the right-hand side of Figure 23.3 indicates, support balanced decision-making within frameworks of shared values. The process of balanced decision-making is dissensual. Dissensus is important. As the examples from mental health given below will illustrate dissensus underpins the respect for diversity of values on which values-based practice is premised. It is best understood by contrast with consensus. Consensual decision-making involves one conflicting value giving way to another. Codes of ethics for example often include rules for when respect should give way to transparency. With dissensual decision-making, by contrast, the values in question (represented by the relevant framework of shared values) all remain in play to be balanced sometimes one way and sometimes in other ways according the particular circumstances of each case.

Values-based practice in surgery

That role of values-based practice in medicine is illustrated by the following case history from orthopaedic surgery. The story is presented in three episodes.

Mrs Jones's knee – 1) dealing with the disease

Mrs Jones (aged 60) had been referred to an orthopaedic surgeon for knee replacement surgery for a painful arthritic knee. The surgeon explained that all operations carried some risk but knee replacement surgery was now done routinely and had excellent outcomes; eighteen months from now Mrs Jones would in all probability have a pain-free knee.

To this point the clinical decision-making in Mrs Jones's case has followed conventional disease-oriented processes of diagnostic assessment based on a well-developed lesion-theory of the causes of Mrs Jones's painful knee and a well-established evidence base for the effectiveness of knee replacement surgery in getting rid of the pain. Mrs Jones was initially very pleased with this outcome. She had feared that the surgeon might decide she was too old for surgery or that her GP (who had referred her) had got the diagnosis wrong.

Mrs Jones's knee – 2) values-based practice

As Mrs Jones got up to leave she turned to the surgeon to say how glad she was that she 'would be able to garden again'. The surgeon immediately looked up from his notes and asked her to sit down again inviting her to tell him a bit more about her gardening. Mrs Jones explained that the reason she wanted something done about her knee was that she could not bend it well enough to do her gardening. The pain was unpleasant but bearable if only she could get back to her garden. The surgeon explained that while she would very likely be pain free after her operation she would be no more mobile and possibly less so with the artificial joints currently available. The result was that after a few minutes further discussion they agreed to see what could be achieved with conservative management (anti-inflammatory medication and physiotherapy).

This stage in Mrs Jones's story illustrates much that is important about values-based practice. The surgeon showed excellent communication skills: as is so often the case this meant listening attentively to what his patient had to say and continuing to listen after the formal part of the interview was finished. Picking up on the cue about gardening allowed the surgeon to make the crucial move past the 'assumption of sameness' (above) and, in discussion with Mrs Jones, to find out that unlike most people with arthritic knees what really mattered to her was not pain relief but restoration of mobility.

The decision (to go for conservative treatment rather than surgery) was thus put on a secure values-base reflecting Mrs Jones's values as a unique individual. But the evidence base was also crucial. It was the surgeon's specialist training and expert knowledge that allowed him to pick up on the significance of Mrs Jones's comments about gardening and to advise her on the options available.

Mrs Jones's knee – 3) from health to well-being

Conservative management worked. Eighteen months later Mrs Jones's mobility was sufficiently restored that she was able to garden again. Her knee was still painful but as she said to the surgeon on follow-up, that was 'a small price to pay'.

In Mrs Jones's story as in all areas of values-based practice the relevant science (including a well-developed disease theory) stands side-by-side with the relevant values (centrally those of Mrs Jones). However, had the decision been based on the science alone, while Mrs Jones's disease (her painful arthritic knee) would have been cured, her well-being would have been in consequence reduced rather than enhanced. The key values-based point is that Mrs Jones's well-being was not anyone else's well-being. For most people with arthritic knees their well-being is enhanced with the relief of pain delivered by a prosthetic joint. But Mrs Jones was not most people.

Mrs Jones's story illustrates a further point about values-based practice summed up in the third of its three principles linking science with evidence, the Science-Driven Principle (see Figure 23.4). The opportunity for a values-based decision resulting in an improvement in her well-being was science driven in the sense that it was the science that opened up the treatment options available. That a similar opening up of options is being delivered by science across an increasingly wide range of conditions is why values-based practice is being developed alongside evidence-based practice in areas such as surgery (Handa et al., 2016).

Values-based practice in mental health

Values-based practice was developed first in mental health (see Further information and websites below). This might appear to contradict the Science-Driven Principle given that disease theories are less well developed in mental health than in areas such a surgery. The need for values-based practice in mental health derives however from the fact that the diversity of values arising in bodily health through advances in medical science, is already present in mental health by virtue of the areas of human experience and behaviour with which it is concerned.

Mrs Jones's painful arthritic knee makes the point. Pain, like most other symptoms of bodily disease, is values-simple in the sense that for most people most of the time it is a bad thing: this is why the surgeon concerned had assumed that Mrs Jones was like most people with arthritic knees in wanting to get rid of the pain. But the experiences with which mental health is concerned are not like pain in this values-simple respect. Mental health is by its very nature values-complex. It is concerned with areas of human experience and behaviour – like emotion, desire, volition, motivation, belief and identity – in which unlike pain our values differ widely. An example of the practical impact of the values-complex nature of mental health is what has become widely known as the recovery movement.

Recovery in mental health

The recovery movement grew out of disenchantment with disease theories in mental health. It had been known for many years (see for example Rogers, Pilgrim and Lacey, 1993) that people with long-term mental disorders were more concerned about finding a job, establishing a home and making friends, than with symptom control. Yet mental health services have remained focused on symptom control even where this involves using medications with socially disempowering side effects.

Recovery practice thus means refocusing the aims of care away from symptom control and towards recovering a good quality of life (Slade et al., 2014). There are of course different ways of deciding just what is meant by a good quality of life. Crucially in recovery practice, 'good' means as defined by the values of (by what matters to) the person concerned. This is why values-based practice has a role to play in recovery. And as with Mrs Jones's knee in surgery, values-based recovery in mental health is about the aims of care being shifted from curing disease to enhancing the well-being of the person concerned.

Compulsory psychiatric treatment

Mental health though is also the one area of healthcare where treatment may in certain circumstances be given to an adult and competent patient in direct opposition to their express wishes. Not only that but compulsory treatment, as it is called, extends to situations in which (in contrast with for example compulsory treatment for an infectious disease) the intervention is justified not to protect others but in the interests of the person concerned.

Compulsory psychiatric treatment so described may seem in flat contradiction to the principles of values-based practice. Recall, though, that values-based practice is about balanced decision-making between conflicting values. Compulsory psychiatric treatment is thus open to a dissensual approach similar in principle to that adopted in any other area of healthcare.

It was this dissensual approach that was line adopted in a training programme produced by the UK's Department of Health to support implementation of revised legislation on compulsory psychiatric treatment, the Mental Health Act, 2007 (Fulford, Dewey and King, 2015). Figure 23.5, which is taken from the training materials (available as a pdf from the Collaborating Centre website, see below), shows the basis of the approach. The five circles represent five 'Guiding Principles' (Purpose, Respect, Participation, Resources and Least Restrictive Alternative) governing the use of the Act. These Guiding Principles were derived from an extensive consultation carried out in the run-up to the launch of the new legislation. The consultation as such was deeply contentious. Opinion was sharply divided along values-lines. On the one hand were those – mainly patients and clinicians – united in support of autonomy. On the other were those – mainly politicians and the wider public they represented – concerned more about saving lives. But there was wide agreement

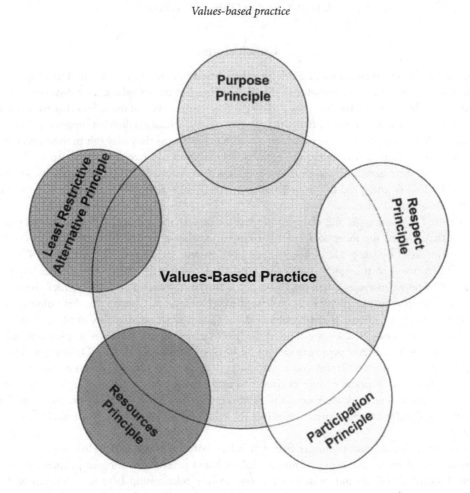

Figure 23.5 The Guiding Principles as a framework of shared values

among those consulted on the values reflected in the five Guiding Principles. The Guiding Principles therefore formed a framework of shared values as the basis for a dissensual approach to decision-making under the Act. This is why they are shown not as a list but as a 'round table' in Figure 23.5.

The challenge for practice, though, was that the Guiding Principles, although indeed representing values shared by all those concerned, are, like the shared values considered earlier in the chapter, individually complex and jointly conflicting. The Principle of Respect, for example, is a complex value in the sense defined above (of meaning different things to different people). Respect is also a value that comes into conflict with other Guiding Principles. It is for example necessarily in conflict with the Purpose Principle (which is about treatment that in being compulsory fails to respect the patient's wishes).

This is why 'values-based practice' is shown at the centre of the round table of Guiding Principles in Figure 23.5. It is the skills and other process elements of values-based practice that support stakeholders in interpreting and balancing the Guiding Principles on a case-by-case basis in the use of the Act. Where there is a high suicide risk, for example, the Purpose Principle would outweigh Respect for the patient's wishes. In another case, with similar features except that the risk of suicide is minimal, the balance would come out the other way. The required balance is thus dissensual. Whatever the balance in a given case, the framework of Guiding Principles as a whole remains in play to be balanced one way in some cases and quite differently in others depending on the particular circumstances presented.

Conclusions

This chapter has described the emerging role of values-based practice in healthcare. The chapter opened with an interactive exercise that highlighted three challenging features of values: their diversity, the surprising extent of this diversity, and the complex and conflicting natures even of the values that we share. Values-based practice, as was then described, offers a process (based on learnable skills) that supports stakeholders in responding in a balanced way to these challenging features of values as they play out in their everyday practice. In being process rather than outcomes focused, values-based practice is a partner to evidence-based practice. Examples were given of how values-based practice works out in the (relatively) values-simple area of surgery (Mrs Jones's knee) and the (more) values-complex area of mental health (recovery practice and compulsory treatment).

As anticipated at the start of the chapter, one way to understand the role of values-based practice in healthcare is that it shifts the focus of decision-making from disease to well-being. Mrs Jones's well-being was actually enhanced by using a less effective (conservative rather than surgical) treatment of her disease. Values-based practice is to this extent well-being-practice. Consistently with this understanding there are clear continuities between values-based practice and work on well-being described in other chapters in this book. Nordenfelt's philosophical work on quality of life (Nordenfelt, Chapter 16, this volume) is a clear case in point: recovery practice in mental health is about recovering a good quality of life as defined by the values of the person concerned. Other continuities are reflected in the resources of phenomenology for raising awareness of the values of people in various healthcare situations (Dahlberg, Dahlberg and Ranheim, Chapter 14; Eatough Chapter 17; and Galvin and Todres Chapter 30; this volume). The training methods employed in values-based practice were derived originally from analytic philosophy of values (Fulford, 1989 and 2014) but recent work has shown the extent to which the two kinds of philosophy, analytic and phenomenological, offer complementary resources for values-based clinical care (Stanghellini, Bolton and Fulford, 2013).

There are though also discontinuities between values-based practice and well-being. One such discontinuity is in their respective scopes of interest. Values-based practice has focused primarily (though not exclusively, Fulford, 2014) on individuals in the one-to-one relationship between clinician and patient characteristic of contemporary practice. Work on well-being, by contrast, has extended from the individual to the social (Knowles, Chapter 6, this volume) and embodied (Bullington, Chapter 5; Lamont-Robinson, Chapter 26; Hemingway, Chapter 20, this volume) aspects of experience and includes geographical, cultural, historical dimensions and identity dimensions (for example, Seamon, Chapter 10; Rapport, Chapter 2; Darvill, Heaslip and Barrass, Chapter 11; Smith, Chapter 22, this volume). In focusing on individual decision-making values-based practice is concordant with standards of best practice in person-centred medicine as reflected medical guidance (General Medical Council, 2008) and law (Herring et al., 2017). But there are well-grounded criticisms – philosophical (Venkatapuram, 2014), ethical (Dickenson, 2013) and indeed scientific (Marmot, 2006) – of this individual-centred approach. This is an area then in which values-based practice has much to gain from the extended range of work on well-being. It has much to gain too from work in areas that although not traditionally within the scope of healthcare are inseparable from it in practice. Consonance between individual and corporate values, for example, has been shown to be important for well-being at work (Lord, forthcoming) and in the context of professional training (Cohen et al., 2013).

Paul Gilbert writes of well-being in terms of our primitive preconceptual experiences of being at home, contrasts examples of feeling out of place, unfamiliar or intrusive things or even disruptions, and points to our desire to function well in our contexts and activities without impediments. There are modes of activity that fail to succeed in conducing to well-being because of tone or the way in which the activity is engaged in; we long for 'well-functioning' or a feeling of home (Gilbert, Chapter 1, this volume). This is a powerful metaphor. But the metaphor points to a paradox. The issue is this: Value-based practice starts from respect for diversity of values and aims to support balanced dissensual decision-making in which this diversity is sustained. As such it is an irreducibly pluralistic approach. But as the moral and political philosopher Isaiah Berlin pointed out over fifty years ago (Berlin, 1958), writing in the shadow of National Socialism, when it comes to values our default position is monism not pluralism. Most people shy away from the challenges of choosing between values, preferring to be given 'the right answer'. You may have experienced this default to monism if you were tempted to look at the answers given in Figure 23.1 to the 'three words' exercise before committing yourself by writing down your own answer. The default to monism has certainly proved to be a major challenge in implementing values-based practice (Fulford, Dewey and King, 2015). So the paradox is this: The contribution of values-based practice to well-being is in Paul Gilbert's metaphor to make us feel at home, in multifaceted ways, negotiating our place effortlessly, with the plurality of our values. But plurality of values if Isaiah Berlin is right is more likely to make us homesick.

References

Berlin, I. (1958) *Two Concepts of Liberty*. Oxford: Clarendon Press.

Cohen, D., Winstanley, S., Palmer, P., Allen, J., Howells, S., Greene, G., and Rhydderch, M. (2013) *Factors That Impact on Medical Student Wellbeing – Perspectives of Risks*. School of Medicine, Cardiff University: Individual Support Programme.

Dickenson, D. (2013) *Me Medicine vs. We Medicine: Reclaiming Biotechnology for the Common Good*. Columbia: Columbia University Press.

Fulford, K.W.M. (1989, reprinted 1995 and 1999) *Moral Theory and Medical Practice*. Cambridge: Cambridge University Press.

Fulford, K.W.M. (2014) Living with Uncertainty: A First-Person-Plural Response to Eleven Commentaries on Values-Based Practice. Ch 13 in Loughlin, M. (ed) *Debates in Values-Based Practice: Arguments for and Against*. Cambridge: Cambridge University Press.

Fulford, K.W.M., Dewey, S., and King, M. (2015) Values-Based Involuntary Seclusion and Treatment: Value Pluralism and the UK's Mental Health Act 2007. Ch 60 in Sadler, J.Z., van Staden, W., and Fulford, K.W.M., (eds) *The Oxford Handbook of Psychiatric Ethics*. Oxford: Oxford University Press.

Fulford, K.W.M., Peile, E., and Carroll, H. (2012) *Essential Values-Based Practice: Clinical Stories Linking Science with People*. Cambridge: Cambridge University Press.

General Medical Council. (2008) *Consent: Patients and Doctors Making Decisions Together*. London: General Medical Council.

Handa, I.A., Fulford-Smith, L., Barber, Z.E., Dobbs, T.D., Fulford, K.W.M., and Peile, E. (2016) The importance of seeing things from someone else's point of view. *BMJ Careers on-line Journal* (published in hard copy as 'Learning to Talk about Values'). http://careers.bmj.com/careers/advice/The_importance_of_seeing_things_from_someone_else's_point_of_view

Herring, J., Fulford, K.W.M., Dunn, D., and Handa, A. (2017) Elbow room for best practice? Montgomery, patients' values, and balanced decision-making in person-centred care. *Medical Law Review*, 25 (4), 582–603.

Lord, A. (forthcoming). Enhancing Well-Being and Motivation for Staff Working with Patients Who Have Inconsistent or Challenging Engagement in Services. Ch 17 in Hadler, A., Sutton, S., and Osterberg, L. (eds) *The Wiley Handbook of Treatment Engagement*. London: John Wiley & Sons Ltd.

Marmot, M. (2006) Health in an unequal world: social circumstances. *Biology and Disease. Clinical Medicine*, 6, 559–572.

Rogers, A., Pilgrim, D., and Lacey, R. (1993) *Experiencing Psychiatry: Users' Views of Services*. London: The Macmillan Press.

Sackett, D.L., Straus, S.E., Scott Richardson, W., Rosenberg, W., and Haynes, R.B. (2000) *Evidence-Based Medicine: How to Practice and Teach EBM* (2nd Edition). Edinburgh and London: Churchill Livingstone.

Slade, M., Amering, M., Farkas, M., Hamilton, B., O'Hagan, M., Panther, G., Perkins, R., Shepherd, G., Tse, S., and Whitley, R. (2014) Uses and abuses of recovery: implementing recovery-oriented practices in mental health systems. *World Psychiatry*, 13, 12–20.

Stanghellini, G., Bolton, D., and Fulford, K.W.M. (2013, March) Person-centred psychopathology of schizophrenia: building on Karl Jaspers' understanding of the patient's attitude towards his illness. *Schizophrenia Bulletin*, 39(2), 287–294. doi:10.1093/schbul/sbs154. Epub 2013 Jan 11.

Venkatapuram, S. (2014) Values-Based Practice and Global Health. Chapter 11 in Loughlin, M. (ed) *Debates in Values-Based Practice: Arguments for and Against.* Cambridge: Cambridge University Press.

Further information and websites

For a general introduction to values-based practice illustrated through a series of clinical cases see Fulford, Peile and Carroll (2012).

The website of the Collaborating Centre for Values-based Practice at St Catherine's College, Oxford is at: www.valuesbasedpractice.org

The website gives a detailed Reading Guide and downloadable PDFs to support training and other developments in values-based practice. These include:

- The Handbook for Values-based Surgical Care (this is linked to an on-line Teaching Resource Library that includes example responses to the three words exercise similar to those given in Figure 23.1).
- The Foundation Module for the training programme supporting implementation of the Mental Health Act, 2007 (from which Figure 23.5 is derived).

For both documents, go to *http://valuesbasedpractice.org/more-about-vbp/annotated-index/* and scroll down the table of contents.

The NICE statement cited in the text linking values with evidence is given at: www.nice.org.uk/guidance/cg181 (and scroll down the page to the statement 'Your Responsibility').

The *Montgomery* Supreme Court judgment on consent is at:

Montgomery v Lanarkshire Health Board (judgment delivered March 11, 2015) www.supremecourt.uk/cases/uksc-2013-0136.html

PART 3

How is well-being manifest in human life? The aesthetic nature of well-being

24

CREATIVITY AND AESTHETIC THINKING

Toward an aesthetics of well-being

Dorthe Jørgensen

Aesthetics of existence and competence development

Many people talk about seeing themselves and their lives as a work of art. This thought builds on the post-modern idea that 'the grand narratives' about, for example, God, reason, and truth have collapsed. All the values that were seen to be absolute in the past have lost their credibility, and 'the subject,' which used to be the seat of moral knowledge and action, has dissolved. The identity of post-modern man is thus unclear and his existence uncertain. According to thinkers like Michel Foucault these problems can be solved by developing what he calls an *aesthetics of existence*, and this 'aesthetics' is precisely about regarding oneself and one's life as a work of art (Foucault, 1991: 350–351). Foucault links the aesthetics of existence and the problems to which it is a response to the ancient Greeks. He believes that Greek ethics were focused on 'the problem of personal choice,' and that these ethics were a reaction to problems similar to those we are experiencing today with our loss of faith in religion-based ethics and our distaste for our private lives being controlled by law. Foucault is manipulating history, however, for actually Greek ethics were closely linked to mythology, in other words the religiosity of the time. These ethics found their cohesion, their effect, and their credibility in references to the sphere of absolute values that the Greek gods still represented in mythological form at the time of Plato and Aristotle. In fact, the preference of Foucault and other post-modern theoreticians for reflecting ethical questions in aesthetics does not derive from antiquity but from the 18th century. More specifically, it is related to a phenomenon known at the time as 'the beautiful soul.' Admittedly, the beautiful soul does refer back to antiquity, to the Greek ideal of a beautiful-and-good person, but when old ideas are taken up again, they generally result in something new. This also happened to the beautiful-and-good person, when it became the beautiful soul, and the same is happening now when the beautiful soul has become 'me as a work of art.'

Early in antiquity, beauty-and-goodness consisted of external attributes, such as a well-proportioned body, expensive clothes, and a high-class name, all of which were regarded as evidence of qualities of an intellectual and moral nature. Gradually beauty-and-goodness came to be seen as something more internal that needed to be *trained* into being, and the Greeks began to consider what they themselves could *do* to become beautiful-and-good. Nonetheless, this internalization was nothing compared to the sentimentality and sensitivity later linked to the beautiful soul of the 18th century. Furthermore, it is the self-encirclement of this sentimentality that has now been massively superseded by the individualism in the post-modern aesthetics of existence. In the 18th century, people still felt duty bound to a common morality that had general validity, whereas today this would be incompatible with post-modern thinking. The present-day idea of seeing oneself and one's life as a work of art is merely the individual's personal project, nursed for one's own benefit. It is an expression of an individualistic idea of self-realization that chimes in with the current interest in competence development. Many workplaces now expect 'personal competences,' and many employees view courses on competence development as an opportunity to 'realize themselves.' In reality, however, the desired competences are often something as impersonal as 'being flexible and ready for change,' while 'action competence' so highly regarded by 'competence educators and educationalists' amounts to no more than the ability to make use of one's knowledge and skills in areas different from those in which they were acquired. Where qualifications have value in themselves and retain that value over time, competences are opportunistic: they are an answer to something else, ultimately the prevailing trend of society, to which they have to adapt in order not to depreciate. That is why there is always a need for yet another course, and the effort of 'realizing oneself' is not only never-ending, but also futile.

The present preference for competences rather than qualifications shows how the focus has moved from the *content* of knowledge to its *usefulness*. This is in line with the instrumental way of thinking in our knowledge society, in which knowledge is no longer a goal in itself, but only a means for growth and control. Thus knowledge plays a different role today than in the past, and simultaneously the concept of knowledge has shrunk considerably. The interest today is solely in the *particularized* knowledge produced by highly *specialized* fields of science or appertained to specific competences. Formerly there were a number of different concepts of knowledge, and wisdom, the Greek *sophia*, was seen as the highest form of knowledge. To be more precise, wisdom was not seen as the opposite of knowledge but embraced all the other forms of knowledge. If there is still a focus today on anything from those days, it is not on *sophia* but on *phronesis*, that is, the practical knowledge of how to act in a given situation and how to act 'wisely' in life. Wisdom has been left to the new religious movements; modern research and society in general are only concerned with scientific understanding and general life knowledge. The result is a neo-positivism in the human and social sciences, and a competence development of an increasingly aggressive psychological kind. Souls are formed on an assembly line, not for the benefit of the individual, but in order to increase efficiency and maximize profit. This is the purpose of competence development, for in the knowledge society nothing is more profitable than people who can get on in the world, who can see the possibilities and exploit them for personal gain; this does not demand qualifications, but competences. The competent person is a wily person – different from the thinking person. The wily person moves around and helps to run the engine room in a society allegedly giving priority to 'creativity and innovation.' He stages himself and is his 'own work,' whereas the thinking person questions and perhaps ponders over what a 'work' actually is.

Reason and wisdom

Can modern people do no more than acquire knowledge and meet the demands of their surroundings? Is there no potential for reason, or is it simply taboo because post-modern theoreticians have made reason suspect? The Enlightenment philosopher Immanuel Kant was not afraid of reason, but he also distinguished between reason and understanding. Although according to him enlightenment is about using one's own understanding, he was fully aware that understanding is not enough.[1] Understanding operates with cause and effect, it calculates and finds explanations, and it is oriented toward usefulness. Without understanding we would not survive; but it is not the understanding and its way of thinking that graces us as human beings. On the contrary, the peculiar quality of the human being is its ability to ponder on its impressions, put a perspective on its knowledge, and reflect on its thoughts and behavior, for which it needs reason, not understanding. Reason differs from understanding in that it does not simply subordinate empirical data to general concepts in order to state something – for instance, that this is a flower, and this flower is called a 'violet.' Instead, reason forms and finds its orientation in ideas of that which cannot be observed empirically, and which we therefore know nothing exact about, such as God, the soul, and the world as a whole.

Human reason can therefore only flourish where there is room to refer to more than just pragmatic facts, not least to something larger and more comprehensive than the human itself. The good life has as a premise that we can give reality to our striving for such a reference, traditionally known as metaphysical truth, and the higher insight that this striving facilitates, and which was previously called wisdom. If we are to live optimally, we must add to the way of thinking controlled by understanding, a further way of thinking based on reason. There must be room for the 'holistic' way of thinking, which is characteristic of reason and is the precondition for us pursuing not just knowledge, but also wisdom.

This line of thought may seem strange today, but it was a matter of course from antiquity until recently. It is not the thought that wisdom as well as knowledge, both reason and understanding, are necessary that is strange. It is we who are strange if we believe that as the single exception in world history we can ignore this thought. As late as in the 1700s and 1800s one could become professor of 'world-wisdom' (*Weltweisheit*). With Plato in mind this may seem rather ambitious, since he himself warned that only gods can be wise, whereas humans must be satisfied with simply *striving* for wisdom. Nevertheless, Plato did not want to stop the human desire for wisdom, but to encourage further thinking, even after one believes that one has found the truth. The point was not that one should be interested only in knowledge, but that in one's search for wisdom one must be aware that one cannot possess it, only long for it. This was also the task for those people who were given professorships in world-wisdom in the time of Kant, and Kant himself even differentiated between 'school philosophy' and 'philosophy understood as world-wisdom' (Kant, 1998: A 838–839, B 866–867). School philosophy is philosophy carried out as a technical discipline concerned only with those questions of an analytical kind that interest experts in this discipline; questions which they are likely to believe they each have solid answers to. World-wisdom on the other hand is philosophical thinking that is concerned with what in principle is of interest to us all, such as existential and ethical questions, and deals with its subject in the free, open, and questioning way that was originally characteristic of philosophical thinking. In many cases the professors of world-wisdom in the real world have probably not handled this task particularly well, but it is worth holding on to the principle. The message is to reflect on questions of general interest – being attentive to people's experiences and to the universal in the personal – and to do so in such a way that we not only gain knowledge, but also strive for insight of a more comprehensive kind.

Linked to the narrative of the knowledge society is also the story about globalization. In analogy to the narrowness of the concept of knowledge in the knowledge society, the truth about globalization is probably ambiguous. Even so, it is a fact that many problems of, for example, a social, economic, political, or environmental nature, must be seen in a global context to be understood properly. Globalization may not be total, but in many areas it is a reality, and what can be more relevant in the age of globalization than world-wisdom? The relevance is already given in the expression itself, *world*-wisdom, and it is supported by the semantic meaning of the word: to have comprehensive insight into issues that concern the particular, but are simultaneously of general interest. Furthermore, many people will probably think that we grow in knowledge day by day, since the level of education is increasing all the time, and our educational courses are becoming more and more academic. Today we 'study' to become whatever, a hairdresser for example, and the number of university-style colleges has exploded. However, in reality the consequence is *not* more wisdom, not even 'practical wisdom' (life knowledge), because there is far more theorizing than philosophizing, even at the institutes of philosophy. This does not mean that we need more academic philosophy, for as Kant said of school philosophy, it is just a technical speciality for experts, that is: theorizing. There is rather a need for more of the free, open, and questioning reflection that philosophy was originally defined to be – thinking that is not determined from without but has its purpose in itself, and thinking that reflects on what that means. This philosophical thinking is a prerequisite to avoid narrow-mindedness and to comprehend the complexity of, for example, political and ecological issues of a global scale. Such world-wisdom has never been more necessary than in the knowledge society with its highly specialized expert cultures and growing demand for global interaction.

Intermezzo

The post-modern way of thinking contrasts unity and diversity only to give priority to *diversity*. In contrast, when we think philosophically, we try to recognize *unity* in diversity. From the post-modernist side philosophical thinking is therefore accused of *reducing* diversity; it is blamed for 'essentialism.' However, when philosophy is of the free, open, and questioning kind, as it was originally expected to be, that is, when it is seeking *wisdom*, it does not erase all empirical differences in order to replace them with a single common denominator. Philosophical thinking does not aspire to simplification, but rather to finding something that unites. It aims to find harmony between what is different – not between what is similar. Since philosophy seeks not only knowledge but also wisdom, it allows for both understanding and reason to blossom. In so doing it manages to create a link between unity and diversity, moreover in such a way that diversity is not made subordinate to unity or vice versa. Today however, the words 'reason' and 'understanding' are used as if they mean the same, because most of us have forgotten all about the ability to think 'holistically,' which was the original meaning of the word 'reason.' Our time is controlled by the approach managed by understanding that is known from modern research, which focuses on aspects of cause and effect, and from modern politics, which give priority to the utility value of things. We think not only *with* the understanding but also *without* support from reason, and we therefore think theoretically and altogether unphilosophically. We are inclined to contrast things, we often end up with either-or instead of both-and, and this bad habit is legitimized by the post-modern ideology that it is inadvisable to seek anything that unites because then diversity is violated. It is therefore necessary to put *thinking* on the agenda, more precisely the thinking based on reason, and this will in fact mean *aesthetic thinking*. For what is it about thinking that potentially lets it find a form so that it strives for both knowledge and wisdom? What creates the display of reason that makes it possible to reflect on something from various perspectives? Already Kant asked these questions, though with other words, and his answer was: the aesthetic judgment's expanded way of thinking. When we judge aesthetically we not only decide whether something is nice or not, and our aesthetic judgment is not solely concerned with art. The expanded way of thinking appertained to aesthetic judgment is the very precondition for all the cognitive abilities of the human being to combine – from sense perception to reason – so that the highest of them, reason, can come into play. This so-called aesthetic way of thinking is required for reason to carry out its characteristic transcending of the empirical, without losing its ground connection: to form and to orientate itself toward ideas about what we can neither register with our senses nor grasp with the understanding, yet ideas that concern us as human beings.

Aesthetic thinking

The word 'aesthetics' has long been on the lips of many people, including many post-modernists, but a change of paradigm is necessary to understand it correctly. Today the word 'aesthetics' evokes associations toward art theory or theories about the aesthetization of everything from politics to consumerism, but when it was introduced in the mid-18th century by Alexander Gottlieb Baumgarten, it was used to define a new discipline in philosophy (Baumgarten, 1954: §116; Baumgarten, 2007: §1). This discipline had the aesthetic experience as its crucial issue, and it did not see such experience as anything particularly sensuous, but as a kind of cognition. The latter is important for our understanding of how we can operate with a concept such as aesthetic thinking. It is precisely as a way to *cognition* that the aesthetic experience has an importance for philosophy, understood as thinking of the free, open, and questioning kind. Furthermore, in the 18th century people were aware that there are various kinds of aesthetic experiences, for example, both the satisfaction in what tastes good and the sublime pleasure in the incomprehensible. However, they were also aware that it is the experience of beauty that is the epitome of aesthetic experience and that it is not just a question of whether something is nice or not. The experience of beauty is far more comprehensive, and this, as well, is of vital importance to an understanding of how aesthetics and thinking are linked, for it says something about what kind of cognition it really is that we achieve through aesthetic experience. Rather than being about whether something is nice or not, the experience of beauty is the experience that something has a value in itself, and of being part of something larger (Jørgensen, 2006; Jørgensen, 2015). It facilitates a feeling of belonging to this world, and it is thus an existentially important experience of cohesion and meaningfulness. The experience of beauty throws an unusual light over what is a given; it is hard to understand, and it is thought-provoking. Nevertheless, it is communicable, and even though it is always individually manifested, it is not private, but on the contrary is available for all.

According to Kant, the source of the experience of beauty is our aesthetic judgment, whereas it is understanding that produces conceptual cognition, while reason expresses itself in moral action. The difference between conceptual cognition, moral action, and the experience of beauty stems from the fact that they are products of three different ways of thinking (Kant, 2000: §40). Understanding's way of thinking, which results in conceptual cognition, is distinguished by lack of prejudice. This is what is expressed in Kant's dictum that enlightenment comes from following one's own understanding. In contrast, reason's way of thinking, known from the moral imperative about never wanting to do anything that one does not wish to see elevated into a universal law, is characterized by consequence. Whereas judgment's way of thinking is qualified by being expanded, because it follows the principle of placing oneself at the standpoint of everyone else and thus considering many views without subjecting oneself to any one of them. In other words, the expanded way of thinking is characterized by sympathetic insight, and precisely for this reason judgment is not merely about deciding whether something is nice or not. As mentioned, Kant believed that the expanded way of thinking is of fundamental importance for the activity of reason – both for its practical execution of moral actions and for its theoretical creation of, and orientation toward, ideas such as that of 'the common good' which is a prerequisite for moral action. With the expanded way of thinking, particular individual interests are left behind in order to benefit the common good, and it is therefore the crucial precondition for making the moral imperative of reason real. If we were devoid of aesthetic judgment, we would not be able to act morally, and thus ethics rests on aesthetics. However, this thought presupposes of course that the word 'aesthetics' is understood correctly and not as today where aesthetics is simply reduced to art theory or to theories concerning the aesthetization of everything from politics to consumerism.

While Kant is explicit about the ethical implications of the expanded way of thinking, he is more unclear concerning the cognitive ones. He did indeed have an eye for the experience of beauty as that which leads to comprehensive insight. However, he would not call this cognition, because cognition for him was per definition conceptual, and the experience of beauty is by nature without concept.[2] Nonetheless, it is the absence of concept that provides for this type of experience to transmit important insight, and it is thus precisely what brings together aesthetic experience and thinking, and thus also wisdom. When experiences are aesthetic, that is, concerned with beauty, a free and harmonious interplay is felt in one's mind between understanding and imagination. The freedom and harmony stem from the fact that in the aesthetic experience there is no pre-existing concept about *what* is experienced, but there is a *search* for a concept, and thus there is reflection, albeit of a searching kind. In the aesthetic experience the link to the concrete and to the sensuous is intact, because thanks to the absence of concept the particular (the object) is not subordinated to anything general (a concept). Yet a kind of reflexivity is practised whereby 'thinking' is carried out as well, because a search process is happening – namely for a concept, which nevertheless is not found. Thus the thinking that is taking place when there is an aesthetic experience is itself aesthetic, in the sense of being expanded, namely due to the expanded way of thinking appertained to judgment. This also means that when we are thinking in the aesthetic way we are doing exactly what many philosophers used to expect from reason: we are reflecting in a free, open, and questioning way and are striving not just for knowledge but for wisdom as well. Such genuinely philosophical thought is hard to expect from reason at a time where reason has been reduced to understanding, but if we nevertheless want both knowledge and wisdom, we can encourage one another to more aesthetic thinking.

The creative person

Aesthetics is first and foremost about the experience that there is something that has a value in itself and of being part of something larger: it is about beauty. The post-modern aesthetics of existence has nothing to do with aesthetics, but is an expression of aestheticism. It is not aesthetic, but aestheticistic to look upon oneself and one's life as a work of art, as this project is empty of all ideas of morality and truth that are of a common and binding quality. Yet this individualism does not mean that as a countermeasure we are forced to forget all about the idea so popular today of being 'creative.' We just have to understand it properly, that is, to interpret creativity more broadly and see the individual as part of something larger. In the knowledge society, creativity is regarded as a question of innovation: to have new ideas that can increase both efficiency and profit. However, if we take the word 'creativity' seriously, it is not a question of novelty value or profit; it is about *creating*. Furthermore, this creation is not only about what was once the focus, namely the concrete shaping of a material, which is what an artist does, for instance. Nor is it just about generating new ideas, a process that is rated so highly today, not least when the ideas are of a so-called useful nature. On the contrary, human creativity is essentially the ability to transcend that characterizes humans: to be able to imagine something that is not there – that does not exist in a tangible state. This ability not only plays a role for the religious person's belief in a god who cannot be seen, or the novelist's production of literary characters that are also difficult to measure and weigh; it is also the premise for a historian's work if he wishes to contribute to the interpretation of history and not just file historical data. Similarly, natural scientists must be able to transcend the empirical to formulate hypotheses, while politicians without imagination will be criticized for being without vision and thus without the ability to act.

Human beings are by nature creative, but that does not mean that what graces them is controlling nature (recreating it in their own image) or producing useful ideas (being a frictionless pawn in the machinery of the knowledge society). That humans by nature are creative denotes that they are aesthetic, which means that they can undertake expanded thinking. It is precisely thanks to this ability that we can transcend what is given, and imagine what is not there. The expanded way of thinking is as mentioned characterized by sympathetic insight, and the implied empathy is employed not only when putting oneself in the position of the other. Something similar is the case when one imagines a god, a character in a novel, a past event, a possible result of an experiment, another state of society, and all the other things that come into our minds, and without which we would be cultureless – and thus would not be human beings. The knowledge society and the post-modern way of thinking jeopardize what is human about the human being and put at risk what is cultural in culture. For despite all the talk about creativity and innovation, the knowledge society's narrow concept of knowledge and its 'utilitarianism' reveal a thinking controlled by understanding, which throws suspicion on imagination and is the cause of the neo-positivism we find in the present-day Humanities, for instance.[3] Similarly, post-modern anti-metaphysics throws suspicion on the ability to transcend, and this is precisely why post-modernism is stuck in a dualistic pattern of reflection that forces it to contrast unity and diversity in an unphilosophical way. The aesthetics of existence and the competence development must therefore be replaced by the process of formation which the ambition to acquire a beautiful soul could be, provided this is not just interpreted sentimentally as a question of increasing one's sensitivity and enjoying one's aesthetic experiences. It should rather be considered a question of holding the ethical and cognitive implications of beauty in respect: the message of the experience of beauty that there is something of value in itself and the coherence between what would otherwise be kept separate, established by the expanded way of thinking.

The point is to be able in thought to be present in more than one place at a time and to be able to reflect on things at different levels without contrasting the thoughts thus produced. This is necessary to be able to make a link between, for example, the historical and the meta-historical, tradition and the new, or the local and the global. It is thanks to this way of thinking that we can lift ourselves up above our private needs and desires to consider the common good, so necessary in a time marked by individualism. It is also this way of thinking that makes it possible to gather without reducing what is different to what is the same: to think of the universal without losing a sense of what is unique about the particular. This is what is needed in a society marked by fragmentation and globalization. Furthermore, aesthetic thinking is necessary in order to recognize the kinship between human and natural science. They both presuppose creativity, are both dependent on imagination, are both at a loss without expanded thinking, and both relate to the world in an aesthetic way – that is, sympathize with their object instead of holding it at arm's length – when they have substantial cognitive realizations. Similarly, it is also aesthetic thinking that is needed for the formation of character as a world citizen, because this demands that one acknowledges oneself as the holder of not just one, but two 'citizenships,' namely the national as well as a global, without feeling split and at odds with oneself. To 'realize oneself' as a beautiful soul of a non-sentimental and non-aestheticistic, but truly of the *beautiful* kind – that is, one who can think in an expanded way – is therefore not just an issue for aesthetes or specialists. On the contrary, it is something we should all be involved in and concerned about, not only in theory but also as a practical skill. Or it will be if we want a society where we don't just chase knowledge but also show the will to wisdom, and where we thus demonstrate that in spite of everything we still lay claim to reason.[4]

Translated by Dorthe Jørgensen and Hanna and Edward Broadbridge

Notes

1 In his call for enlightenment (Kant, 1996), Kant does not distinguish literally between 'reason' (*Vernunft*) and 'understanding' (*Verstand*), but he makes use of this distinction in other important works, including his aesthetics (Kant, 2000).
2 The word 'concept' here and in what follows refers only to understanding's kind of concepts. The experience of beauty is not without an idea, by Kant also called a concept of reason.
3 See Jørgensen (2017) for the history and meaning of the notion 'imagination,' including the importance of imagination for aesthetic thinking.
4 This chapter was first published in Danish: Jørgensen, Dorthe (2008). 'Hvordan vi tænker: Om vejen til visdom' [How We Think: The Path to Wisdom], in J.T. Bertelsen et al. (eds.), *Viljen til visdom* [*The Will to Wisdom*]. Aarhus: Slagmark, pp. 100–109.

References

Baumgarten, Alexander Gottlieb (1954). *Reflections on Poetry: Meditationes philosophicae de nonnullis ad poema pertinentibus*. Trans. and eds. K. Aschenbrenner and W.B. Holther. Berkeley: University of California Press.
Baumgarten, Alexander Gottlieb (2007). *Ästhetik 1–2*. Trans. D. Mirbach. Hamburg: Felix Meiner Verlag.
Foucault, Michel (1991). 'On the Genealogy of Ethics: An Overview of Work in Progress,' in P. Rabinow (ed.), *The Foucault Reader*. London: Penguin Books, pp. 340–372.
Jørgensen, Dorthe (2015). 'Sensoriness and Transcendence: On the Aesthetic Possibility of Experiencing Divinity,' in S.A. Christoffersen et.al. (eds.), *Transcendence and Sensoriness: Perceptions, Revelation, and the Arts*. Leiden: Brill Academic Publishers, pp. 63–85.
Jørgensen, Dorthe (2006). *Skønhed – En engel gik forbi* [*Beauty – An Angel Passed By*]. Aarhus: Aarhus University Press.
Jørgensen, Dorthe (2017). 'The Philosophy of Imagination,' in T. Zittoun and V.P. Glăveanu (eds.), *Handbook of Imagination and Culture*. New York: Oxford University Press, pp. 19–45.
Kant, Immanuel (1996). 'An Answer to the Question: What Is Enlightenment?' in I. Kant, *Practical Philosophy*. Ed. and trans. M.J. Gregor. Cambridge: Cambridge University Press, pp. 11–22.
Kant, Immanuel (1998). *Critique of Pure Reason*. Trans. P. Guyer and A.W. Wood. Cambridge: Cambridge University Press.
Kant, Immanuel (2000). *Critique of the Power of Judgment*. Trans. P. Guyer and E. Matthews. Cambridge: Cambridge University Press.

25

COLLABORATIVE DRAWINGS

Blue-prints of conversation dynamics

The role of images and image-making processes in improving communication and well being – a series of workshops at the National Portrait Gallery

Deborah Padfield

Well-being

Despite periodic calls for its revision, and many networks and conferences, the World Health Organization's definition of health and well-being has remained the standard since 1946, 'Health is a state of complete physical, mental and social well-being and not merely an absence of disease or infirmity' (Clift and Camic 2016).

Many experts, including within this volume, have put forward alternative notions of well-being (Stickley et al. 2017; White and Blackmore 2015; Atkinson and Scott 2015; Chatterjee and Noble 2013; Galvin and Todres 2013; Carr 2004). This chapter does not attempt to repeat what has already been said but aims to build on the notion of well-being not confined to the absence of disease or illness.

With an ageing population and a rise in chronic health-related conditions, well-being can and must exist within a range of conditions. There are dangers in making an equivalence between health and well-being as Sarah Atkinson (2013) and others have highlighted. Framing discussions of well-being solely within that of healthcare focuses on individual experience at the expense of the relational. Creativity however, is one means of exploring improving well-being as both an individual and relational experience. Images and image-making processes have a role to play within healthcare, in promoting improved trust and rapport between those with long-term health conditions and their healthcare providers – more urgent than ever before and of equal value to both. This chapter will focus on ways in which collaborative drawing and image-making processes can trigger discussion of significant experience and personal narrative often felt to be 'not medical' or 'not relevant' by both clinicians and patients and thus frequently omitted from medical discussions, when their very omission is detrimental to well-being.

In the words of facial pain specialist Joanna Zakrzewska (2011):

Too often have we divided the mind from the body. The two go together and it is about fusing them back together again. The functional imaging [fMRI] . . . is showing more and more how these psychological factors are influencing pain; our perception of pain, our readiness to accept pain, and I think having some physiological basis to be able to explain to patients that these things are important and do have an impact opens up the discussion a lot more. I would consider it medical but a lot of people wouldn't as they have shut the door on the psychological aspect. I think every illness, particularly chronic illness has a psychological component. Often . . . clinicians don't want to go there.

Khetarpal and Singh (2016) identify the power inherent within concepts of health, illness and disability and the contribution language makes to continuing divisive constructs. The same divisive power could be ascribed to the ways in which well-being is described and conceived. They describe language as:

> A powerful instrument that can mould our thoughts even about ourselves, our near ones and the world in which we dwell. Phrases, clichés and anecdotes are used to describe identities. . . . The phrases and anecdotes work towards objectifying disabled persons, and converting them into lessons, learning experiences and something that carries hidden messages, rather than viewing them as human beings with their own desires, needs, aims and goals.
>
> (p. 162)

When we discuss well-being, whose definition are we accepting? Embracing the power of language itself raises questions around how we conceive and frame well-being as much as around how we view disability. It is an apposite moment to review the role images can play in advancing nuanced concepts of health and well-being, learning from those whose well-being is challenged, encouraging toleration of ambiguity, of living and finding well-being within the way we adapt and embrace challenge and difference – ways in which we accept that which we cannot change and build on and flourish through that which we can and that which we are.

There is a physicality, a livingness, an unpredictability to which we have to respond, within the creative process. Artist Jenny Saville describes this as follows:

> When I'm in the process of working an area of the painting, in my head I have an idea of a sequence of marks I'd like to try. Usually it doesn't work out like I planned – sometimes it's better and more suggestive than I'd imagined, but often it feels like a potential disaster and I panic. Adrenaline sets in, as a kind of rush where you're pulling all these paint strings to articulate something and you have to hold your nerve. Just one mark can start to pull together something that has no structure. It's a weird game of control – trying to get to it – to suck it out of yourself and out of the painting. There is a moment when the painting starts to breathe, it gets a kind of presence.
>
> (Saville 2012, p. 318)

Artist and psychoanalyst Patricia Townsend highlights the ways in which Saville is speaking of the developing artwork

> as a living, breathing being as if it has become another person. She is engaged in a 'game of control' in which there is an attempt to coerce it into the shape she has (consciously) imagined whilst at the same time she is responsive to its own suggestions, learning from her medium as well as imposing her will on it.
>
> (Townsend 2015, pp. 121–122)

The process of art making can be seen as similar to the process of building on and responding to the physiology one has been dealt, embracing and changing with its inner and changing dynamics rather than resisting it. Evolving with ill health or pain, breathing through and with it – can be seen as a process of resilience and growth contributing to the evolution of self.

There are many projects where images have been generated by those living with illness or pain in order to process, understand and communicate the most distressing aspects of their condition (Closs et al. 2015; Oliveira and Oliveira 2013 cited in Christenson 2013, also Main 2012; Henriksen, Tjornhoj-Thomsen, and Ploug Hansen 2011; Geller 2011; Collen 2005) to others as well as themselves, and descriptions of the many benefits of phototherapy and photo-elicitation techniques in a range of contexts (Dennett 2011;

Radley, Hodgetts and Cullen 2005; Radley and Taylor 2003; Martin and Spence 1987; Spence 1986) alongside renewed interest in the value of creativity for well-being through social prescribing with cinema on prescription, arts on prescription and museums on prescription gaining current traction. However it is the potential for photographic images and collaborative drawing processes to act as stimuli to mutually beneficial two-way conversation between patients and healthcare providers that this chapter will focus on, drawing on a series of art workshops offered to pain patients and clinicians to attend together at the National Portrait Gallery and University College London Hospital (UCLH)'s artificial hospital in London in 2009 as part of the *face2face*[1] project. The aim of these workshops was to stimulate a type of discussion between those living with facial pain and those who treat facial pain using images and image-making processes to minimize traditional hierarchies and expand dialogue and interaction beyond what is normally possible in the clinic. It could be argued that the well-being and resilience of individuals increased in parallel with the collective well-being of both cohorts.

Face2face

The *face2face* project explored how photographic images co-created with pain patients could expand pain dialogue in the consulting room to include aspects of experience frequently omitted using traditional measures such as rate your pain on a scale of one to ten. The project had many strands: art workshops for clinicians and patients to attend together; the co-creation of photographs with facial pain patients reflecting their experience at different points in their treatment journey; the creation of an image resource developed as an innovative communication tool for clinical use and piloted in the clinics of ten pain experts and an artist's film, *Duet for Pain*, focusing on doctor-patient dialogue and the role of narrative.

Developing on from this the *Pain: Speaking the Threshold*[2] project was launched at University college London (UCL) to bring together a multidisciplinary team to analyse the material produced during *face2face*. The project aimed to evidence ways in which photographs of pain placed between patient and clinician could trigger more negotiated dialogue in the consulting room, democratising the encounter and improving the quality of medical dialogue – arguably improving well-being for both those in pain and those treating it. Accessing Prof. Zakrzewska's clinics, I co-created with patients over 1,000 photographic images that reflected and symbolised their pain. From this material we developed a pilot pack of 54 pain cards trialed as a communication tool in clinical consultations at University College London Hospitals NHS Foundation Trust (UCLH). Video recordings were made of 20 baseline/control consultations, without images, and 20 study consultations with images. Many strands of the project have been covered in other publications (Padfield et al. 2017; Semino et al. 2017; Padfield et al. 2015; Padfield 2013; Padfield 2011) so this chapter will focus on the National Portrait Gallery workshops and ways in which collaborative drawing and photographic processes acted as catalysts for improved understanding and communication between patients and clinicians.

The National Portrait Gallery was a particularly apposite venue as most of those attending the workshops, whether patient or clinician were from the facial pain management teams and so for many of them the face was a charged arena. Facial pain has all the difficulties associated with musculo-skeletal pain as well as additional ones specific to the face. The canvas most of us use to express pain is the face, so when that canvas is itself in pain, it is difficult to express in a way which others can read accurately. This impact of pain on identity and interaction was strongly reflected in the discussions during the workshops and the need for it to be heard and acknowledged by clinicians was a major factor in improving a sense of well-being amongst the patient group.

Art workshops at the National Portrait Gallery
for clinicians and patients

Four two-hour workshops were held, two at the National Portrait Gallery (NPG) and two at the Education Centre, University College London Hospitals NHS Foundation Trust (UCLH) during October and

November 2009 for clinicians and patients to attend together. Fifty people attended the workshops made up of patients, carers/relatives, clinicians and other NHS Staff. Some of the participants had not visited the National Portrait Gallery before. Each workshop was complete in itself but built on the previous one to form a series. Sessions were facilitated by myself with artist Mark Woodhead from the NPG and art-psychoanalyst and film maker Helen Omand. Activities involved looking at, discussing and drawing from work in the NPG collection, creating photographic portraits in pairs using objects along with discussion of contemporary photographic practice, quick mark-making exercises, collaborative drawing and an intro-duction to the portrait and to the work of Henry Tonks by art historian Dr Emma Chambers (previous Leverhulme Fellow, NPG). In the quick drawing and photographic exercises an attempt was made to pair healthcare providers with patients by asking participants to work with someone they didn't know. This was another way of facilitating a two-way flow of ideas and knowledge between healthcare providers and service users. All sessions involved a mix of discussing contemporary portraiture either through examples in Pow-erPoint slides or those in the National Portrait Gallery collection to stimulate discussion, practical creative activities and a review at the end of each session on emerging themes from the process and outcomes of the workshop. The sessions were audio recorded and transcribed, evaluation forms were completed by all par-ticipants (n = 50) and the work produced was photographed and documented. The qualitative data was ana-lysed thematically (for a discussion of the challenges and advantages of qualitative analysis see Mason 2007).

Results

The main themes emerging from the free comments in the evaluation forms and workshop transcripts were: the necessity of negotiation, the importance of the group and the value of exchange and interaction. In answer to the question, 'what did you enjoy?' participants wrote:

'The interchange between the participants'

(respondent 50)

'Sharing ideas and doing artwork together and being in a studio. . . . I don't feel so alone about all of this now'

(respondent 40)

'The exchange with a totally unknown person. It was amazing!'

(respondent 46)

'Working in a group discussing art'

(respondent 9)

Increased mutual understanding and two-way discussion were core aims for the workshops. This was re-enforced by the comments from pain sufferers on how they valued clinicians attending these sessions. For example to the question 'What would you like to see included in future workshops?' respondent 16 answered: 'More time and more clinicians'.

The strong desire for clinicians to participate (on an equal footing) correlates with the sentiments repeated by so many patients attending pain clinics that doctors do not hear or understand them, 'what do I need to do to make them understand?' (Padfield 2003, p. 86). Academic and psychologist Dianna Kenny in her review of doctor-patient interaction in pain clinics identifies the challenge to communication when healthcare providers and patients have different expectations and different agendas (Kenny 2004). Articu-lating these and providing a space where they can be explored and shared contributes to the consultation satisfaction and thus the well-being of both patient and clinician.

In the National Portrait Gallery workshops being outside the hospital setting neutralized the institutional hierarchy, but there was still a strong need expressed by pain patients for doctors to hear their perspective and to appreciate the impact of pain on their lives.

The individual words which appeared most frequently in the workshop transcripts and evaluation forms also reflect the importance of effective communication and the dangers of miscommunication. These were: reflections, mirror, sharing, identity, communicate and express. Examples are:

'Share perceptions'

(respondent 5)

'A reflection of the soul, the essence of the person'

(respondent 9)

'In rare moments a mirror of the soul'

(respondent 30)

'An object? Of expression of self mirror reflection . . . image personality'

(respondent 31)

'Communication, expression, identity'

(respondent 39)

'Crucial in identity, expression of emotions and needs of patients'

(respondent 10)

'To show expression/emotions'

(respondent 12)

Mirroring

Mirroring in the sense of looking and being looked at, of projecting onto/receiving from another became focal in the discussions and when there were disconnects and misunderstanding within these processes, suffering and isolation were described as the result. Miscommunication with others emerged during the *face2face* project as a whole as a key factor increasing intensity of suffering and the sense of isolation for facial pain patients.

Several individuals commented on the experience of being given permission to really look at someone's face for a long time, 'Permission to study another person' (respondent 24).

Perhaps the power of art workshops to address disconnects in communication is due to the fact that when we are drawing or photographing, we look in a different way to how we do in the rest of life, usually, though not always, without judgment. We get absorbed into the forms, the tones, the colours rather than into a series of moral or personal judgments. 'The intimate and *un*mediated sensation that occurs between body, gesture and material is particular to drawing, and is what continues to make drawing a radical and potent method of thinking, feeling and enquiry' (McCausland 2016).

The hope is that this approach to looking and accepting can be paralleled in the consulting room. This could be one of the ways in which the legacy of the *face2face* project could work to increase well-being amongst patients and clinicians more widely. Luce Irigaray identifies respect for and confidence in both each other and the self as essential qualities for shared dialogue.

It is necessary to listen to the saying of the other, and to discover a saying that could be fitting for the two. This saying cannot already be foreseen by a previous discourse: it arises from mutual listening, from the sense that is discovered thanks to the confidence of two subjects in one another, from the search for words that correspond to this reciprocal abandon.

(Irigary 2008, p. 6)

The process of looking together and drawing together cements this.

Revealing, perceiving, exposing, concealing

The importance of the schism between self and other, the complex relationships between revealing, perceiving, exposing and concealing and how these are negotiated within communication was evidenced by the discussions triggered when participants were shown a slide of the logo image from *face2face*, Figure 25.1.

If you've got a broken limb you can show that you've got pain through the face, you don't show it through your broken limb necessarily, whereas here you've got to try and show your emotion and pain through the same medium and perhaps you're trying to layer it or not show it sometimes and that's why you've got different faces which you are trying to peel away to try and get to the bottom of it. Perhaps you don't want to show some people part of it and want to hide it from people.

(workshop participant with pain)

Whether or not what they felt was their 'authentic' self was expressed through the face, (whether or not such a thing exists is a different question) and whether this was accurately or inaccurately understood by other people was uppermost in the minds of facial pain sufferers. The words 'broken limb' is repeated twice in a short phrase, reminding us of the metaphors of injury equating invisible pain with physical injury, correlating with one of the three main categories, X-Ray/Anatomy, Mirror, Weapon, David Biro identifies as core pain metaphor categories (Biro, 2010 and 2014) and the category of injury metaphors identified by Semino et al. (2017). Emotion and pain appear in the same sentence, very close to each other, posited as discreet and separate layers, 'emotion and pain', which it is suggested are in turn peeled to reveal or layered to conceal. There is a distinction made between depth and surface paralleling a distinction between the mask and the inner or 'authentic' self, but you could also turn this on its head within the framework of 'different faces' which 'hide' or 'show'.

In the short extract above the word show appears five times within two sentences, suggesting notions of 'showing' and 'hiding' are pivotal to the statement, and ability and/or inability to express, a locus of significant suffering. It might also suggest the need to evidence experience, sensation and pain. Whichever way these are interpreted, there is a tension between emotion and pain felt, and emotion and pain understood by/communicated to others, which increases suffering and by inference increases pain. The image, (Figure 25.1) which literally layers a negative print onto a positive print, re-photographing them to become one, acted as a trigger for these discussions of sensation. I believe it was a trigger only because it resonated with an already existent and deeply rooted element of pain experience, bringing this to the surface of consciousness via language. This ability to permeate below the surface, to bring back material from memory to be discussed via language is a key characteristic of photography and one on which much has been written, from Benjamin to Berger (Benjamin 1936; Berger 1972, 1980; Berger and Mohr 1982. See also Seremetakis 1994).

Looking

Many of the comments in the discussion on facial pain resonated with those voiced during the previous project *perceptions of pain* on musculo-skeletal pain, for example:

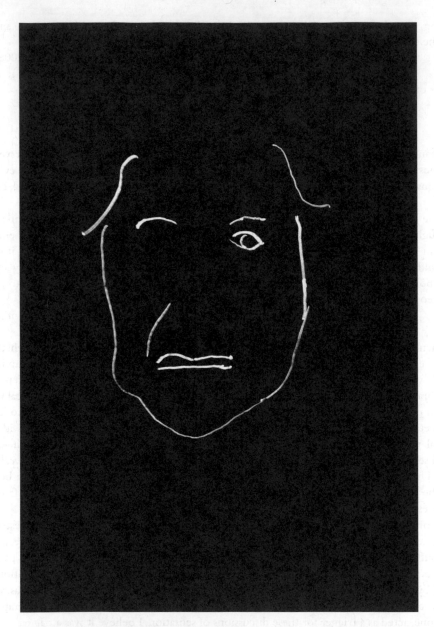

Figure 25.1   Deborah Padfield with Nell Keddie from the series perceptions of pain 2001–2006, Silver Gelatin Print
© Deborah Padfield, reproduced by kind permission of Dewi Lewis

I have a feeling that it's another face looking into the face. Two perspectives of the same person. One is looking inward towards himself, trying to see.

(participant with pain in response to Figure 25.1)

This idea of looking/being looked at, of performing/witnessing, of splitting has resonance not only for pain dialogue, but for portraiture.

The original sufferer with whom I made the image in Figure 25.1 described how she:

> didn't realise until [she] saw the photograph but it is about having the inner and the outer experience at the same time. It is because you have inserted the collage between my face and my hand. It is about touch. It is about having two sensations at the same time, normal and abnormal, It is almost as if my face were in positive and negative. It is about presence and absence.
>
> (Keddie 2001, shortened version in Padfield 2003, p. 113)

The processes of revealing/hiding and showing/masking through discourse catalysed by other images were evidenced as important issues with which pain sufferers struggled; for example one participant said of a self portrait made by another participant during the third workshop:

> Perhaps it shows a way, of coming to terms with this pain, and finding ways to cope with it, because, not showing the eyes to me is like hiding, and hiding is a place of refuge, finding a place of refuge, finding this refuge place in childhood, in the happy times, and be able to recover perhaps, a little bit of that carefree-ness. . . . As children, when we are hurt, we stop what we are doing, and be with the hurt, and that in itself is part of the remedy.
>
> (W3, Transcript of Workshop 3 NPG)

It appears that although there are issues specific to facial pain many of them also thread their way through all pain experience, and through discourses on photographic portraiture for example: the process of visibility – looking/being looked at; of pain behaviour – performing/witnessing, revealing/masking, the construction of identity of another, the loss of identity to the gaze of another, loss of identity from the self. Portraiture and facial pain both raise questions around the representation and/or communication of a cohesive or 'authentic' self and notions of identity as continually evolving rather than as fixed or stable. Aldersley-Williams writes 'We are not only our skin, colour, sex, our professional reputation, the sum of our possessions. We are simultaneously and quite possibly contradictorily, many other things as well' (2009, p. 15). He asserts that identity is always formed partly in response to social surroundings, not by the individual in isolation, which suggests that improvements in individual well-being might only be achieved through improvements in the well-being of the group. He expands: 'The question "who are you?" invites the riposte "Who wants to know?" long before it leads onto the more reflective question, well yes, who actually am I?' (p. 15). This strengthens the argument that creative workshops and any interventions aimed at improving the well-being of patients should also involve those who care for them and that the well-being of both cohorts is relational and mutually interdependent.

Identity

The aim of the third workshop was to explore notions of identity specifically and the impact pain has on sense of self. Participants were asked to represent their identity not through the face but through objects, in the hope of capturing identity and individual experience at the intersect between language and object. This would remove the face as the locus of identity and contestation. Clinicians and patients were asked to bring in objects with which to create photographic self-portraits and work in pairs to photograph them during the session. The resulting conversations happening around the process revealed many aspects of facial pain experience, the most significant of which was that pain, like identity, has a longitudinal arc, resonating not only with the present but with what has come before and what will come after. This correlates with part of the IASP definition of pain: 'Each individual learns the application of the word through experiences relating to injury in early life' (Merskey and Bogduk 1994). Pain is given significance by earlier experiences and colours the anticipation of future experience. Referencing her photograph of two dissimilar stones, workshop participant (study code W2) stated:

> This would be in the background, it's shrunk, there is not much of me left. But this one is me, this is all pervading, because I feel like I've lost part of my face, I feel like I've lost part of my soul and that there is a massive great big cleft going down me and it's destroying me. . . . But that's me, that symbolises everything about my identity now, and my identity in the past, which I crave, because I'd love not to feel so fractured and in pain. . . . I used to be a geologist.
>
> *(face2face* participant, Study Code W2)

Her words not only highlight the fracturing effect pain has on identity, but through reference to stones and geology, reference time – the longitudinal nature of identity and pain. They also reference her own identity as a geologist. The way in which she moves between describing the stones and herself is reminiscent of some of the dialogue in *perceptions of pain* (see the extract below; Padfield 2003, p. 100). It suggests that for some people with facial pain the complex layers of identity can be reflected and represented more fully or more freely via objects and discussion of objects than via their face or a traditional self portrait. For example, looking at the images we had made together, one pain sufferer from INPUT (pain management unit, St Thomas Hospital) taking part in the *perceptions of pain* project and who had found it very difficult initially to describe her pain in words, described herself through description of the sunflower in the photographs we had made together:

> It is just in agony by the look of it. I caught it on a bad day. I didn't have a very good day that day. The head is down, it just seems as though it has ended its life, but what it will do this year is it will shoot back up again. The roots are strong. It varies with me. This one will come up again.
>
> (Padfield 2003, p. 100)

Another significant aspect of pain referenced in W2's description quoted above, is the equation of pain with loss. In the *face2face* project this is emerging as a critical feature of pain experience. It is an element re-occurring in almost every strand of the project.

The shadow metaphor alluded to by W2 integrates both loss and identity.

> That will be massive, and that will be shrunk into the background, and this will cast a massive shadow, and that sounds really horrible, but that's how I feel.
>
> *(face2face* participant, Study Code W2)

It is an image which did not occur so often within *perceptions of pain*, suggesting that it has more resonance for those with facial than with musculo-skeletal pain.

It was not only pain sufferers but clinicians who made photographic self-portraits using objects. This allowed the perspective of those witnessing pain to be discussed alongside those living with pain and thus for two-way exchange and learning. Noticing unexpectedly a small image of a face reflected in the silver foil within her 'self portrait', Figure 25.2, one pain specialist observed:

> there is a little face there. It's me looking at faces, and faces looking at me and observing, which fits in with me liking art and liking looking at things . . . and my job as a doctor . . . looking at people. . . . But there's something else hidden underneath, . . . that people discover when they look a bit deeper. That's why I loved finding that face in the middle, because suddenly you find

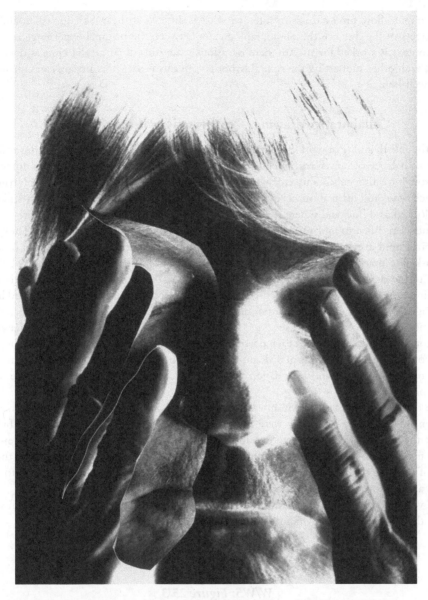

Figure 25.2 Photograph by participant A (clinician) from NPG workshop, digital print, 2009

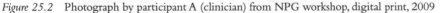

something extra in there that you didn't think was there to begin with. We didn't see it until we looked at the photograph, . . . until we photographed it.

> (*face2face* workshop participant, Study Code A)

Once again the process of looking/being looked at and witnessing/disclosing were central to the discussion and once again stimulated by photography. It could be argued that the distance the photograph provides allows us to recognise and share experiences which are difficult to articulate, just as clinical detachment might allow professionals to listen to what is difficult to hear. Sontag (1978, 2003) reminds us of the dangers of the distance the photograph creates between the original experience and the viewer but in this context it worked for us. Are there occasions when this distance and clinical detachment can complement each other supporting the central hypothesis of this work – that images can enhance dialogue and mutual well-being?

Collaborative drawings – conversations through drawing

The aim of the fourth and final workshop was to untangle some of this further confronting and addressing the inherent in-balance of power within clinical dialogue. Like pain, the communication process is largely invisible. Through treating collaborative drawing as conversations the exercises aimed to construct a process through which we could learn about its dynamics and patterning. Could we observe how and where dialogue gets blocked, and how and where it moves freely between agents in a shared manner?

Participants were asked to find a partner by sitting opposite someone they didn't know. They were given a sheet of transparent acetate, a black pen and were asked to create collaborative portraits (two per pair). They were asked to draw one line of a portrait of their partner and then to exchange sheets before adding another line to the drawing they had been passed, this time as a self portrait (as the image they had been given by their partner would now be of them). Then they swapped back again and drew a third line in what was beginning to be a portrait of their partner, and so on and so forth until they had two portraits they felt finished. Participants were not given a specified time or number of lines to complete the drawings in, but asked to negotiate when they thought each portrait was finished. Treated as conversations through drawing, the process could be seen as a process of dialogue broken down into visible sections. Issues of manipulation, compliance, resistance, control and negotiation were revealed and exposed, all of which have relevance to doctor-patient exchanges.

The type of negotiation enacted within each pair differed wildly, varying levels of awareness, relationships and dynamics evolving. Not only were these parallel relationships found in the clinic but the characteristics of the resultant images – demonstrating a direct fit between outcome and process. Are there implications in this for medical dialogue and the well-being of interaction in the clinic? Does the quality of the process of dialogue parallel the success of the outcome of that dialogue? If so it is crucial to understand its dynamics and explore ways in which it can become more mutually satisfying.

After the workshops the acetate drawings were used to make photograms in the darkroom which were exhibited in the exhibition at the Menier Gallery in 2011[3].

Some examples

W/W5: Figure 25.3

The drawing process for partnership W and W5 was slow, each retaining control of their own part of the drawing without entering into much dialogue with that of their partner; the final drawing having the appearance of being unfinished. There was a sense they had not found any resolution to their exchange by the time the exercise was finished. It was notable that W (pain clinician) partnering W5 (pain patient) said he 'went for symmetry and imposed it within the development of the thing'. Both W and W5 drew few and simple lines, neither engaging with nor looking at the other. W said he realised he was looking at the page rather than at W5 and noticed he was doing so. Most significant of all, he confessed with the drawing he drew what he expected rather than what he saw. W5 said very little. This is a fascinating expose of some doctor-patient dynamics, (to which pain consultations are particularly susceptible) where both participants come bringing their own agendas and language, in the form of standardised questions and crystallised stories, which are then imposed onto the consultation. If dialogue has a tendency to go along anticipated

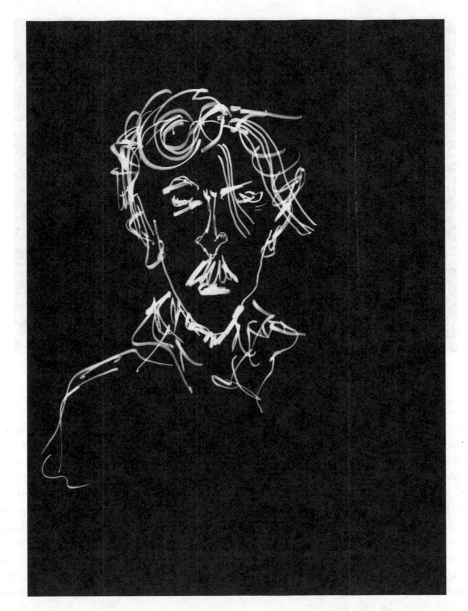

Figure 25.3   Photogram from collaborative drawings on acetate by NPG workshop participants W and W5

patterns, it is arguable that images inserted into it can shift it into the present, encouraging the unexpected and encouraging speakers to engage with what is actually being said in the present, rather than what they expect to be said.

X/Y: Figure 25.4

Partnership X/Y revealed levels of manipulation possible in dialogue, highlighting another common characteristic of medical dialogue. X (medical student) was partnered with Y (relative of person

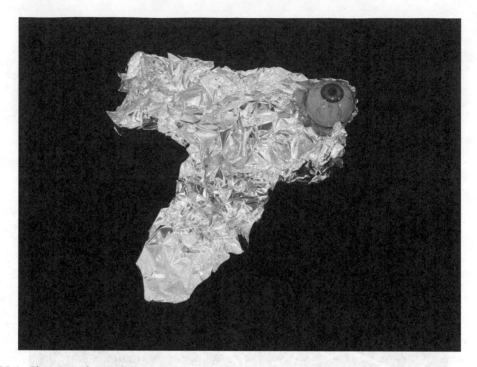

Figure 25.4 Photogram from collaborative drawings on acetate by NPG workshop participants X and Y

with pain). Y ended up feeling unsatisfied with the portraits produced describing how he felt he was being compelled to fill in between the lines he was given, and that it made him feel he was being controlled – which he didn't like, but acquiesced in. X, a medical student, acknowledged she had consciously laid down lines which she had been hoping Y would follow, and admitted being glad when he did. X seemed surprised that Y had noticed he was being manipulated as she hadn't thought he would! Is it important that patients do not feel they are being manipulated, and that when they feel they are, they can voice this recognition? Equally how many times do clinicians feel manipulated by patients, and is there space for them to articulate this without fear of destroying doctor-patient trust? It is a common occurrence in pain consultations for both doctor and patient to enter the arena with different agendas. It is the task of effective and shared communication to shift these, reconciling conflicting aims. Manipulation is an obstacle to mutually acceptable solutions emerging, but recognition of its limiting effect can help avoid it.

W4/W3: *Figure 25.5*

W4 and W3 were both people living with pain. The sudden destructive turn in their exchange was a stark reminder of the potency of images and image-making processes, and the importance of keeping these safe for all participants. It was also a reminder that this cannot always be within anyone's control; the same may be true of the consulting room. Images, though able to catalyse emotional disclosure are, by the same token, able to trigger unexpected and spontaneous emotional reactions. They work at a deep level sometimes revealing what needs to be brought to the surface and into the consulting room to be discussed as part of the pain experience. They also need to be accompanied by recognition of the depth of emotion they can evoke.

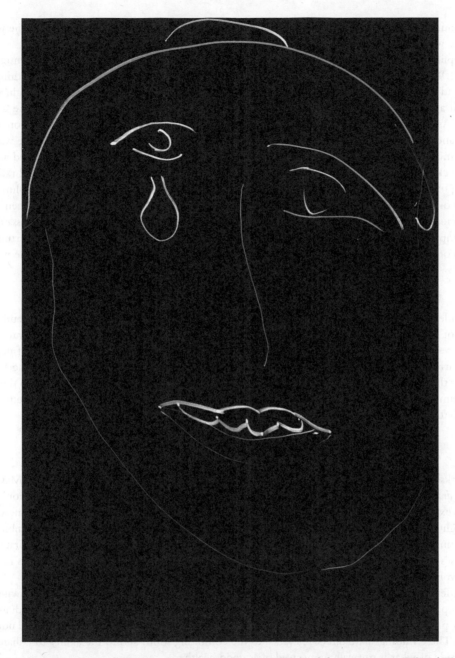

Figure 25.5 Photogram from collaborative drawings on acetate by NPG workshop participants W3 and W4

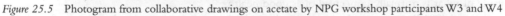

The exchange between W4 and W3 became heated when W4 said she was getting impatient as she felt she was 'more lenient' on W3 then W3 was on her.

Look at those frown lines! They must've taken three goes to do.

(W4)

W4 continued her assault on W3 by saying she thought that W3 had deliberately brought out the weakness in her face whereas she herself had tried to depict and stay with the lightness of W3.

W3 replied very quietly that she was only trying to convey the determination and concentration she saw in W4. W3 then tentatively observed that 'to create we destroy . . . in order to create something new'.

This had a placatory effect on W4 – it was very gently asserted – and W4 went on to admit to the group that at first she 'felt very sad and unbearable' while drawing and then described how she 'started to have fun'. As W4 smiled, W3 said she was seeing W4's teeth for the first time. A smile arose spontaneously from W4 and W3 said how courageous she felt W4 was. The tension eased between them, there was laughter – the moment of conflict had been smoothed over. It could quite easily not have resolved anywhere near as quickly. W3 had responded spontaneously to what was being thrown at her by W4 and rather than remaining fixed in a position of conflict had used adaptability and sensitivity to facilitate a resolution. W3's comment on destroying 'to create something new' was also a reminder of the proximity between destruction and creation, which resonates with discourses around pain. With pain, the self has been assaulted and identity impaired or destroyed; conversely images and image-making processes can offer opportunities for new ways of relating to the world and the self to be created, new ways of being well within the world.

G/V: Figure 25.6

This pair identified 'negotiation' as central to their process. They evidenced awareness of the inbuilt frustrations of not being able to control the whole image simultaneous with a fluid and straightforward negotiation. The resultant image reflects this simplicity and clarity. G/V demonstrated the benefit of negotiated dialogue, arriving at images both were happy with through a process both were equally engaged in. Is it significant that neither of these participants were pain sufferers? Is there something intrinsic to the experience of pain that can skew democratised dialogue as much as the difficulties of inherently unequal power relations within a medical setting?

Concluding thoughts

In her workshop on sensational drawing at the Encountering Pain Conference (2016), artist Onya McCausland described *drawing as* 'engaging collaboration and dialogue to exploit verbal language and interaction' and 'as a vehicle to explore how gaps between words, meanings and marks on paper can open cracks into new experiential insights'. She focused on the interaction 'between subtle tangible sensations through a combination of shared communications and imagination' rather than seeing drawing as purely optical. The collaborative drawing exercises at the NPG, part of the *face2face* project, engaged participants from different cohorts in a shared process involving sensation and the physical body as much as perception or language.

The different processes of negotiation visible within these pairs of collaborative portraits/drawings could be seen as paralleling those that happen within communication in the consulting room. The drawn 'conversations' provide a visual mapping illuminating the dynamics of both spoken conversation and non-verbal exchange. These findings have direct relevance to the consulting room and to the ability to enhance wellbeing outside of what is normally conceived of as good health.

Giovanni Rosti (2017) states that 'Improving patient-physician communication is an area of medicine that deserves greater attention'. He describes how

> current medical practice is dominated by evidence-based medicine, [which] dictates what therapies the clinician will offer in a given circumstance, ideally supported by (evidence-based) guidelines. However, when taken alone it tends to decentralize the patient. There are many different approaches that can be used to understand the patient and what he or she is experiencing as a result of their illness.

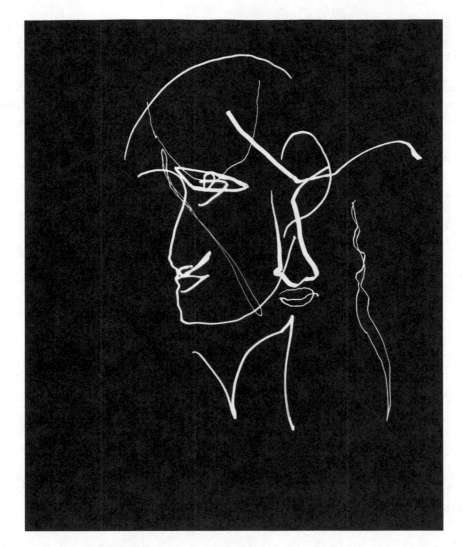

Figure 25.6   Photogram from collaborative drawings on acetate by NPG workshop participants G and V

One way in which I believe images and the image-making process can aid clinicians' understanding of what their patients are experiencing and be transformative to patient clinician interaction and well-being is in effect a shared space in which to reflect together, a space which encourages negotiated dialogue to come into being. Images can expand a space to accommodate the unknown, or the not yet consciously known – which might be fundamental to an individual's pain and fundamental to their well-being – but neither voiced nor heard yet in a clinical space. Voicing difficult sensation and embarking on a shared communication process where deeply personal insights are heard, engaged with and valued are key to participation in recovery and well-being.

In an interview for a new film *Pain under the Microscope* (Padfield and Omand 2016) screened at the Encountering Pain Conference 2016,[4] psychologist Dr Amanda Williams said

It is hard to think about what people need to communicate without saying that to do so there must be someone who listens, and not just one person who listens but a listening world . . . and I don't think that listening understanding world is there.

This throws the emphasis back on all of us to help create a listening environment, erode disbelief and improve understanding. There are many components of health and well-being but feeling understood and acknowledged by others is one. Creative exchange is one step towards building that listening understanding world and increasing well-being whether or not it is accompanied by 'health'.

Figure 25.7 Deborah Padfield with Linda Williams from the series face2face, 2008–2013, Digital Archival Print

© Deborah Padfield

Notes

1 For further information on *face2face* please see: www.ucl.ac.uk/encountering-pain/past-projects and www.ucl.ac.uk/slade/research/mphil-phd/deborah-padfield
2 For further information on *Pain: Speaking the Threshold* please see: www.ucl.ac.uk/encountering-pain/past-projects and www.ucl.ac.uk/slade/research/projects/pain-speaking-the-threshold
3 For further information on the *Mask: Mirror: Membrane* Exhibition at the UCH Street Gallery and the Menier Gallery, London, please see Padfield (2012).
4 For further information on the *Encountering Pain* conference held at UCL in 2016, please see www.ucl.ac.uk/encountering-pain

References

Aldersey-Williams. in: Aldersey-Williams H., Arnold K., Gordon M., Kotsopoulos N., Peto J. and Wilkinson C. (eds) Identity & Identification. 2009. London, Black Dog Publishing.
Atkinson S.J. Beyond components of wellbeing: the effects of relational and situated assemblage. *Topoi*. 2013;32:137–144.
Atkinson S.J. & Scott K.E. Stable and destabilised states of subjective wellbeing: dance and movement as catalysts of transition. *Social and Cultural Geography*. 2015;16:75–94.

Benjamin W. 'L'œuvre d'art à l'époque de sa reproduction méchanisée' in: Alcan, F. (ed) *Zeitschrift für Sozialforschung*. 1936. Jahrgang V, Paris, pp. 40–68.

Berger J. *Ways of Seeing*. 1972. London: Penguin.

Berger J. *About Looking*. 1980. London: Writers and Readers Publishing Cooperative Ltd.

Berger J., Mohr J. *Another Way of Telling (on Photography)*. 1982. New York: Pantheon.

Biro D. *The language of pain. Finding words, compassion and relief*. 2010. New York: WW Norton & Co.

Biro D. 'Psychological Pain: Metaphor or Reality?' in: Boddice R. (ed.) *Pain and Emotion in Modern History*. 2014. Basingstoke: Palgrave Macmillan, pp. 53–65.

Carr A. *Positive Psychology*. 2004. Hove: Brunner-Routledge.

Christensen G. Conceptualizing the arts as tools for medicine and public health. *Journal of Applied Arts & Health*, 2013; 4(3):247–264.

Chatterjee H., Noble G. *Museums, Health and Wellbeing*. 2013. London: Ashgate Publishing.

Clift S., Camic P. (eds) *Oxford Textbook of Creative Arts, Health and Wellbeing*. 2016. Oxford: Oxford University Press.

Christensen G. Conceptualizing the arts as tools for medicine and public health. *Journal of Applied Arts & Health* 2013: 4(3):247–264.

Closs S.J., Knapp P., Morely S., Stones C. Can pictorial images communicate the quality of pain successfully? *British Journal of Pain* 2015: 9(3): 173–180.

Collen M. Life of pain, life of pleasure: pain from the patients' perspective – the evolution of the PAIN exhibit. *Journal of Pain & Palliative Care Pharmacotherapy* 2005;19(4):45–52.

Dennett T. Jo Spence's auto-therapeutic survival strategies, in: Bell S. and Radley, A. (eds) 'Representations of illness and disease'. *Health*, 2011;15(3):223–239.

Galvin K., Todres L. *Caring and Well-Being: A Life-World Approach*, 2013. Abingdon & New York: Routledge.

Geller B. The PainT project. *Pain News* 2011; Winter:42–43. www.britishpainsociety.org/bps_nl_winter_2011.pdf

Henriksen N., Tjornhoj-Thomsen T., Ploug Hansen H. Illness, everyday life and narrative montage: the visual aesthetics of cancer in Sara Bro's Diary, in: Bell S. and Radley A. (eds) 'Representations of illness and disease' *Health*, 2011;15(3):277–297.

Irigaray, L. *Sharing the World*, 2008; London: Continuum.

Keddie N. Interview 2001 as part of the *perceptions of pain project*. 2001.

Kenny D.T. Constructions of chronic pain in doctor-patient relationships: bridging the communication chasm. *Patient Education and Counseling*, 2004; 52(3): 297–305.

Khetarpal, A & Singh, S. Reintroducing differences linguistically! *Indian Journal of Medical Ethics*, 2016;1(3):162–166.

Main, S. Picturing Pain: Using creative methods to communicate the experience of chronic pain, *Pain News*, 2012; 1:32–35. www.britishpainsociety.org/bps_nl_vol12_issue1.pdf

Martin, R. & Spence, J. New portraits for old: the use of camera in therapy, in: Betterton, R. (ed). *Looking on: Images of Femininity in the Visual Arts and Media*. 1987. London: Pandora.

Mason, J. *Qualitative Researching*. 2007. Thousand Oaks, CA: Sage Publications.

McCausland, O. *Encountering Pain Conference Programme* abstract. 2016.

Merskey, H. & Bogduk, N. (eds) *Classification of Chronic Pain*, Second Edition, IASP Task Force on Taxonomy. 1994. Seattle: IASP Press. pp. 209–214.

Oliveira, J. & Oliveira M. Depicting depersonalization disorder. *American Journal of Psychiatry*, 2013; 170(3):263–264.

Padfield, D. *Mask: Mirror: Membrane: The Photograph as a Mediating Space in Clinical and Creative Pain Encounters*. University of London Thesis. 2013.

Padfield, D. Mask: Mirror: Membrane, *PAIN NEWS*, 2012; 10(2):104–109.

Padfield, D. *Perceptions of Pain* (Monograph). 2003. Stockport: Dewi Lewis Publishing.

Padfield, D. Representing the 'pain of others', in: Bell, S. and Radley, A. (eds) Another way of knowing; Art, disease and illness: *Health*, May 2011;15(3):241–258.

Padfield, D., Chadwick, T. & Omand, H. The body as image: image as body. *Lancet*, 2017; 389(10076):1290–1291.

Padfield, D., Zakrzewska, J.M. & Williams A.C. de C. Do photographic images of pain improve communication during pain consultations? *Pain Research & Management*, 2015; 20(3):123–128.

Radley, A., Hodgetts, D. & Cullen A. Visualising homelessness: a study of photography and estrangement. *Journal of Community and Applied Social Psychology*, 2005; 15:273–295.

Radley, A. & Taylor, D. Images of recovery: A photoelicitation study on the hospital ward. *Qualitative Health Research*, 2003; 13:77–99.

Rosti, G. Role of narrative-based medicine in proper patient assessment. *Support Cancer Care*, 2017; DOI 10.1007/s00520-017-3637-4

Saville, J. Interview with Simon Schama, 2005, in: Stiles, K. & Selz, P. (eds), *Theories and Documents of Contemporary Art*, pp. 316–318. 2012. Berkeley, Los Angeles, London: University of California Press.

Semino, E., Zakrzewska J.M. &Williams A.C. de C. Images and the dynamics of pain consultations. *The Lancet*, 2017; 389:1186–1187.

Seremetakis, C.N. *The Senses Still, Perception and Memory as Material Culture in Modernity*. 1994. Chicago: University of Chicago Press.

Sontag, S. *On Photography*. 1978. London: Penguin.

Sontag, S. *Regarding the Pain of Others*. 2003. London: Hamish Hamilton Ltd.

Spence, J. *Putting Myself in the Picture*. 1986. London: Camden Press.

Stickley, T., Parr, H., Atkinson, S., Daykin, N., Clift, S., de Nora, T., Hacking, S., Camic, P.M., Joss, T., White, M. & Hogan, S.J. Arts, health & wellbeing: reflections on a national seminar series and building a UK research network. *Arts & Health*, 2017; 9:14–25.

Townsend, P. Creativity and destructiveness in art and psychoanalysis. *British Journal of Psychotherapy*, 2015;31(1):120–131.

White, S.C. & Blackmore, C. *Cultures of Wellbeing: Method, Place, Policy*. 2015. London: Palgrave Macmillan.

Zakrzewska, J.M. Interview in the film *Duet for Pain*. Padfield. 2011.

Acknowledgements

Some of this work was completed as part of my PhD thesis under the primary supervision of Prof Sharon Morris, Slade Deputy Director, Slade School of Fine Art and the secondary supervision of Prof Joanna Zakrzewska, facial pain consultant, University College London Hospitals NHS Foundation Trust. My PhD was funded by the Arts and Humanities Research Council UK (AHRC).

I am grateful to the Slade School of Fine Art for their support for the process and projects and to the dept of Education at the National Portrait Gallery for hosting us.

I would like to thank all of the participants who attended the workshops and gave of their time outside normal working hours as well as those who co-facilitated the workshops: Mark Woodhead and Helen Omand and Dr Emma Chambers for her fascinating paper on Henry Tonks.

Competing Interests

I have no conflict of interest to disclose.

Funding

Arts & Humanities Research Council (AHRC) and Arts Council England (ACE).

I was supported by the AHRC and by a Centre for Humanities Interdisciplinary Research Fellowship (CHIRP) from University College London (UCL) and Joanna Zakrzewska was supported by the National Institute for Health Research University College London Hospitals (UCLH) Biomedical Research Centre while carrying out this research.

Additional support for the workshops was kindly provided by the National Portrait Gallery, London and additional support for the exhibitions by UCLH Arts, the Derek Hill Foundation Trust, LAHF and Paintings in Hospitals.

26
EMBODIED CONNECTIVITY THROUGH THE VISUAL AND TACTUAL ARTS

Catherine Lamont-Robinson

Drawing on rich languages of sensory engagement in the visual and tactual arts across both medical student and patient communities, the following chapter proposes an alternative version of well-being where participatory manifestations of embodiment shape thinking and reveal joint insights around what it is to be human.

At the University of Bristol School of Medicine we believe that an holistic and philosophical approach to embodiment enhances both medical students' own well-being and their clinical education. Opportunities to develop and integrate ways of observing, processing and knowing through the arts are provided across the curriculum.

Trevor Thompson, G.P. and champion of arts and humanities within Bristol medical school initiated and led the development of the interactive website (Out of Our Heads) launched in 2009. As the curator, I was invited to draw from an archive of medical arts over several years. These creative pieces were subsequently grouped into categories which emerged directly from students' lines of enquiry and reflect diverse aspects of clinical and life learnings. In this regard, Will Duffin represented the medical student community as a critical friend. In addition to showcasing diverse examples of reflective practice, the website is an established peer-learning resource in medical education and continues to host arts pieces from Bristol students, staff and external contributors.

We have published both the evolution of this medical arts interface co-designed and programmed by medical student and website programmer Danny van de Klee (Thompson et al., 2010b) and also the paradox of 'compulsory creativity' as a curricular requirement with colleague Louise Younie (Thompson et al., 2010a).

An example of how the place of aesthetic engagement within the curriculum both externalizes thought and extends students' potential to process and integrate multiple dimensions of living with illness is evident in first-year Rebecca Wood's animation employing time-based media to share her interpretation of the lived experience of a stroke following a memorable home visit. She reflects:

> I have tried to capture Mr Barnes' experience of cognitive disturbance after the stroke within a short animation, using his own words amongst the images. The layers of transparent paper and blurred, unfocused illustrations intimate the haze separating Mr Barnes from the real world, preventing him recognising common things or connecting with his environment. The disjointed, skipping of the music and images references the way that time moved strangely within his mind. This film aims to give the audience a direct sense and understanding of the experience he

shared – allowing us a privileged snapshot into the subjective experience of his stroke as opposed to the outward signs and symptoms.

(Wood, 2013)

Arts contributions from patient-participants in well-being groups are valued resources in small-group sessions at Bristol. In this regard, Louise Younie, a medical educator and GP, leads a Creative Arts for Health elective where second-year medical students are invited to directly engage in the arts practice within workshops which fore-front the role of the arts in clinical contexts (McIntosh and Warren, 2013).

A recent addition to the Out of Our Heads website is the inclusion of creative works from patients in well-being groups and also medical student artworks responding to these pieces:

Following a small-group seminar with the focus of 'Patients as Teachers', second-year student Caitlin wrote:

> I found the theme of what is unseen by doctors fascinating in this week's session. The patient artwork with the tree flowering below ground, the rich tapestry covered by the curtain of depression, the speck of blue amongst the tumult of colours. . . . You feel as if you are being taught to see more in lectures, to make new connections and think of the many possibilities to reach the diagnosis but perhaps this is not the case, perhaps I see less now. Again one of the patient artworks brought this home to me – when they drew what they wanted from a doctor, they drew a hand. When I see a patient and I look at their hands I'm looking for clubbing, I'm checking for capillary refill time, nicotine stains and any other clinical clues. . . . Maybe we as doctors should see more like this, I'm so taken up with lists of questions to ask and signs to look for, that when I see a patient I doubt I see with the kind of penetrating eyes that the patients drew for doctors, that could see what was left unsaid, the flowers in the tree roots so to speak.
>
> (McDonnell, 2011)

Caitlin's aesthetic sensitivity to unfamiliar, idiosyncratic visual languages is by no means rare across the medical student community. Students continue to be surprised by a direct connection with art by their peers and patients. In workshops creative pieces and hands-on engagement from both communities become both primary resources and method in explorations around well-being.

Collected works in the website category (visceral encounters with the blood and guts and beauty of embodiment) not only focus on patients' embodiment but also that of students (Bone Deep).

Internalizing the 2016 curriculum focus on Resilience in her first year (Whole Person Care), Emma writes:

> Having been diagnosed with Type 1 Diabetes aged twelve, it could be argued that I had to act resiliently with regards to my own health earlier than most. When I was younger I used to look to drawing and other artistic mediums as an outlet, but as I got older I felt I didn't have the time for it anymore . . . therefore I decided to use this as an opportunity to engage in some art myself to remind myself of how I could use this as a coping mechanism. I feel like I have a better understanding of my body than most, given that I have to control my blood. This led me to create this piece of work which I've called Sweat, Blood and Tears. It is inspired by the concept of a connected system but of things we don't necessarily think of at first as being linked. On looking at the piece it may look disjointed, why would the heart be connected to the eye? I've tried to link everything together with vessels of the heart connected to the eye, sweat creeping up from the bottom left and curling round the heart and then with strings and chains heading out of the picture symbolising links to everything else that is important in this system. Sweat, blood and tears might not mix and originate from completely different parts of the body but they can all be linked by

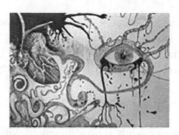

Figure 26.1   Sweat, Blood and Tears

the fact that their presence increases when you are in a stressful emotional state: sweat is secreted, blood flow is increased and (if you are anything like me) tears flow. I will now definitely have a greater consideration for mind-body medicine as a doctor but I will also look to integrate the principles I have discussed here into my daily life in order to really try to master resilient thinking.

(Ferreira, 2016)

Identifying with one's own and acknowledging others' diverse embodiment through creative engagement is also integral to a number of student placements in community contexts. Electives such as 'At Sea with Disability' provide opportunities for Bristol students to undertake a week-long tall-ship experience sailing with the Jubilee Sailing Trust. A wedge of light on a moon-lit sea inspired a third-year to muse on her shifting perspectives:

This particular photograph summed up for me the whole learning experience on the voyage. This was taken during my 12 am watch, when the moon cast its reflection into the still waters beneath it. I was struck how similar to an ultrasound of new life it was, and thought it a great metaphor for the knowledge gained at sea and the formation of new opinions regarding disability.

(Thompson et al., 2016)

Sensory knowledges as dynamic resources: an artist-educator's perspective

Guy Claxton suggests that we underestimate our body's intelligence and habitually dampen our 'interoceptive awareness' (Claxton, 2015).

My particular fascination as an artist-facilitator lies in multi-sensory and holistic engagement through arts materials. The invitation to take a sensory walk and produce an informal diary prior to an arts-based workshop is often acknowledged by the students as a valuable experience in terms of enhancing observation skills in general and embedding 'being fully in-the-moment' both in clinical and every-day contexts.

Auto-biographical material drawn from texts which illuminate idiosyncratic, sensory meaning-making following traumatic bodily disruption often triggers in-depth hands-on enquiry in small-group contexts.

One such lived experience highlights the complexity of privileging sensory knowledge. Johanna Uotinen, an autoethnographic researcher, documents a destabilizing shift from analytic to multi-sensory processing following several days as a patient in an Intensive Care Unit:

Unbeknown knowing is unfiltered, raw knowledge that is produced by our body and senses. At the same time, it is inevitably fuzzy, vague, and difficult to reach or analyze. Bodily knowledge is constantly produced, but when we are in our normal condition it remains hidden, avoids analyses and significations, and it is difficult for us to become aware of, even if we wanted to. . . . When

I contemplated the depths of my sense-based unbeknown knowledge, I was surprised at how strong my need for conscious knowing and understanding was.

...This proves how strong the position of our intellectual and conscious knowing is compared to our bodily knowledge, and how difficult it is to believe in the latter until we find evidence for it in the former.

(Uotinen, 2011, p. 1313)

A collaborative clinical and academic case-study is now presented with a particular focus on how we may build upon new readings of the complexity of embodiment. The integrative potential of the arts in terms of cognitive and sensory processing and also enhancing patients' well-being is scrutinized in this regard.

The HeART of Stroke creative interventions

Caroline Ellis Hill and colleagues Life-Threads Model (Ellis Hill et al., 2008) investigating the impact of stroke on identity was the foundation stone of an NHS-funded RCT trial named the HeART of Stroke (Ellis Hill et al., 2015) across two research sites. Following Caroline's vision and in collaboration with her colleague Fergus Gracey, a creative intervention was developed and later offered to randomized post-stroke patients in Bournemouth and Cambridgeshire as an alternative to traditional rehabilitation programmes. The arts sessions were designed to support general well-being, self-esteem, confidence, sense of belonging and purpose following a stroke and full details of this collaborative intervention are gathered on the Bournemouth University HeART of Stroke website (HeART of Stroke study, BU Research, 2015).

Current research into arts for well-being communities suggests that field research has been relatively neglected as a means of investigating the experiential dimensions and impact of arts participation. Artist-researchers such as Sarah Desmarais (Falmouth University, 2014) have become increasingly attentive to the value of observing nuanced bodily presence within groups in terms of scaffolding individual aesthetic practices, and welcome the opportunity to internalize and process somatic qualities which will inform patients' selection of physical, sensory and conceptual materials.

It is this elastic and complex dynamic between the materials, the body-mind and the collaborative context, which sits at the core of the following phenomenological case-study from the perspective of myself as the artist-facilitator for the HeART of Stroke interventions in Bournemouth.

Workshop context

The remit of the HeART of Stroke sessions was open and emergent – implicitly welcoming a range of arts-based responses from participants including improvisational, observational, metaphorical and conceptual. The ten sessions of two hours were planned to offer informal opportunities for holistic, multi-sensory and collaborative engagements.

Session materials

The materials provided included a core of traditional fine art media, fabrics, papers, clay and natural forms supplemented weekly by additional materials, objects, texts and visual references in response to emerging interests and practices. Sketchbooks as informal creative journals were provided from the outset and they became reservoirs of ideas, references and experimental studies.

Session provocations

Starting points were designed to complement the deficit-focused rehabilitation clinical model – acknowledging past experiences positively, whilst providing opportunities to fold in new, visceral and imaginative engagements:

One of the early sessions began with the invitation to engage in tactual explorations of sensory materials. These diverse forms and textures triggered connections, memories and experimentation combining materials.

In a collaborative drawing we used soft graphite sticks and pastels on a large sheet of paper to experience responsive materials and highlight the influence of grip, rhythm and pressure. Later, responding to the diverse qualities of others' mark-making, participants were invited to elaborate on characteristics of each other's drawings.

Another early provocation was a visualization of a walk through landscape where I used neutral words as a guide. This visualization was aimed to reveal rich individual imaginative reservoirs and highlight which senses we and others privilege in daily life. Powerful multi-sensory connections with the land – often infused with family memories emerged – 'standing on a bridge listening to the voices of my children playing happily in the stream below float up to me', swimming through mercurial warm waters, a family visit to the thundering Niagara Falls, a Spanish monastery above the clouds, a mesmerizing cello concert in a local cathedral. The will to retrieve, explore and share aspects of these personally charged locations over-rode anxieties around artistic abilities and further, provided a treasure-trove of shared references.

As confidence builds in studio practices I may introduce images, music or texts which provide participants with complementary or parallel perspectives. Later, tangible references to artists with shared motivations working in diverse creative practices often provide a catalyst for the whole group in terms of use of materials, techniques and enquiries.

One such example is a first-year medical student's textile collage which mirrored many of the participants' positive re-framing of the past:

> I chose pieces of material from past sewing projects to represent how in many ways our resilience is a product of our past experiences. This made me reflect on the challenges I have faced, for instance due to my dyslexia, which has meant from a very young age I have been challenged by reading, spelling and a slow processing speed. I have never let my dyslexia hold me back. In the previous projects, where the pieces of fabric came from, there were challenges too, however the finished product always came out well and helped me learn techniques for the next project. This process also helped me consider that it is important to recognise that patients too have different experiences which they have learned from and which have shaped them.

Other artist references which resonated with the groups included unmannered works by artist Alfred Wallis whose spontaneous style, impulse to work with whatever materials were immediately to hand joyfully liberated an initially tentative participant from the notion that there was a 'right way' in studio practices.

After the first two or three weekly sessions, the workshops began to fall into a spontaneous structure. The groups would initially informally share sketchbooks, objects, forms and images gathered or developed during the week. General observations were exchanged and the session would then shift into participants pursuing individual art practices 'going into the zone' as both groups referred to this focused time.

Embodied responses to the lived experience of a stroke

Whilst collected as a group of emergent artists – irrespective of the clinical factors that had brought the participants to the sessions, the group's shared knowledge of bodily disruption surfaced in the first weeks:

During the first workshop Joan pointed out the green crackled image of a sun-dried plastic notice on a fire-door and shared – 'that's how my brain feels!' this observation led to an animated conversation around challenges in processing information directly following a stroke. I made reference to Guy Claxton's concept of 'Hare Brain, Tortoise Mind' (Claxton, 1998). Joan was very taken with the notion of honouring this slower mode of thinking, often repeated this phrase aloud in workshops and playfully fashioned a tortoise in clay.

In the second week, Ken rhythmically painted a sequence of waves across a length of paper – moving from the depiction of choppy water to a sea calm enough to hold the reflection of the sun. He later described this use of materials and selected imagery as representing the transition from erratic and intense brain-waves initially following his stroke to gradually re-adjusting to his surroundings.

Music and song-writing was a long-standing part of Len's life and he was fascinated by the impact of music on the nervous system. Len brought in an image of a neuron responding to music and shared his interest in how these microscopic structures helped enable the brain to respond and reshape.

Losses and gains: the role of materials

Barbara Bolt suggests that 'materials are not just passive objects to be used instrumentally by the artist, but rather the materials and processes of production have their own intelligence that come into play in interaction with the artist's creative intelligence' (Bolt, 2006).

In well-being groups the artist aims for a sensitive balance between challenge and support for participants to work at the edge of their evolving creative potential (Broderick, 2011). For some participants who attended sessions early in their recovery there was an inevitable deficit positioning regarding dexterity and focus. However, as the weeks continued, physical competencies often returned to some measure and new capacities and interests were forged.

Diana had little grip and sensation in her dominant hand at the beginning of the workshops yet was drawn to the delicate fine art materials. The desire to portray glowing stained glass windows through fluid watercolour and to later glaze ceramic vessels drove Diana's intention to take her spontaneous and responsive practice forward. She gradually developed highly individual techniques to adeptly handle a wide range of materials and express emerging fascinations with increasing subtlety, delicacy and accomplishment.

Michael joined the group agitated and frustrated by his loss of dexterity and sensation in one hand – the tightrope between the desire to regain skills and confronting abilities which had receded was starkly apparent. Michael's professional life had revolved around intricate manual work. In the second session, the introduction of paper-clay, a particularly responsive material, encouraged a fluid, simultaneous, two-handed interaction which Michael relished, creating a stream of three-dimensional forms. Once tactile sensitivity began to return, Michael continued to challenge himself with increasingly demanding materials both at home and in the sessions, for example, painting detailed renderings of wild birds on layered gauzes.

Diana and Michael were drawn to particular materials and driven by particular subject-matters early on in the workshops. Informally training themselves in bodily competencies which served their artistic motivations became second nature. For others such as Ann however, this process took several twists and turns and personal satisfaction was hard-won. Ann joined the group already skilled in two-dimensional graphic imagery and was an impressive calligrapher. Despite the aim to 'extend my horizons', after several weeks experimenting with diverse materials, Ann's attention was captured by a swan's feather and decided to represent this delicate form in white gouache on a dark brown background. The quality of her observations and already-honed dexterous abilities combined to produce an exquisite spontaneous representation of this natural form whereas her original intention had been to create 'experimental and abstract artwork'. The rhythmic expression of re-creating each delicate strand of feather by a line of paint triggered a desire to revisit her late husband's pencil drawings, one of which she had previously shared with the group – 'now *he's* the artist...!' Ann completed the sessions with the firm intention to continue this new-found engagement with the visual arts by closely studying her husband's drawing techniques and in parallel, to develop her own styles of responding to natural forms through close observation.

Sarah felt the loss of being unable to continue fine needlework acutely, yet with encouragement, was open to handling textiles on a larger scale.

She began by composing fabrics on a small mannequin, later around her body, then as composite arrangements combining fabrics, wools and threads alongside other textually rich materials. Sarah developed many ingenious ways to extend her esoteric ideas into tactile forms without stitch. An established appreciator of the visual arts already, it was fascinating to note how her confidence as an artist grew as Sarah shifted her perspective from observer to practitioner and relished the symbiotic dynamic between touch and intention (Wilson, 1999).

Discussion

The above examples of workshop engagements are provided to highlight the unique creative journeys undertaken by participants across the sessions as they developed confidence in their observations, reflections and practices through arts materials in a collaborative setting. In order to consider the potential impact of these sessions on the participants' well-being, then draw out potential transferability, it is perhaps relevant to consider some recurring themes across both groups.

Enhanced relationship with the body-mind

Bearing in mind that many of the group were gradually regaining physical abilities following a stroke, attunement with materials within these workshops perhaps re-positioned the body-mind as a creative companion. There was a palpable degree of re-enchantment with perceptual engagements – one of the group articulated how they had begun to see the world with fresh eyes – 'I'm seeing things now I have never noticed before – I can't stop it!'.

Participants also shared that outside of these sessions they were becoming increasingly confident to follow new interests. One gentleman presented a list of the gardens he and his wife had recently visited and suggested this was down to the positive impact of the group.

Improvisation and philosophical enquiry

Running hand in hand with emerging experiential confidence was the invitation to improvise, embrace complexity and ambiguity. Individual enquiries provided the underlying creative spark in the emerging artworks – to give a few examples:

Len's detailed explorations of natural forms beyond the visibility of the human eye such as the fragile forms of water crystals and snowflakes culminated in a painting he titled 'The Source', an elemental and dynamic dreamscape.

'Summer Vision' by John, took form rapidly during one of the sessions. He began with a large-brushed sweep of blue sky and below rhythmically composed a staccato flurry of dotted meadow blooms in intense hues on a dry-brushed backdrop. Several of the group later made reference to the quality of John's focused attention and shared their delight in observing this spontaneous image emerge. Ingold, (2011, p. 60) writes – 'For there to be rhythm, movement must be felt. And feeling lies in the coupling of movement and perception that, as we have seen, is key to skilled practice.' This artwork was triggered by John's growing fascination with multiple interpretations of 'reality'. Inspired by Paul Arden's text, 'Whatever You Think, Think the Opposite' (Arden, 2006), John informed the group that after reading this 'mind-bending' book, life would never be the same again.

Ken's artworks also fused philosophical and experimental enquiries. Re-visiting the experience of a much-cherished music concert following his stroke, Ken created a reclining cello-figure bathed in coloured light surrounded by ancient symbols and spent many weeks experimenting with visual metaphors as this work evolved.

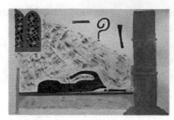

Figure 26.2 Meditation

Identity and impact as artists

Sketchbooks were much used by the participants between sessions and several of the group mentioned with a degree of pride that their friends and families now referred to them as 'artists'. Several participants in the RCT have joined a workshops led by the experienced and inspirational artist-facilitator Pauline Stanley (Artisan – Community Art Studio).

The Bournemouth HeART of Stroke group's artwork across the sessions has recently inspired stroke clinicians at a national conference to engage in hands-on enquiry responding to their unique art forms. This arts dialogue between communities is currently being documented.

Group context

Parker Palmer suggests that only in community can the self exercise and fulfil its nature: 'Lacking opportunities to be ourselves in a web of relationships, our sense of self disappears' (Palmer, 2008).

The group was characterized by an open, democratic and inclusive manner following what Hernstein-Smith refers to as 'the circle of reciprocal effectivity' – which privileges material bodies, experiential histories and ongoing social interactions (Smith, 1997).

The commitment to arts interventions as potential sites of positive identity re-construction and well-being was also championed by the research team from the outset – giving rise to art workshops for stroke clinicians and academics before the research began and open studio events across the trial. Now several months after the research phase is completed, I continue to receive images of artworks from Catherine Ovington the senior research nurse Mary Grant, the principal researcher who was profoundly inspired by the participants' studio processes and insights. As an artist, I was also was influenced by these workshops and later shared with the participants a series of layered images highlighting how their practices and perspectives have become embedded in my outlook as an artist.

Completing the circle

William Viney and colleagues make the case for critical medical humanities models which invite entanglement and consolidate new forms of inter-disciplinary and cross-sector collaborations both within medical education and clinical practice (Viney et al., 2015).

One such example of joint exploration across philosophy, medicine and the arts was a collaboration with philosopher Havi Carel to informally pilot her Phenomenological Toolkit for Patients (Carel, 2012). Along with Havi, Louise Younie, a fourth-year medical student Libby Wilson, myself as an artist-facilitator and six patient-participants shared perspectives through arts engagement and reflection (Carel, 2013). A visual piece which emerged during this collaboration drew inspiration from the fragment of a shattered, antique tea-cup. Alongside this delicate drawing of a finely decorated china form, Gail, a patient participant wrote 'Something that is broken can still be beautiful and useful'. This drawing has subsequently touched a nerve across patient, student and academic-clinical groups. Following a recent inter-disciplinary workshop a clinician reflected on Gail's drawing and reflected 'I wonder if we can be free not to 'repair' or to 'transform' and what that would mean for us ... is there a place for such a being-in-the-world?'

The art practices selected for discussion in this chapter represent fleeting co-ordinates of fragility, strength and insights on the continuum of lived experience. Connecting these unique and complex experiences of well-being in participatory contexts provides a matrix which points to a more unified and democratic model of embodiment.

References

Arden, P., 2006. *Whatever You Think: Think the Opposite*. Portfolio, New York, NY.

Artisan – Community Art Studio. http://thecommunityartstudio.blogspot.co.uk/ (accessed 2.14.17).

Bolt, B., 2006. Materializing Pedagogies. Working Papers in Art and Design. Work. Pap. Art Des. 4.

Bone Deep [WWW Document], *Out of Our Heads*. www.outofourheads.net/oooh/handler.php?p=search&genre=&category=theme%3Dbone_deep (accessed 2.14.17).

Broderick, S., 2011. Arts practices in unreasonable doubt? Reflections on understandings of arts practices in healthcare contexts. *Arts Health*, 3, 95–109. doi:10.1080/17533015.2010.551716

Carel, H., 2012. Phenomenology as a resource for patients. *The Journal of Medicine and Philosophy*, 37, 96–113. doi:10.1093/jmp/jhs008

Carel, H., 2013. *Illness: The Cry of the Flesh*. Routledge, Oxford.

Claxton, G., 1998. *Hare Brain, Tortoise Mind: Why Intelligence Increases When You Think Less*. Fourth Estate, London.

Claxton, G., 2015. *Intelligence in the Flesh: Why Your Mind Needs Your Body Much More Than It Thinks*. Yale University Press, New Haven.

Ellis Hill, C., Gracey, F., Thomas, S., Lamont-Robinson, C., Thomas, P.W., Marques, E.M.R., Grant, M., Nunn, S., Cant, R.P.I., Galvin, K.T., Reynolds, F., Jenkinson, D.F., 2015. "HeART of Stroke (HoS)", a community-based Arts for Health group intervention to support self-confidence and psychological well-being following a stroke: protocol for a randomised controlled feasibility study. *BMJ Open*, 5, e008888. doi:10.1136/bmjopen-2015–008888

Ellis Hill, C., Payne, S., Ward, C., 2008. Using stroke to explore the life thread model: an alternative approach to understanding rehabilitation following an acquired disability. *Disability and Rehabilitation*, 30, 150–159. doi:10.1080/09638280701195462

Falmouth University, 2014. *Beyond the Toolkit: Understanding and Evaluating Crafts Praxis for Health and Wellbeing*: An Arts and Humanities-Funded Symposium Organised by Falmouth University and Arts for Health Cornwall and Isles of Scilly 19th and 20th February. https://www.falmouth.ac.uk/research-case-studies/beyond-the-toolkit

Ferreira, Emma, 2016. Sweat, Blood and Tears. Out of Our Heads. www.outofourheads.net/oooh/handler.php?id=742 (accessed 2.14.17).

HeART of Stroke study | BU Research. https://research.bournemouth.ac.uk/2015/08/heart-of-stroke-study/ (accessed 2.14.17).

Ingold, T., 2011. *Being Alive: Essays on Movement, Knowledge and Description*. Routledge, London; New York.

McDonnell, Caitlin, 2011. Finding the Pain. Out of Our Heads. www.outofourheads.net/oooh/handler.php?id=563 (accessed 2.14.17).

McIntosh, P., Warren, D., 2013. *Creativity in the Classroom: Case Studies in Using the Arts in Teaching and Learning in Higher Education*. Intellect, Bristol.

Out of Our Heads. www.outofourheads.net/oooh/handler.php?p=homepage (accessed 2.11.17).

Palmer, P.J., 2008. *A Hidden Wholeness: The Journey Toward an Undivided Life*, 1st ed. Jossey-Bass, San Francisco, CA.

Smith, B.H., 1997. *Belief and Resistance: Dynamics of Contemporary Intellectual Controversy*. Harvard University Press, Cambridge, MA.

Thompson, T., Lamont-Robinson, C., Williams, V., 2016. At Sea with Disability! Transformative learning in medical undergraduates voyaging with disabled sailors. *Medical Education*, 50, 866–879. doi:10.1111/medu.13087

Thompson, T., Lamont-Robinson, C., Younie, L., 2010a. "Compulsory Creativity": rationales, recipes, and results in the placement of mandatory creative endeavour in a medical undergraduate curriculum. *Medical Education*. Online 15, 5394. doi:10.3402/meo.v15i0.5394

Thompson, T., van de Klee, D., Lamont-Robinson, C., Duffin, W., 2010b. Out of Our Heads! Four perspectives on the curation of an on-line exhibition of medically themed artwork by UK medical undergraduates. *Medical Education*. Online 15, 5395. doi:10.3402/meo.v15i0.5395

Uotinen, J., 2011. Senses, bodily knowledge, and autoethnography: unbeknown knowledge from an ICU experience. Qualitative Health Research, 21, 1307–1315. doi:10.1177/1049732311413908

Viney, W., Callard, F., Woods, A., 2015. Critical medical humanities: embracing entanglement, taking risks. *Medical Humanities*, 41, 2–7. doi:10.1136/medhum-2015–010692

Wilson, F.R., 1999. *The Hand: How Its Use Shapes the Brain, Language and Human Culture.* Vintage Books, New York.

Wood, Rebecca, 2013. My mind is not my own. Out of Our Heads. www.outofourheads.net/oooh/handler.php?id=676 (accessed 2.14.17).

27

POETRY AND/AS WELLNESS

Monica Prendergast and Carl Leggo

How can we live well in the world? How can we learn to live with wellness? Writing poetry is creatively connected to health and healing. In *The Slow Professor: Challenging the Culture of Speed in the Academy* Maggie Berg and Barbara K. Seeber (2016) present a trenchant critique of contemporary academic culture and call for a deliberate commitment to slowing down. They claim that "research does not run like a mechanism; there are rhythms" (p. 57). We attend to poetry as a way of learning how to live with wellness because, as Berg and Seeber understand, "slowing down is about asserting the importance of contemplation, connectedness, fruition, and complexity" (p. 57). In our poetry we linger with the possibilities of language, especially the central energies of poetry that Jane Hirshfield (1997) identifies as "the concentrations of music, rhetoric, image, emotion, story, and voice" (p. 7), in order to linger with the possibilities of wellness.

In this chapter we weave two poems by Carl Leggo with Monica Prendergast's (what we are calling) *abstract found haiku* from a peer-reviewed journal search on the terms "poem, poetry, wellness, health, well-being". The first autobiographical poem by Carl Leggo reflects on the over-busy-ness of contemporary life, in particular the life of a 21st century academic faced with too many tasks and too little time. Leggo's second poem offers an abecedarian that considers how poetry invites meditation and contemplation, a playing of attention and a heartful/healthful way of being. Prendergast has crafted found haiku in previous works (Prendergast, 2016; Prendergast, Gouzouasis, Leggo, Irwin & Grauer, 2009) and has explored this highly constrained Japanese poetic form's potential for effective/affective *crystallization*, to use Laurel Richardson's metaphor for creative analytic practice (Richardson, 2000). Found poems are poems created from pre-existing prose texts, in this case limited to the abstracts of journal articles on the intersecting topics of poetry, health and wellness. All words in the haiku are found in the source abstract, although word endings are occasionally changed for ease of reading and one parenthetical interjection (yes!) has been added by the poet for effect. Haiku titles are words also pulled from abstracts. Not surprisingly, many of the articles selected are from the *Journal of Poetry Therapy* that is dedicated to these interdisciplinary practices of arts and healing. However, there are research studies shared here from other journals and sources. It is our intention to point readers to this scholarly material via the evocative and fragmentary representation of found haiku, a form that both invites and challenges interpretation.

Abstract found haiku: part I

Resilience

in the face of loss,
poetic intervention.
instillation: hope

(Kreuter & Reiter, 2014, p. 13)

Masculinities

disabilities
re-authoring self
helping men as men

(Thompson, Furman, Shafi & Enterline, 2012, p. 105)

Caregivers

depressive symptoms.
after writing poetry?
self-transcendence (yes!)

(Kidd, 2010, n.p.)

Gerontology

"problems" of aging?
older poets write love, change,
death, dying . . . aging well

(Sheets & Liebig, 2011, p. 129)

★★★★★★★★★★★★★★★★★★★★★★★★★★★★★★★★

What I did on my summer vacation

or

What I didn't do on my summer vacation

or

What I wish I had done on my summer vacation

or

What my Facebook friends (apparently) did on their summer vacation

(a poem in search of a title)
or
(a title in search of a poem)

though everything I write is nothing more than an allegory
emblem fragment gasp metaphor parable similitude
I still continue to write, even with hope

this summer, I (the real deal me,
not the lyrical I, the personified voice
of this rambling poem)
attended 40 meetings
assessed 31 portfolios
read 16 master's papers
responded to 15 submissions for a book
edited 12 articles for a journal issue
wrote 10 reference letters
reviewed 7 dissertation drafts
judged 6 AERA proposals and journal submissions
penned blurbs for 2 colleagues' book manuscripts
Skyped, phoned, and texted countless colleagues,
commuted, Cyborg-like, in the summer maze of Vancouver road construction,
and gobbled up e-mail messages like a ravenous Pac-Man
with an indomitable will to thrive amidst the *EEEEE* in e-mail
like the eerie scratch of a teacher's fingernails on an ancient blackboard

I did not dilly dally but diligently daily drove
the daunting dragon of desire and demand

while my Facebook friends (apparently)
        while my Facebook friends (apparently)

did push-ups, ran effortless marathons, hiked tangled trails,
displayed tight, defined, ripped abs, not theirs, usually Bieber's,
waterskied, scuba-dived, skateboarded, biked, hiked, bowled,
painted their fingernails, picnicked, hung out, chilled, relaxed,
danced the salsa, drank beer, consumed photogenic lunches,
practiced karate and Karaoke and kayaking, rescued turkeys
and drowning horses, Trumped Trump with self-satisfied selfies,
expressed enough romance to make Nicholas Sparks blush,
made music, dyed their hair, got tattoos, and grew mustaches,
canoed and canoodled, cruised and chewed cashews,
some played horseshoes, a few even mentioned world news,
posted photos of puppies and pooches, celebrated births, birthdays,
engagements, weddings, even Facebook friendships as old as a year or so,
updated their profile images with daily diligence (I'm still using
the photo from over a decade ago because I will never look
that good again), laughed and laughed with lollygagging lunacy

I don't have a lot of Facebook friends, I don't even have a lot of friends
(a poet's occupational hazard), but my posse of friends visited
every country on the planet that begins with M, except Madagascar

my friends promoted intriguing books I know I will never read
(I can't keep up with Facebook – what chance do I have with books?),
found inner serenity, the sweet tangy taste of strawberry wit beer,
10 essential gelato flavours, and 6 solutions for world peace,
not to mention aphorisms, maxims, and proverbs for loving living
(You might be given a cactus, but you don't have to sit on it.)

my Facebook friends smiled a lot, ate a lot, drank a lot,
laughed a lot, poked people, and pondered Pokemon,
posted images of Jesus in Portuguese buns, made
funny faces with false teeth, and composed the world
with the domestic nostalgia of Laura Ingalls Wilder

the one thing, the one thing none of my Facebook friends
did all summer was work – they were entirely idle,
indolent, languid, lethargic, lost in luxury and licentiousness

at 32 years old, Mark Zuckerberg
is the fifth richest person in the world
(probably stays up nights thinking about Bill and Warren)
every time one of my friends posts another image
of the sumptuous spaghetti and clams in olive oil and garlic
they are savouring on a summer patio in some exotic corner
of England Thailand Australia or Saskatchewan
Mark Zuckerberg marks another chunk of change
he claims he has more to give away

I don't know what to make of Zuckerberg, I am too busy
liking my friends' posts to attend creatively and critically
to Zuckerberg's vision and ambition, drive and desire

like Columbus Cortes Cabot Cook Cartier Coronado
Zuckerberg confesses, "The thing I really care about is
the mission, making the world open"
the mission, making the world open

in August I visited my mother in Newfoundland
if I had posted images of my mother,
I would have smiled, she probably
would have smiled too, though
she doesn't like smiling for a camera,
and if I had posted such a photo
you would never guess how the hours
I spent with my mother this summer
were mostly spent wondering, Who
is this woman I have known for more
than 63 years and still don't know?

the son's sad sense of persistent befuddlement
cannot be expressed on Facebook
where the facetious reigns, where
faces are rendered glamourously
with Hollywood's superficial gloss and alchemy,
an aging son's lingering angst is no story for Facebook

or I could write about Terry, my childhood friend,
who died with a stroke or an aneurism, not sure,
or Paul who died with ALS, all too sure,
or Uncle Bud who wonders if bungee jumping
might have caused his creeping dementia

I could tell you many stories that broke my heart
in the month of August alone, but those stories
will remain unspoken – who can receive them –
an old man's sadness is best hidden
like yellow toenails and wrinkled body parts
not even old men can think about

Mark Zuckerberg is the only one of my friends
who wants me to be open but since Mark Z. is
not really my bud, I will continue to eye Facebook
with suspicion and author only the stories authorized by

Butler's performativity
      Baudrillard's hyperreality
Cixous' dreams
      Deleuze's rhizomes
Haraway's posthumanism
      Derrida's différance
Irigaray's mimesis
      Foucault's panopticon
Kristeva's semiotic
      Levinas' ethics
Sedgwick's neologisms
      Barthes' mythologies

(so glad I can write wonderful gibberish
to confound Facebook friends wallowing in
their images of animal antics and foodie passions?)

in a poetic spell of word-making
where language will not languish
in the anguish of APA authority

I continue to embrace

alphabetic adventures
biophilic biography
coherent composition
dramatic denotation
energetic errors
fecund fictions
gregarious grammar
haunting holiness
incendiary idiolect
joyful journaling
kinetic knowledge
ludic language
meandering murmurations
noumenal narration
organic orations
poetic playfulness
questing questions
ruminative representation
sensual savouring
textual truth
urgent ululation
vibrant verbs
whimsical witnessing
xylophonic xerography
yearning yammering
zestful zeugmas

What did I do on my summer vacation?

this summer, I (the real deal me,
not the lyrical I, the personified voice
of this rambling poem)
attended 40 meetings
assessed 31 portfolios
read 16 master's papers
responded to 15 submissions for a book
edited 12 articles for a journal issue
wrote 10 reference letters
reviewed 7 dissertation drafts
judged 6 AERA proposals and journal submissions
penned blurbs for 2 colleagues' book manuscripts
Skyped, phoned, and texted countless colleagues,
commuted, Cyborg-like, in the summer maze of Vancouver road construction
and gobbled up e-mail messages like a ravenous Pac-Man
with an indomitable will to thrive amidst the *EEEEE* in e-mail
like the eerie scratch of a teacher's fingernails on an ancient blackboard

I did not dilly dally but diligently daily drove
the daunting dragon of desire and demand

and I wrote this poem

all that remains is the obligatory
selfie of the poet reading his poem
for posting to Facebook

★★★★★★★★★★★★★★★★★★★★★★★★★★★

Abstract found haiku: part II

Windows

schizophrenia:
morbid/insight poetry
illness/inner world

(Bakare, 2009, p. 217)

Findings

"ethical crafting":
aesthetic attention is
ethical practice

(Sjollema & Yuen, 2016, p. 1)

Yeats

Asclepius, god
of healing and poetry:
life-affirming writing

(Merritt, 2009, p. 235)

Exploration

homeopathy:
consultation is poem
deep, deeper healing

(Mardon, 2006, p. 20)

Explanatory

language as a field
of energy – playfully
shaping how we feel

(Soter, 2016, p. 161)

★★★★★★★★★★★★★★★★★★

Twenty-six meditations on living with poetry

a

like a poet
the bumblebee,
ironically named,
full of grace,
hovers over
the hibiscus,
eager for delights
in this summer
soon to end

b

poetry is fired
in the alchemy
of the alphabet
where letters know
our stories steeped
in autumn's hope

c

may our scholarship
sing with the vital voices
of poets in love, longing
for the possibilities
of words for translating
each day's demands

d

can poetry save us?
or at least help show the way?
or encourage us there is still hope?
can poetry offer an antidote to hate?

e

what might happen if politicians were poets?
what might happen if poets were politicians?

f

with only an imagined memory
of last night's black moon
I now anticipate with longing
October rhythms brimming
with cacophonous colour

g

if I could bend
this line lightly &
remember how
you laughed loud
in the summer sun
I might know how
love holds us fast

h

like a line of poetry
seeking its apt shape
on the page, may you
follow the light
of poetry calling you

i

if all the poets & all the poetry
in the world suddenly
disappeared, how would
the world be different?

j

each day is a line
full of wild poetry
beyond imagination
in the spell of grammar
with no punctuation

k

a poem is a magical evocation
of creative possibilities

l

poetry is a way of leaning
into the world with enthusiasm,
possessed by words!
poets cannot be polite!
poets ought to be political!

m

poetry emerges from the lively
intersections of light & shadow,
sound & silence, action & stillness,
heart & mind, always refuting binaries

n

what is the relationship between mastery &
mystery, between mastering language &
living creatively in the mystery of language?

o

how powerful are words?
what is more powerful than words?

p

the iamb, a metrical foot composed
of an unstressed syllable & a stressed syllable,
reminds me of the heart's beat, the poet's claim:
I am

q

we just need to speak & write
the words that are calling us &
trust that somebody somewhere
will be glad for the words

r

a poem is a way of breathing,
a way of attending to the rhythms
of each day's possibilities

s

even in a busy day of meetings, I continue
to seek the poetic in the midst of the prosaic,
sure that the poetry is everywhere

t

what is the difference between:
anybody
everybody
nobody
somebody?

u

poetry enthuses & sustains
the imagination, spirit, heart, & body
poets need to call out with
renewed vision & hopeful language

v

what might happen if poets wrote
only about what most fired their
imaginations & hearts calling
out with hopeful & truthful abandon?

w

whether writing poetry or not writing poetry,
each day is full of poetry

x

the first poets are children,
full of wonder for the world & for words

y

how is poetry pedagogically powerful?
why don't more people read poetry?
what might happen if more people read poetry?
how does poetry help imagine &
sustain the spirit of a community?

z

poetry invites attention & intention
without the contentious tension
that fires so many conversations

★★★★★★★★★★★★★★★★★★★★★★★★★★★

Abstract found haiku: part III

Disaster

evacuated
"Nobody came to help me"
older adults' fears

(Miller & Brockie, 2015, p. 103)

Recovery

hearing and listening
living with mental illness
story told and "heard"

(Saunders, Usher, Tsey & Bainbridge, 2016, p. 1)

Therapeutic

poetic justice:
the chronically ailing poor
heal mind and body

(McGee, 2009, n.p.)

Restoration

"art of medicine"
not to lose sense of personhood
a way to learn, know

(Brueggemann, 1985, p. 370)

Benefits

serious illness
"something to hang my life on"
increased wellbeing

(Ricketts, Greive & Gordon, 2011, p. 265)

Lingering thoughts

In our poetry we understand Jean-Luc Nancy's (2006) claim that "poetry refuses to be confined to a single mode of discourse" (p. 5). And like Nancy we know that "poetry is at ease with the difficult, the absolutely difficult" (p. 4). We write poetry and we experiment with different kinds of poetry because we know that language and rhetoric help compose the world. We agree with Gregory Orr's (2002) view that "poetry can have enormous transformative power" (p. 6). Orr understands that the world is "disorderly and chaotic" (p. 16). We only need to read the daily newspaper to know that the world is full of challenging and complex stories. In writing poetry, we create a sense of order that infuses us with hope for the kind of change that can foster well-being.

References

Bakare, M. O. (2009). Morbid and insight poetry: A glimpse at schizophrenia through the window of poetry. *Journal of Creativity in Mental Health, 4*(3), 217–224.

Berg, M. & Seeber, B. K. (2016). *The slow professor: Challenging the culture of speed in the academy.* Toronto, ON: University of Toronto Press.

Brueggemann, J. G. (1985). Poetry and medicine. *Perspectives in Biology and Medicine, 28*(3), 370–373.

Hirshfield, J. (1997). *Nine gates: Entering the mind of poetry.* New York, NY: Harper Perennial.

Kidd, L. I. (2010). *The effect of a poetry writing intervention on self-transcendence, resilience, depressive symptoms, and subjective burden in family caregivers of older adults with dementia* (Unpublished doctoral dissertation). Case Western Reserve University, Cleveland, OH, USA.

Kreuter, E. A. & Reiter, S. (2014). Building resilience in the face of loss and irrelevance: Poetic methods for personal and professional transformation. *Journal of Poetry Therapy, 27*(1), 13–24.

Mardon, J. M. (2006). Poetry and homeopathy: An exploration. *Homeopathy, 95*(1), 20–27.

McGee, R. S. (2009). *Poetic justice – Writing for health and emotional freedom: Creating a therapeutic writing program for the chronically ailing poor* (Unpublished doctoral dissertation). Drew University, Madison, NJ, USA.

Merritt, R. (2009). W.B. Yeats: Poet as healer. *Journal of Poetry Therapy, 22*(4), 235–247.

Miller, E. & Brockie, L. (2015). The disaster flood experience: Older people's poetic voices of resilience. *Journal of Aging Studies, 34*, 103–112.

Nancy, J.-L. (2006). *Multiple arts: The muses II.* (S. Sparks, Ed.). Stanford: Stanford University Press.

Orr, G. (2002). *Poetry as survival.* Athens: University of Georgia Press.

Prendergast, M. (2016). Found haiku from Laurel Richardson's "Writing: A method of inquiry". In J. White (Ed.), *Permission: The international interdisciplinary impact of Laurel Richardson's work* (pp. 123–126). Rotterdam: Sense.

Prendergast, M., Gouzouasis, P., Leggo, C., Irwin, R., & Grauer, K. (2009). A haiku suite: The importance of music-making in the lives of secondary school students. *Music Education Researcher, 11*(3), 303–317.

Richardson, L. (2000). Writing: A method of inquiry. In N.K. Denzin & Y.S. Lincoln (Eds.), *SAGE Handbook of Qualitative Research* (2nd ed., pp. 923–948). Thousand Oaks, CA: Sage.

Rickett, C., Greive, C., & Gordon, J. (2011). Something to hang my life on: The health benefits of writing poetry for people with serious illnesses. *Journal of Australasian Psychiatry, 19*(3), 265–268.

Saunders, V., Usher, K., Tsey, K., & Bainbridge, R. (2016). If you knew the end of a story would you still want to hear it? Using research poems to listen to Aboriginal stories. *Journal of Poetry Therapy, 29*(1), 1–13.

Sheets, D. & Liebig, P. (2011). The moon day poets: Creative expression and aging. *International Journal of the Humanities, 8*(11), 129–147.

Sjollema, S. & Yuen, F. (2016). Evocative words and ethical crafting: Poetic representation in leisure research. *Leisure Sciences: An Interdisciplinary Journal, 38* [published online]. http://dx.doi.org/10.1080/01490400.2016.1151845

Soter, A. O. (2016). Reading and writing poetically for well-being: Language as a field of energy in practice. *Journal of Poetry Therapy, 29*(3), 161–174.

Thompson, R., Furman, R., Shafi, N., & Enterline, M. (2012). Poetry, masculinities, and disability. *Journal of Poetry Therapy, 25*(2), 105–114.

28

THIRTEEN WAYS OF LOOKING
AT A CLINIC

Jennifer Schulz

This is a story about the clinical internship year I spent ten years ago in a community medical clinic working as a therapist-in-training with chronically mentally ill and economically impoverished adults. I came to this internship after teaching in the university for years as a creative writing and literature professor, and thus, I was accustomed to writing and interpreting stories. However, becoming oriented to a new clinical career within the disorienting national context of increasingly managed care and alarming federal cuts to Medicare, Medicaid, and Social Security, I found it impossible to draw conclusions or find definitive explanations about the often confusing and contradictory dynamics I witnessed within and surrounding the clinic during those ten months. Instead, I took the stance that year with which, in fact, I was most comfortable: that of speculation. Thus, this is a story that resists conclusions and explanation. It is a story without convention: without protagonist, identifiable conflict, rising action, climax, or resolution. It is a story, primarily, about seeing and it is a story that attempts to see. Neither chronological, nor teleological, this story is, instead, phenomenological and speculative. In the words of philosopher Hans-Georg Gadamer (1960/1998), this story is a "coming to an understanding" (p. 469).

As Gadamer works to describe the speculative quality of language and the "speculative element" of the hermeneutical dialectic, he uses "speculative" to imply the opposite of dogmatic and "the realization of meaning, as the event of speech, of mediation, of coming to an understanding. Someone who speaks is behaving speculatively when his words do not reflect beings but express a relation to the whole of being" (p. 469). For Gadamer, this kind of speculative language is most vividly experienced in the poetic word – where

> I and the world meet. If poetry shows people in conversation, then what is given in the poetic statement is not the statement that a written report would contain, but in a mysterious way, the whole of the conversation is as if present.
>
> (pp. 474, 470)

Transcribed here are a series of conversations (if not the "whole" conversation), where I and a particular clinic met in a particular moment in history.

Telling a story of the clinic, rather than a "written report," necessitates a dialogal structure and a "speculative" form. Thus, as I considered the form and method for the telling, I turned to Wallace Stevens's poem "Thirteen Ways of Looking at a Blackbird" as a model. The stanzas that preface each section of this story, *present* reality rather than *represent* reality as the blackbird emerges in thirteen ways as an unfixed being, rather than a fixed object of interpretation. Each section of the story offers its own specific perspective (by means of anecdote, case story, memo, or footnote) on the clinic while also drawing from and re-seeing the section that precedes it, and anticipating, or setting a context for, the next. The blackbird is neither subject nor object but *both* observer and observed. Indeed, the first time we see the blackbird, it is its "moving eye" that we see, not the bird itself. Does it see us before we see it? As it carries us between and among the various sections of this story, the blackbird, like the clinic, emerges as observed and observer in constantly shifting forms. Staff, administration, patients, even the physical space of the clinic, all at different times occupy the role of Stevens's blackbird. My story, like Stevens's poem, is an attempt to present the whole of the being of, in this case, the clinic. However, the whole of being, as Gadamer would argue, should not imply an exhaustive or totalizing study, but rather an opportunity to see the clinic in the lived experience of the clinic.

My hope is that this story will invite further speculation on what is possible for treating the mentally ill in terms of the whole of their beings and in the lived context of the spaces explicitly designated for treatment; indeed, perhaps we can find more creative possibilities as they emerge in stories.

I

Among twenty snowy mountains,
The only moving thing
Was the eye of the blackbird.

On the first day of my internship in September I walked through the front clinic doors feeling fraudulent and frightened. When Linda, the transsexual receptionist, asked on that first day, without looking up from her piles of paperwork, if she could help me, I told her I was the new intern and I was looking for my supervisor. She glanced up at me and with no change in her expression picked up the phone and rang his extension. We stared at each other while I could hear from her receiver two rings, three rings, four rings, then a voice mail message. Linda hung up. "I don't know where he is. Ask Anna," Linda said, looking back down at her work.

"Who's Anna?"
Linda sighed, "Oh right. . . . Um, let me call her."

Although she didn't know me, I recognized Linda as a long-time clinic staff member from some volunteer work I had done years before with one of the clinic's local foundational sources of financial support. Back then, in the mid-nineties, I knew the clinic as a progressive community clinic dedicated to serving the most marginalized downtown populations: prostitutes, homeless men and women, homeless men and women with tuberculosis and AIDS, crack and heroin addicts, street alcoholics, the transgendered, transsexuals, and transvestites who had, at times, been violently targeted. I had always idealized the unique integration of the surrounding urban community with the clinic. It was one of the reasons I wanted this internship. And it was one of the reasons that, as I stood waiting at the front desk with Linda periodically glancing up at me, I wondered if I (certainly not marginalized) belonged here at all.

Minutes later a woman in a long African print skirt, brightly colored tank top and Birkenstocks walked through some heavy doors on the other side of the lobby (from what I remembered as the mental health wing). Anna, the Clinic Manager – she introduced herself. "He's not here," she said.

Something sank in my already nervous stomach.

"Gee, he must have forgotten that you were coming." By now Linda was looking at me again, and so were the patients in the waiting room. I felt hot and confused.

Anna smiled and said, "Here, come back to his office and you can write him a note."

I followed her, feeling conspicuous and childish as I passed people who, I thought, might someday soon come to me for therapy. I tried to pull my head up and look self-assured.

Anna let me out the back staff door, for which I was grateful.

I was on the bus and nearly home when my cell phone rang.

He was livid. "I was in a meeting in the administrative offices. Anna told me that she forgot. . . . So – look, can you come back? I would like you to co-lead a couple of groups with me this year and one of them meets today at one. They're expecting you."

I got off at the next stop and turned around.

My supervisor was waiting for me in the alley and he unlocked the staff door for me. I was thankful not to have to walk through the lobby again.

"Group's starting in five minutes. You made it just in time. Are you ready?"

I was hot, out of breath, tired from my sleepless night before, from the back and forth on the bus and from nerves. "Sure."

We walked into the group room and sat down at the tables that took up the center of the room. "Let's see, I guess you could call this the bi-polar group," he said. "Most of the members are bi-polar, several deal with psychosis and I think all of them have or are recovering from addictions. Do you know what kinds of cases you would like to start out with?"

I looked at him wide-eyed and silent in part because the group members had begun filing into the room. Most of them sat across the table from me or on the other side of my supervisor. He introduced me as clinician-in-training, the new co-facilitator of the group, and potentially someone they would come to see in individual therapy. It was quiet as the group members, all men except one woman who sat directly across from me, looked at me and mumbled some hellos.

After a pause, the one other woman in the room, Sheryl, said, without taking her eyes off me, "I'll start I guess. I'm going to kill the mother."

As she continued to stare at me, I swallowed hard. My mind raced (Do you have a plan? A weapon? – why wasn't I trained for this?) and I sat silently, feeling not only Sheryl's unflagging stare but also the eyes of everyone else in the room seeing right into and through my fear and utter sense of disorientation.

When I walked into the clinic lobby on that first day I was looking for orientation, for supervision. Having moved from one discipline as a literature professor defined by relatively clearly prescribed university infrastructure, into another discipline as a clinical psychology student/therapist-in-training, I was, I suppose, anticipating structure, technique, rules, guidance.

I longed for this structure even after embracing (within the familiar walls of the classroom) the hermeneutical approach of Heidegger (1962) and Gadamer (1960/1998) – wherein understanding becomes an intersubjective creative and dialogical process, irreducible to technique – that drew me to existential and phenomenological psychology in the first place and, frankly, that drew me to the kind of clinic that seemed to be able to create its own cosmos ("The Island," as one patient would later describe it to me).

There was, however, something about Sheryl's pronouncement in that first moment of group that made me forget to consider her in terms of "being in the world," of Heidegger's Dasein. Sheryl was going to kill someone (the mother, *her* mother?); she was telling me this quite directly, and there must be something to do. It became impossible in that moment to recall some of the very words that drew me to this work – Rollo May's (1983) application of Heidegger to therapy:

> Our Western tendency has been to believe that *understanding follows technique*; if we get the right technique, then we can penetrate the riddle of the patient. . . . The existential approach holds the exact opposite – namely, that *technique follows understanding*. The central task of the therapist is to seek to understand the patient as a being and as being in his world. All technical problems are subordinate to this understanding.

(pp. 151–152)

I had not shifted careers to become trained as a technician in human interaction. I had made this change because I thrived on the experiences of human interaction and on the creativity of being in genuine dialogue. Nevertheless, the "technical problems" that May subordinates to "understanding," did not seem to cover matricide. And "all technical problems" did not seem to cover the larger problem of my supervision that, if read through a literary vein, was foreshadowed during my first moments standing at Linda's desk when my supervisor was nowhere to be found and when the Clinic Manager denied his presence at the clinic that day. In November, two months into my internship – just as I was beginning to build up a caseload of patients, just as Sheryl was beginning to accept my presence as co-facilitator in group and had stopped threatening to kill me or her mother, just as I had finally gained full access to the clinic's EPIC computer database and my own staff-entrance keys – my supervisor was fired.

II

I was of three minds,
Like a tree
In which there are three blackbirds.

While this is, in some ways, a story about my own transition from the work of university teaching into that of psychotherapy, this is mainly a story about a community clinic – by all accounts one of the last clinics in the city – finally beginning its painful and inevitable transition toward a managed care model of integrated medical and mental health care. It is about what made this clinic resist a national, legislatively and economically coerced trend for so long and what made this transition uniquely fraught with pain and uniquely full of potential. This is a story of staff members and patients. It is a story about the myths and realities surrounding the clinic and its history, myths, and realities that had invested the brick-lined walls of the lobby with the sense of (and hope for) an unshakeable stability – *maybe this will be the one place that will maintain its mission, maybe this will be the one place that will actually stay in place, will continue to catch all those who "slip through the cracks" of all the other places.*

I stepped into this landscape at the pre-dawn of what was to become a constant series of upheavals (disrupting all corners of the clinic) over the course of the next ten months. Stevens's three blackbirds, and the "three minds" of the speaker, emblematize the multiplicity of voices, agendas, desires, and needs that were competing within the clinic and within my own lived experience during those months.

This story of the clinic is, thus, inevitably, unavoidably about how the process by which the clinic began evolving into a new kind of clinic coincided with my process of learning to be a clinician. Without my former supervisor, and without consistent supervision until sometime in the middle of the winter (six months into my internship year), I experienced a kind of unmediated access to the clinic. My caseload rapidly grew when I inherited several of my former supervisor's patients immediately after his departure (and was called to witness their grief and their anger with the clinic administration), I took part in leaderless mental health team meetings held behind closed doors and at the level of whispers (if the team lead could be fired without warning, what was going to happen to the rest of the team, and what would happen to our patients? – my colleagues wondered), and I rapidly developed daily relationships with the medical doctors, the staff in the accounting office, and the Clinic Manager – all of whom had a direct impact on my relationships with my patients.

For the most part, I sat with my patients behind my closed office door or behind the closed door of the group room, yet the clinic was all around us and together we learned how to see it and be in it in creative and, often, improvised ways – as the clinic continued to "see" my patients, to "see" me, and to "see" us in ever-changing disciplinary ways. Throughout that year I was coming to a lived understanding and practice of an intersubjectivity that included and, simultaneously, extended beyond the therapist-patient dyad.

Theorists such as Stern (1997) and Orange, Atwood, and Stolorow (1997) describe intersubjectivity in the clinical situation as a creative process. It

> is not so much a theory as it is a sensibility. It is an attitude of continuing sensitivity to the inescapable interplay of observer and observed. It assumes that instead of entering and immersing ourselves in the experience of another, we join the other in the intersubjective space.
>
> (Orange, Atwood, & Stolorow, 1997, p. 9)

These theorists were not writing about the shared geographic, political, cultural, and physical space of a clinic but about "the psychological field located at the point of intersection between two subjectivities . . . generated by the interplay between transference and countertransference" (Atwood & Stolorow, 1984, p. 6). My story is an attempt to broaden the scope of these theorists' field by looking at the interplay among all the various subjectivities (staff, patients, and administrators) within the clinic in psychological terms of transference and countertransference and also in terms that take into account this broader context: discipline and creativity.

This clinic, like most clinics today, was structured or organized according to, in Michel Foucault's (1995) terms, panoptic mechanisms of constant surveillance (by means of patient charts, computerized registration and scheduling, and administrative hierarchies). For Foucault, the clinic, along with the prison, the factory, and the university, provide an architectural and infrastructural manifestation of the ways in which panopticism functions as "a generalizable model . . . a way of defining power relations in terms of the everyday life of men" (p. 205). Although the Executive Director of this clinic (who single-handedly fired my supervisor as just the beginning of a series of radical "personnel changes") emerged again and again as the locus of seemingly unchallenged and unilateral decision-making power, the disciplinary mechanisms at work could neither be identified with nor localized in one source of power, as became apparent when *he* was suddenly fired by the relatively invisible Board of Directors in the early spring. Over time I came to understand the disciplinary mechanisms at work as also a part of an intersubjective process – taking place in everyday interactions as well as in more formalized procedures of, for example, charting and scheduling.

But in the context of these intersubjective disciplinary practices, other kinds of practices emerged as well that seemed to open up spaces for creativity. In his response to Foucault, Michel de Certeau (1988) writes,

> If it is true that the grid of "discipline" is everywhere becoming clearer and more extensive, it is all the more urgent to discover how an entire society resists being reduced to it, what popular procedures (also "miniscule" and quotidian) manipulate the mechanisms of discipline and conform to them only in order to evade them, and finally, what "ways of operating" form the counterpart, on the consumer's (or "dominee's"?) side, of the mute processes that organize the establishment of socioeconomic order.
>
> (p. xiv)

De Certeau characterizes his project as "analogous" to Foucault's in his attempt to "perceive and analyze the microbe-like operations proliferating within technocratic structure and deflecting their functioning by means of a multitude of 'tactics' articulated in the details of everyday life" (p. xiv). In this way, de Certeau resonates the potentiality that Heidegger identifies in everydayness. In *Being and Time*, Heidegger (1962) writes that "the basic kind of Being which belongs to everydayness. . . [is] the *'falling'* of Dasein" (p. 219). He identifies "idle talk, curiosity, and ambiguity" as the "everyday manner" of Dasein, which is a kind of concealment of our authentic selves within the distraction of Das Man, an inattention to the potentiality of our being and the being of others. His response to "fallenness" is to postulate "authentic existence [as] . . . not something which floats above falling everydayness [or transcends the disciplinary structures]; existentially, it is only a modified way in which such everydayness is seized upon" (p. 224). That is, inherent in the everyday practices of moving through physical space and engaging in conversation is the potential encounter with one's own authentic beingness.

As I moved further and further into the landscape of the clinic, and settled into an everyday in the clinic, in addition to seeing and not-seeing the subtle disciplinary mechanisms in which I was implicated, I came to see how in other kinds of everyday interactions (mostly in interactions with my patients) we were engaging in tactics of improvisation, resistance, and creativity – intersubjectively uncovering our authenticity.

If the implicit conversation between Heidegger and de Certeau helped me to remember that creativity and resistance inheres in the everyday (and, consequently, helped me to remain present and hopeful – or, at least, present – with my patients in the midst of profoundly disillusioning "policy-making" and "personnel adjustments" in the clinic around us), Gadamer (1960/1998) helped me to come to a new kind of understanding of what was happening in the intersubjective spaces of the clinic. This understanding emerged in the interstices of technique, diagnosis, and procedure. This was a kind of understanding that inhered in dialogal revisionings and rehearsings, a shared experience – even (and often) a form of play – between my patients and me and among staff members. At least three different sets of voices, at least three different sets of actors, all of at least three different minds: how could I tell a linear story?

III

The blackbird whirled in the autumn winds.
It was a small part of the pantomime.

The departure of my first supervisor early on in my internship coincided with New Year's, a clinic holiday. After New Year's, I walked past the men sobering up on the steps down from Avenue and stuck my key into the lock of the Staff-Only entrance with some trepidation. (I was not even certain that I still had an internship.) I stepped inside the doors and gasped audibly. "Christ!"

The Clinic Manager, sitting in her tiny corner office, rolled her office chair backwards so she could see me. "I know, I know. They're bright, aren't they?"

"Are we going to do some dissections in the staff meeting today?" I asked.

She laughed and said, "Things are changing quickly around here, aren't they?"

I looked at the walls, "Why gray blue; I kind of liked the cream."

She said, "We didn't paint; it's just the new lights."

The week that our lighting went "full-spectrum, not fluorescent" (as I heard Anna reiterating to each person who returned from vacation through that door), I met my psychotherapy groups with the remaining two licensed therapists on staff (Alice on Thursdays, Kate on Fridays). The clinic manager had realized that without a licensed social worker in the groups, Medicare would not reimburse the clinic for these sessions. Before group on Thursday Alice found me and said, "Help me take these tables down in the group room. We can't run a group with tables."

I said, "This group has always had tables."

"Well, not anymore. If they miss the tables we can talk about why."

The Thursday group spent forty-five minutes talking about the lack of tables.

Before the Friday group, Kate, my other co-therapist, found me and said, "Let's put the tables up. Haven't you always run the groups with tables?"

The tables were imperative for Friday's group, a hindrance or not. One member had been bringing his pet chinchilla to group and placing her on towels spread out on the tabletop in front of him. Sometimes, another member brought her "Africans" (her afghans), lay them out on the table, and crocheted.

After several weeks, group membership began dropping off, on both Thursday and Friday. Group members started leaving messages on my voice mail asking if they could talk to me in private about group.

Many of the members were my former supervisor's former patients who were now without an individual therapist. I agreed to see two of them in individual therapy, one of which had, in the past five years, a couple of serious suicide attempts. The other had stabbed himself in the chest almost exactly a year ago and was feeling "shaky" about the upcoming anniversary.

I called two others and told them that I could not see them in individual therapy and urged them to continue with the group. I told them that they would be put on a waiting list until the clinic hired another full-time clinician. But I feared that even when the full-time clinician came, they would still be without the kind of therapy they were accustomed to. What I did not tell them was that they were too "well" to get re-assigned to a therapist. There were other patients hanging in limbo who were more "serious" cases.

In the end of January I ran the Friday group on my own. Kate was out of town. I walked in to find Patty (with the "Africans") handing around pictures of her grown children. Matthew was taking "Fluffy" out of her cage. He put her on the towel and reached into his bag. He handed me a rolled-up sketch. Matthew was a very talented artist. I remembered that he told me he would give me a sketch when I finished my internship. I suddenly felt concerned.

"What's going on with the group today?" I asked.

"I'm pissed," Al said. "I used to be friends with Linda at the front desk and now she treats me like a piece of computer data. I refuse to 'check in,' in protest; I don't care if I fuck up the new clinic database."

"Maybe we could look at Linda's behavior as a symptom of the general mood in the clinic these days – all the changes are pretty disorienting," I said. "And imagine Linda's position; she sits out in the open all day. She doesn't even get to close the doors like we do." I pulled the doors to the group room closed.

Al looked at me and waited a beat. "Thank you for that." I knew he meant it. He was not one to mince words. Then he added, "But what's up with these fucking lights?!"

I turned off the overhead lights and pulled an old 1970s floor lamp – the kind with the four bulbs facing in different directions – in from the hallway (designated for the dumpsters). I plugged it in. Matthew switched it on. Worked fine. Best I'd felt in that room all week. All month.

Unfixed and unstable, the clinic taught me how to improvise, to seize upon the everydayness of the space; indeed the clinic became the backdrop and provided the props for impromptu pantomimes that actually helped all of us re-see possibilities for encountering our authentic beings, even in the midst of new bureaucratic policies and practices that constantly threatened to preempt such possibilities.

Later, after group, I filled out encounter forms for all the group members at the front desk. Linda said to me, "Can you please do something about Al? He thinks this is his living room. He doesn't understand that this is a business."

IV

A man and a woman
Are one.
A man and a woman and a blackbird
Are one.

Clay was the first patient I met at the clinic. Over the course of the first week of my internship my supervisor, the outreach nurse, the physicians, and the Head Receptionist (those who had been there long enough to have something to say about him) described Clay to me as "one of our lifers." On my first day my supervisor provided me with just the outline and a few details of the life of this nearly 60-year-old-man, wearing a neatly-trimmed silver beard and mustache and plaid shirt and jeans, who walked into one of the psychotherapy groups I was to co-lead.

Severely abused throughout his childhood, Clay had also survived three suicide attempts, and as many hospitalizations (one of which included electro-shock therapy) throughout his adulthood. Clay had become a "lifer" at the clinic – relatively stabilized on a regimen of psychotropic medications (to modulate his moods and to quiet the voices in his head), weekly group sessions, and bi-weekly individual therapy sessions. "He's one of our success stories," several of the staff members echoed proprietarily throughout that first week.

The next day, standing in my classroom at the university where I was teaching a literature course on twentieth-century narratives of trauma, I was suddenly struck by the incongruities inherent in this particular "success story." I talked with my students about the "impossibility" and "incomprehensibility" of the trauma narrative, about the "refusal" that trauma narratives make of, in Cathy Caruth's (1995) terms, a "certain framework of understanding, a refusal that is also a creative act of listening" (p. 154). I talked about this "creative act of listening" of "new ways of gaining access to histor[y]" in terms of resistance; in this classroom, we were working to resist the dominant fictions, the ideological frameworks by which we are manipulated, enticed, habituated into seeing history as a teleology of progress.

In an era of managed care and budget cuts, wherein putatively "progressive" and "cost effective" clinics are run like businesses and "client/consumers" are efficiently registered, serviced, documented, and sent on their way, the very advertisement of a "clinic lifer" comes to appear as an act of political resistance. Indeed, according to managed care, the "success story" would characterize the patient who had been able, as a result of ten sessions of behavioral modification, in addition to complying with the right combination of medications, to re-assimilate into his or her productive place in society. The ready equation of "clinic lifer" and "success story" further disrupts a more far-reaching narrative of American individualism – the Horatio Alger "pull yourself up by your bootstraps" ethos that has been co-opted by those who understand health care as a business concern rather than a civil responsibility.

The "Clay-as-clinic-success" claim instead enacted an idealized version of a clinic (constitutive of its pre-managed care history) where individuals like Clay could find a "home." Clay had become characterized by the clinic staff as a "lifer," a "chronic patient," who also came to stand in as a "pillar" of a community (emblematizing continuity and stability) that was losing its footing. "He's one of our success stories," I came to see, was, on the one hand, a statement of resistance to managed care mechanisms for prescribing and totalizing our patients and our approaches to treatment. On the other hand, it was itself an act of totalizing or fixing Clay in place – as a way to shore up our own sense of place.

When Clay and I met for the first time, he spoke to me in a dull monotone, as if measuring each word and each inflection, carefully keeping any affect out of his self-expression or, for that matter, self-presentation. He walked slowly, with an equally measured step; if anyone could appear immobile while in motion, this was it. I stood to meet him and I found myself searching to find him underneath what felt like fossilized granite. Nevertheless, his presence was paradoxically warm and inviting and after just a few meetings I found myself working to keep my own emotions that would curiously well up in his presence, in check. My own gestures and expressions became slower, smaller.

In January, Clay's individual therapist of seven years (my supervisor) left the clinic and together he and Clay decided that Clay would become my patient. "He just needs to check in with someone – you know, because of the agoraphobia – maybe even just every other week," my supervisor said. "You can help create a kind of holding environment until he can transition to someone more long-term." At the time, within the first few months of my internship, I did not understand the dynamic quality intrinsic to "holding." In part, I was afraid that Clay would de-stabilize (and for a brand new therapist, this took on many different forms and meanings that could keep me awake at night) and so I heard "holding" in terms of "safety" (read "stasis"). Also, I was becoming keenly aware of a kind of fear, on the part of the staff, of the rapidly de-stabilizing ground upon which the clinic tenuously sat. This fear radiated out into our discussions regarding the patients' well-being (particularly those who, like Clay, had lost their therapist of anywhere from seven to ten years). This fear also took the form of nostalgic historicizing reflections of the "ways things used to be" – when patients and staff alike felt a kind of "living room" atmosphere radiating throughout the clinic and, in particular, in the clinic lobby. My own fear as well as the complicated fear/nostalgia circulating through the clinic contributed to my sense that Clay needed to be held "in place."

Now, years later, I realize that I learned something else from and with Clay that had less to do with keeping him in "place" than in co-creating new intersubjective space. When I met Clay, he was "the clinic's." Our time together, in part because of the clinic, opened up new kinds of spaces – akin to, but also transcendent of, the "intersubjective field" of the therapist-patient dyad (Atwood, Brandchaft, & Stolorow, 1987) as well as of the "intermediate zones" that Winnicott (1971) talks about as the creative spaces for "play" (p. 105).

When we met individually for the first time he expressed a desire to set and work to meet some goals. Before his last hospitalization, he had loved to walk through a local park not far from the clinic. "All the way to the end," he said. "I had my own bench where I would sit and watch the boats. It used to be a very spiritual place for me." We decided that he would build up to a walk to the bench by first walking to and from the entrance to the park.

Weeks passed without him walking so I asked him if we could take that walk down to the park together, wondering, the whole time, if this was therapeutically sound. He looked up at me, his eyes wide. He said, almost sheepishly, "You know, you can take some elevators down to and up from the waterfront. We wouldn't have to actually walk the hills."

"Great," I said. "Let's take the elevator."

He relaxed and smiled, "I really like elevators. I wish I could take them everywhere."

"Me too. Let's take elevators even where there are no hills!"

"Even where the ground is flat!"

"Yes!"

The next time we met he was feeling depressed. He said, "I had a little high weeks ago – which I now attribute to delusions of grandeur." He told me that he was more afraid of the highs than the lows. Then he described the different sets of voices that he hears, mostly when he is feeling manic. "One set is a whole bunch of people angrily arguing – like it was in my house when I was a child. The other is scarier. A commanding voice that orders me to do things – mostly hurt myself."

He was also disheartened, he said, by the clinic. There had been so many staff turnovers in the pharmacy recently that his "Mediset" was never ready for him when he came to exchange his empty box for a full box, as had been his pattern for years. "I have to keep training new pharmacists," he said, and I smiled. What does it feel like, coming to the clinic, having lost your therapist of seven years and now your pharmacists? I wondered out loud. He complained about being treated as a number and feeling as if he had become part of a big factory. "The people at the front desk don't know my name anymore," he said. "Except Linda, but she's always too busy to notice when I arrive," he said.

Feeling my own sense of disorientation and disenchantment with the rapid shifts in policy and culture, but reminding myself that "my job" was to keep Clay "in place," I responded with a platitude, "This clinic is *your* clinic, not some bureaucrats'."

He looked at me, paused, and then said with a little gleam in his eyes, "*My* clinic? Clay's Clinic. Good . . . then I am going to get busy and make some changes around here."

In his chart that day, I noted Clay's "medication compliance" (one of the signs that he was continuing to be a "success"), I noted his depression and his fear of mania but also his ability to be self-reflective, to monitor and talk about his moods ("success"). This note was coherent with the larger template of the treatment plan. The story I left out was the one that was beginning to play out in vivid color in my mind: "When Clay Ran the Clinic."

I was following Clay. Or. We were each leading the other to new kinds of spaces, where our roles as therapist/patient would lose their distinctness, not disappear, but become more flexible. And I had ceased to hold him in place a long time ago. *A man and a woman and a clinic are one.*

I began to think about the distinction that Michel de Certeau (1988) draws between places and spaces. "A place," he writes,

> Is the order (of whatever kind) in accord with which elements are distributed in relationships of coexistence. It thus excludes the possibility of two things being in the same location (*place*). The law of the "proper" rules in the place: the elements taken into consideration are *beside* one another, each situated in its own proper and distinct location, a location it defines. . . . It implies an indication of stability.
>
> (p. 117)

The place ensures certain prescribed roles (therapist/patient, for example) wherein Clay and I existed as distinct beings with distinct boundaries between us that could be mapped out by diagnoses, clinic protocols. By contrast, de Certeau writes that a space

> exists when one takes into consideration vectors of direction, velocities, and time variables. Thus space is composed of intersections of mobile elements. . . . Space occurs as the effect produced by the operations that orient it, situate it, temporalize it, and make it function in a polyvalent unity of conflictual programs or contractual proximities. On this view, in relation to place, space is like the word when it is spoken, that is, when it is caught in the ambiguity of an actualization, transformed into a term dependent upon many different conventions, situated at the act of a present (or of a time), and modified by the transformations caused by successive contexts. In contradistinction to the place, it has thus none of the univocity or stability of a "proper."
>
> (p. 117)

In other words, in the play of our interactions, Clay and I claimed a space that defied the maps of the place.

That is, the "place" in which I was to hold Clay was the clinic as a set of conventions, diagnoses, documentation strategies, and distinctions among the various individuals and sets of individuals who make up the place (from the over-worked Head Receptionist, to the Clinic Manager, to the pharmacists, to the therapists, to the patients, etc.). The "spaces" that Clay and I were traversing criss-crossed, doubled-back on themselves, inscribed contradictions on the very structures that worked to define the place: elevators that carried you along level ground, clinics where the patients ran the show. We were taking words out of context; we were turning the clinic into a space.

This was different from Winnicott's (1971) potential in-between space of play or Atwood, Brandchaft, and Stolorow's (1987) intersubjective field. This was not just between Clay and me. The place of the clinic depended upon Clay to live out his role as "success story/lifer." No one, including me, including Clay, I think, wanted to relinquish our hold on him as a "pillar." Paradoxically, in the very limitations and prescriptions of the role, it was making our space-making, the practicing of this place, possible. And even as he continued to identify with the role, Clay was playing with the space as well.

V

I do not know which to prefer,
The beauty of inflections
Or the beauty of innuendos,
The blackbird whistling
Or just after

One day in the spring, Clay sat down in group and addressed everyone; "I have something on my mind that is kind of troubling me and I just have to get it out while I remember." My co-therapist and I leaned in, the other group members looked concerned. After all of the play, I suddenly remembered "our place." "There is someone talking to me who I don't know," Clay continued in a serious measured tone. Oh no, I thought, is this his psychosis? He looked across the circle at me. "I think she's another therapist in the clinic. She comes up to me in the lobby when I am waiting for my appointment and she just starts talking to me like she knows me." He was smiling now, a little conspiratorially, perhaps? My co-therapist and I asked for a description and, sure enough, it was our colleague. My co-therapist began to explain our "team approach" – that, in weekly staff meetings we all bring in cases to share – and that other clinicians become, in the process, very invested in patients who are not their own. I was looking at Clay at this point thinking, You're ours. You're the whole clinic's. What is that like for you? And I was also starting to see, with some delight, where this was going.

He listened carefully to my co-therapist, considered her words, then said very slowly, "I will just have to say to her the next time, 'Excuse me. I'm afraid I don't know you. Who are you and why are you talking to me? Maybe you need to talk to someone about that.'" By now he was laughing.

Stevens's blackbird whistles in "inflections" and "innuendos" – it is as much the poet as the subject of the poem or the object of the speakers' observations. Clay helped me to see that he, and the other patients in the clinic, were telling this story as much as the staff and the administrators were. And it is through Clay's words that I tell my own story.

VI

Icicles filled the long window
With barbaric glass.
The shadow of the blackbird
Crossed it, to and fro.
The mood
Traced in the shadow
An indecipherable cause.

Throughout the first few months of my internship I got swept up in the stories and practices that emerged out of the clinical staff's team approach: improvised collaborations among doctors, the nurse practitioner, mental health counselors, and the consulting psychiatrist. They felt refreshingly creative (albeit maddening at times), fueled by a moral consensus regarding the unchallenged right of every individual in this city to receive medical and mental health care, particularly with the specter of managed care, budget cuts, and a very expensive war (the misdirected invasion of Iraq following the 2001 World Trade Center bombings) hanging ominously over the clinic. Thursdays at noon we would close the large double doors and the space inside the group room would become thick with stories, descriptions, speculations, diagnoses, and plans (some subversive), and mysteriously, collectively we would begin to take on the presenting symptoms (more often than not, some degree of mania) of our featured patients.

I had been told that, underlying the collaborations, a disciplined hierarchy had always been in place. The psychiatrist ran this meeting; she often held the floor for the first twenty minutes, raising questions about the patients scheduled to see her that day. The physicians and nurse practitioner came next. The medical staff was expected to dispense meds with psychiatric expertise, expertise to which they only had access one hour per week (and by means of the lengthy and thorough assessments the psychiatrist dictated into the chart notes and through their on-the-fly training).

The mental health counselors came last. We informed the doctors (mostly in side conversations) that, in fact, our patients had not been complying with their medications (or had been selling them on the streets), we advocated for changes in dosages (although we were, of course, even less formally trained in psycho-tropic drugs than the internists), and we filled in the gaps in the stories: the patient is or is not psychotic, is or is not suicidal, is or is not a danger to others. These assessments were the moments during which we had the floor and our ability to keep the floor hinged on the words we choose and on which side of the is/is not diagnostic category they fell.

The meetings were an activated set of tactical operations made up of collaborations and play across the levels of clinical staff. I use the term "tactics" here to differentiate the kind of operations that happened during the meetings, as well as throughout the week in other kinds of shared spaces, from "strategies" – those operations that took place at the level of management: structural changes initiated by the Executive Director (and the Board) and enforced by the Clinic Manager, the Head Reception-ist, etc.

This distinction is a manifestation, again, of Michel de Certeau's (1988) theoretical debate with Michel Foucault (1995) around the "battles or games between the strong and the weak, and . . . the 'actions' which remain possible for the latter" (de Certeau, p. 34). A strategy, de Certeau and Foucault would agree, is a calculated exercise of organizational power on the part of those recognizably in control. Strategic power masters places and time "through the foundation of an autonomous place." This place makes possible "panoptic practices" that transforms individuals within that place into "objects that can be controlled and measured" (p. 36). If, according to Foucault, strategies and tactics are mutually reinforcing sets of operations, whereby strategies play out on a global political stage and tactics play out on a local level, for de Certeau, tactics is "an art of the weak."

The Executive Director initiated and worked to enforce the strategies for clinic procedures – ranging from the way patients were registered and tracked as they walked into the lobby (by means of the ubiqui-tous EPIC database), to the way clinicians practiced behind the closed doors of the exam rooms, to, eventu-ally, eliminating as many closed doors as possible. An agent of the "new business model" of health care, the Executive Director spoke for the clinic (in terms of *our* mission and *our* funding needs) in the state capital, while back in the clinic he began to build a seemingly impenetrable structure of disciplinary mechanisms against an "other" that shifted disconcertingly to preempt a unified resistance; sometimes all clinicians were the "others," increasingly, just the mental health counselors were. The patients, on the other hand, although not articulated as such, had most certainly become, for clinic administration, both the "consumers," as well as the "others."

With shifting loyalties, came an atmosphere paradoxically mixed with suspicious subtext (reproductive of the disciplinary mechanisms at work) and surreptitious collaborations (productive of potentialities for resistance). The tactics, which characterize the latter, that we practiced in our weekly meetings crystallized in relationship to the administrative strategies. A tactic, for de Certeau, "must accept the chance offerings of the moment, and seize on the wing, the possibilities that offer themselves at any given moment. It must vigilantly make use of the cracks that particular conjunctions open in the surveillance of the proprietary powers" (p. 37).

Our tactics, mainly dialogal in nature, worked to transform the *place* of the clinic into a *space*. Our con-versations created impromptu infrastructures that, however isolated and momentary, also helped us develop linguistic codes that were translatable across spatial and situational contexts.

The first time I experienced such collaboration first-hand was in the middle of winter. I was on my way back from the chart room, through the lobby, and to my office on the opposite side of the clinic when I quickly opened the chart I was carrying, trying to fill the gaps in a story unfolding around me that just wasn't making sense. One of my patients had been refusing for months to take any psychotropic medica-tions and many of our sessions included some forceful reiteration on his part of indignation about the pres-sure he had received from his medical doctors in the past and pride in his ability to ward off such incessant and, to his mind, utterly "conspiratorial, if not irresponsible, pill pushing." That morning, however, just a half hour or so before my weekly session with him, I had found a note in my box informing me that Richard had lost his recently filled Zyprexa over the weekend and had been given a new prescription by the on-call doctor. I read his doctor's note from two months previous when, apparently, she first convinced him to take the anti-psychotic medication. At first, I felt naïve – why hadn't I been tracking her notes? Then, when I read on, and noticed the complexities of the story.

At our next staff meeting I wrote my name on the board for the first time all year with Richard's name underneath – signifying to the others that I had a priority patient.

"So I realize I could have just looked at the meds chart, but I didn't really even think to doubt him when he said he wasn't taking, and would never take, psychotropic drugs," I said sarcastically and as loudly as I could over the various conversations that ensued after the consulting psychiatrist had finished with her part of the meeting. "I'm talking about Richard K. And the Zyprexa refill."

His doctor, who was sitting across the table looking at me, laughed, "Well, I told him they were stomach meds – you know, for his irritable bowel."

"I know, I read your note."

Other doctors and mental health counselors stopped their conversations and were looking at us. "What?"

By this time, both Richard's doctor and I were smiling at each other. "Hey," she said to me, "Do you know what the taboo word is with Richard?"

Matter-of-factly, I said, "Oh, that's easy, 'chronic.'"

"Shit, why didn't you tell me before? You know, I can't even diagnose this guy with allergies."

"It's in my notes."

The consulting psychiatrist (who I had scheduled Richard to see that day, in the next hour) joined the conversation. (I breathed a sigh of relief; things were going better than expected. I had been hoping to capture her attention – which was always divided among the rest of the clinicians.) "What's his diagnosis?" she asked me.

I said, "He has been variously diagnosed with everything from schizophrenia to Asperger's syndrome. He says that no one has been able to help him."

She looked up from another patient's chart that she had been reading. I suddenly had her full attention; I got serious – I knew I had less than thirty seconds for my "case presentation." "He wants to be 'cured.' Mostly he wants to be 'understood.' He wants someone to tell him 'what he has' and 'who he is' but he cannot bear to hear that he cannot become normal, better than 'normal' – 'exceptional.' He has told me that if he learned he had a 'chronic disorder' it would be grounds for suicide."

The room was quiet for just a split second until another chart emerged in front of the psychiatrist. Before she looked down at it and moved on, she nodded at me and said, "Interesting. So he's on my schedule for. . . ?"

"Today. At two o-clock." I leaned back, breathing a sigh of relief. I looked across the table at Richard's doctor and we raised our eyebrows and give each other a half-smile. In that exchange, we communicated our shared experience of feeling stuck, of asking for help, and of being heard.

Alice, my new supervisor, suddenly added, as an aside to the nurse practitioner sitting near us, "This guy. In group, he is so defensively angry; I feel a little paranoid by the time group ends each week. I feel like I need to go back to my office and lie down afterwards, say soothing things to myself."

"Hey, Alice, maybe you could use some 'stomach meds,'" another doctor across the table joked.

Amidst the "idle talk" and banter I was aware of another level of meaning-making in which we – the staff of the clinic – participated and collaborated, a level at which we revealed our vulnerabilities and those of our patients within the constrictive resources and discourses of the clinic. To an outside observer, we probably would have appeared irreverent and dismissive, but in the quick exchanges of glances, we spoke to each other in an intimate language that I learned without being taught, that I learned out of necessity.

VII

O thin men of Haddam,
Why do you imagine golden birds?
Do you not see how the blackbird
Walks around the feet
Of the women about you?

Staff meeting. A Thursday noon in March. Several clinicians wrote their names on the whiteboard and listed the names of specific patients for priority discussion.

One of the doctors went first. "So I am considering firing Howard J."

Other medical staff groaned.

"Is he the one who was trying to fondle some of the nurses?" the psychiatrist asked.

"Yup. And who made really inappropriate comments to Mary Jane out at the front desk and who is not taking any of his meds."

I mouthed "fire?" to my new supervisor across the table. She shrugged at me then she voiced it:

"Fire him? How do you fire him?"

The new Medical Director nodded with a frown on her face and said, "His doctor will need to write a letter to him warning him that unless he complies with his medications and behaves appropriately he will no longer be able to receive our services."

"I already did that, like you suggested several weeks ago," the first doctor said.

"Oh, okay. Then he's fired."

Most of the mental health staff remained quiet throughout this exchange as the newly implemented (impromptu?) "firing procedure" unfolded among several of the doctors.

"OK – this brings up a long-standing issue that we need to address. Especially now with our shrinking funding and resources," one of the doctors said. "This is a medical clinic. Patients have to be established with a primary care doctor in order to receive mental health care, right?"

Everyone nodded.

"Well, I feel like fifty percent of my job has become mental health care. Look, I understand that the mental health system in this country is broken, but we can't fix it. It's not our job to fix it."

The nurse practitioner spoke up, "I am certain that I could justify checking someone's blood pressure who is depressed. Doing an HIV test. Checking for tuberculosis. And in the process listening to them and, if necessary, referring them to one of our mental health counselors. Isn't that all part of primary care? There are days when I could actually see more people because of no-shows. I'm not going to turn people away because they present with 'just depression.'"

I watched the Medical Director write a note on her pad about filling the nurse practitioner's open slots.

"Speaking of productivity," the Medical Director said, "we have begun the search for the new mental health lead and we are specifically looking for a candidate who can help us implement a new model of integrated medical and mental health care so we can see more people and are not spending all our time on mental health issues. This is a behaviorist model of treatment – a brief consultative model. It is considered to be a wave of the future."

Side conversations among mental health clinicians and among medical clinicians drowned out the rest of her announcement.

We did not get to the rest of the names on the board.

VIII

I know noble accents
And lucid, inescapable rhythms;
But I know, too,
That the blackbird is involved in what I know.

Two days after the staff meeting transcribed in the previous section all clinicians received the following memo (detailing the proposed new model for mental health care) from the Executive Director and the Medical Director. In response, the mental health staff proposed an alternative model that would respond to the medical staff's increased need for access to mental health practitioners but still protect the process of psychodynamic, client-centered, and humanistic psychotherapy that we were all practicing with our clients – most of whom were long-term trauma survivors dealing with mood disorders, personality disorders, and psychoses in conjunction with chemical dependency. Although we acknowledged a situational usefulness of behavioral interventions, we argued that most of our clients were dealing with such a fractured sense of reality or connection to other humans that this model, as a primary source of treatment, would not address the needs of our patient population – and would, in effect, be inefficient.

Additionally, we argued, 15- or 20-minute sessions could not be billed to Medicare and Medicaid.

We raised these concerns to the Medical Director and the Executive Director but they quickly replied that found that our alternative did not really address the most pressing needs of the clinic.

Thus, the following represented the potential new disciplinary eye of clinic administration:

Operational considerations: a memo

Facility requirements

- Behavioral Health Consultants [aka mental health clinicians] are part of the primary care treatment team and work alongside other providers. They use whatever exam room or office space is available to see patients – and this may be a different office space each visit.
- Behavioral Health Consultants should have access to a work-station for charting, phone calls, and messages.
- If space allows, a room or office centrally located in the treatment pod allows easy access to other providers and lessens barriers that would deter PCPs from referring patients.

Provider/patient ratios

- Six hours of Behavioral Health Consultant time per week is needed for each 1,000 unique users.
- For example, a clinic with a total population of 10,000 unique users would need 1.5 FTE's.

(The algebra in this section of the memo never ceased to confound all clinicians – even those who supported the model.)

Patient flow/appointment scheduling

- The BHC's schedule should be set up in 15-minute intervals (30 minute maximum).
- Stagger scheduled appointments to leave open spaces for "curbside consults" and "warm hand-offs" from PCPs.

- The BHC should have an open-door policy encouraging "on demand" consultations with PCPs at any time during the day.
- When consultation is requested in the middle of a current therapy session, the BHC should make immediate contact with the PCP (by phone or in person), resolve the clinical question within 2–3 minutes, or agree to re-contact the PCP at the end of the current session.
- If necessary, an emergency session can be held on top of the normal consultation schedule.
- The primary goal is for the BHC to extend out as far as possible to take care of a problem if a PCP thinks of making contact.

There was nothing in this final statement that seemed clinically sound; even from my limited experience as a mental health counselor I was rapidly learning that "taking care of a problem" was not my role. And yet, from the language of this memo, I got the distinct impression that the medical staff members were the ones we were supposed to be treating. If the authors had their way, the medical staff would usurp the place (and time) of the patients – who were merely "warm" bodies relegated to the "curbside."

When the new Mental Health Lead was hired in late February and began in early March, I could feel a collective "bracing" among the mental health staff. She immediately implemented a new policy that gave the front desk unrestricted access to our EPIC "appointment desks" so they could schedule in our open slots. But we still maintained access to the books as well and could block out times for charting and enter in our recurring appointments. None of us was expected to do twenty-minute consultations; she would "take care of that sort of thing for the time being." We did not like the fact that the front desk had such access to our schedules, but "at least we're not getting the "brief consultative model," we sighed with relief.

This became something of a mantra. Even when the Mental Health Lead started arbitrarily auditing our charts and leaving terse emails for us or, in one case, post-it notes in the charts requiring revisions to the treatment plans, even when we felt ourselves being constantly surveilled by means of EPIC ("I was looking at your appointment book today and I noticed . . ."), we repeated, "At least it's not the Brief Consultative Model."

It wasn't until the announcement that "in the near future patients will be restricted to every-other-week sessions and will be cut off after fifteen sessions" and that non-Medicare (self-paying) patients (including those who were homeless and "outside" the system) would have to start paying $66 per psychotherapy session, that it became more difficult to continue breathing that sigh of relief.

IX

When the blackbird flew out of sight,
It marked the edge
Of one of many circles.

Once a year the clinic closed at noon to observe an all-staff clinic ritual: the annual reading from the clinic's "Book of the Dead." On this day the lead social worker sat in a folding chair right in front of the reception desk with a spiral notebook on his lap, the rest of us sat facing him in the waiting room chairs.

Because there had been such rapid turnover in staff throughout the preceding months (due to the Executive Director's "housecleaning" layoffs throughout the fall, and to the response on the part of other staff members who feared for their own jobs or who were so deflated by arbitrary disciplinary measures that they quit), he introduced and explained the annual ritual in which we were all about to take part.

"Every year we make some space to honor members of our community who have died in the past year. I will say each name and then we should all feel free to speak our memories of any of these individuals." He read a list of about thirty to forty names, pausing for a few beats after each name. Throughout this process, sporadically someone would draw in his or her breath upon hearing a specific name; someone would say softly, "Oh no! Really?" or "I just saw him a few weeks ago!" upon hearing another. There was a collective sighing sound when he came to the end of the list.

For the next forty-five minutes, names got attached to stories – stories that began with the smallest of details: "Who could forget John A. Some days, he would sit right at the end of the reception desk all day, greeting people as they walked in – he wouldn't even have an appointment, but it was rainy or he was tired. He became kind of a fixture here," Linda said, smiling. This initial story would set off a sequence of stories: "Did anyone know that John A. was a professional kazoo player?" one of the doctors said.

"Yes! I used to hear him down at the park – Did you know that he was on David Letterman once?" a social worker added.

The stories continued as staff members who have been in the clinic long enough added their memories or comments like, "*That's* John A.? I never knew his name but I always really liked seeing that guy sitting there."

As the room quieted, someone introduced another name and another set of stories emerged.

When the hour was up, we all dispersed uncharacteristically quietly to our respective stations and wings of the clinic.

That was in January. Months later the social worker and I sat drinking a beer at a nearby pub after work. It was the last week of April and I was nearing the last month of my internship. He seemed more relaxed than I had seen him all year. We met just two weeks after the Clinic's Board of Directors announced the termination, effective immediately, of the Executive Director and we swapped stories about this momentous change of course. But I was looking for a particular kind of story that day: a history.

In the seventies he worked for Mental Health Task Force helping to direct resources into the needs of the downtown homeless community – which at the time was reeling from the de-institutionalization of the mentally ill. He remembered, "All the down and outers on 'skid-row' – who were themselves not so healthy – would talk to me and say, 'Where did all these nuts come from?'" He and another colleague, in the late seventies, raised money and located a site for the clinic, which opened its doors in 1978.

"At the time, the mission of the mental health department (and the clinic in general)," he continued, "was to help connect the core of these people's beings back to the humane. Our patients are nomads on so many levels of their beings, without any 'ekos' – you know the Greek word? – it means home and economy; they are without home and without money. Our patients are butchered, battered, and bereft. They are people whose hurts come from a lack of love, lack of respect, and lack of economics. . . . There is a profound spiritual dimension to what our legacy holds."

He looked me straight in the eye and said, "In the last nine months you have witnessed one of the most wrenching, unpleasant, disastrous periods the clinic has experienced in the last twenty-five years. The technocratic mentality of the now-former Executive Director threatened to disconnect us from the humane legacy, history, and culture of this clinic. I wonder to what extent we can bring back the ethos, the 'ekos,' now that he's gone?"

The social worker reminded me that the ethos of the clinic, like Stevens's blackbird, is never really out of sight even when it seemed that we were "losing sight" or losing perspective. The clinic was also the rituals of history making; the clinic, as the Day of the Dead reminded me, was involved in the very existential beingness of staff and patients alike.

X

At the sight of blackbirds
Flying in a green light,
Even the bawds of euphony
Would cry out sharply.

I had seen Richard K., the 50-year old man who became the subject of the "stomach meds conversation," every week since September. After months of the rigidity and repetition that characterized our sessions, I realized that I was dreading our sessions, that I was constantly in search of a *plan*, a *technique*, something, anything to break through the patterns of obsession and compulsion in which, eventually we were both taking part. The more I searched for tools, I realize in retrospect, the more I found myself, as Stern (1997) puts it, "in the grip of the field" (p. 192). The field to which Stern specifically refers here is the interpersonal field between patient and therapist in which both participants "create, and until it is discovered (over and over again), maintain the states of relatedness that brought the patient to [therapy]" (p. 192). Richard wanted to be "cured" of whatever was keeping him from "making interpersonal connections and from making $100,000" (the two goals he articulated over and over whenever we would revisit his treatment plan). As I searched for this man, for some empathic access to him, I met with wall after wall of repeated phrases and such black/white goals and expectations of therapy.

I got to the point where I would question every question I posed, every activity I "assigned" in terms of its practical efficacy. At some point during each session, Richard would ask me, "Is this going to help? Will this give you a better understanding of my problem? Will this help you fix what's wrong with me?"

Richard would walk from the lobby to my office, head down. If we met another person along the way he would startle and curse under his breath. He would enter my office, sit in his chair and cover the sides of his face with his hands – blocking me out of his field of vision and obscuring any visual access I might have to his face. Then he would rock incessantly in his chair. Perhaps I was "in the grip of the field" because it felt as if there were *no* interpersonal field in those sessions. Between two o'clock and three o'clock every Friday, I felt that I had never before been so isolated. The life of the clinic receded from my consciousness as, what had become a mutual search for an "answer," a "solution," sucked the air and light out of the room.

During our first session, he told me that, although he had been in therapy for almost ten years, up to this point no one had been able to understand him or to help him. He told me that he was "just existing, not living." He was skeptical of my abilities and my potential for insight and each week we ended the session with him saying, "I guess I'll come back for one more week, and then we'll see."

We would sit at a forty-five degree angle and Richard would shield his face and rock. Some days he was sullen and quiet, answering my questions (as I tried to keep the desperation out of my voice) in one-word responses. Other days, he would speak in cliché phrases. I would ask Richard questions about his previous therapy and his relationships with his family members and his responses came to sound tape-recorded (some of which I recognized verbatim from the chart notes covering those ten previous years). There were about a dozen such pronouncements and I got to the point where I could say them verbatim to myself.

So after about three months, I did. He had recently written his father a letter and was spending every session obsessing about what he would say if his father called him. Feeling more than a little nervous, I suggested that we role-play the conversation. I would play his father first, and then we would switch roles. I remember little of the actual content of the role-play. What stood out for me then, and now, was the palpable shift I felt in Richard. During the role-play, his hands dropped from his face into his lap and he looked me straight in the eyes. As I played his father (based on the many and repeated turns of phrase and clichés he had fed me), I saw the hint of a smile pass across his face. As we switched roles, he deftly moved in and out of character with grace and ease, varied his speech to connote different characters, and flashed me a victorious grin when he played his father and I broke out of character once to say, "Man, he is *tough!*"

Gadamer (1998) argues that, "Every experience worthy of the name thwarts an expectation" (p. 356) and that through "real experience" we discover "the limits of power and the self-knowledge of [our] planning reason" (p. 357). Although, on one level, I had been listening to (and expecting) seemingly tape-recorded repetition from Richard, I heard, during this role-play, that there was always more to hear. Playing his father, in an unscripted and unplanned way, Richard and I would share a lived experience. I could become more curious about Richard's responses; what did I (as his father) need to say to him to provoke what had felt like his default hostile, defensive stance? I developed an image of us (as Richard and his father) standing in opposite corners of the ring, coming together to hurl accusations, then retreating to build up more power with which to deliver the next round of blows.

As we transitioned out of the role-play, I heard resonances of my own defensiveness in our sessions. Had we been standing in opposite corners? As Richard hurled expectations (and questions of my competence) at me, was I defending and retreating into technique rather than really listening to him? As he tried to convince me over and over of his helplessness and hopelessness was I trying to convince him otherwise and thus not hearing beneath the repetition to a profound sadness and fear?

Jessica Benjamin (1990) describes these moments of oppositionality in the therapy relationship in terms of a "collapsing of the space of intersubjectivity":

> Characteristically, the dynamic pattern of interaction includes a collapse of the space in which it is possible to think, to work with the difference between my view and yours. In this all too familiar and yet compelling dynamic we are often aware of the felt negation of our or the other's subjectivity. . . . The intersubjective level aims to transform differences from the register of power, in which one partner asserts his or her meaning, will, need over the other . . . to an understanding of the meaning of the struggle . . . the chief commitment of psychoanalysis is to release the psychic hold of the power struggle and to establish the commitment to recognition, the dialogic process itself.
>
> (pp. 203–204)

The role-play was able to open up space for metacommunication where we could look together at the roles we had played (as Richard and his father) and, slowly, tentatively, to look at the parallels between the role-play and our own interactions. We could move into a collaborative space, rather than more deeply into a combative space and, thus, hear beneath the content of our words.

One day, after several weeks of role-playing, I felt as if we were ready to face each other as each other again. I suggested that it was time to put his father in his place (he had been taking up most of our time in sessions) and, it amuses me now to recall, we both automatically looked at the potted plant in the corner of the office. "There?" I asked. He nodded mutely.

The next week he was sullen, his hands covering his face, which was already shadowed by a large-brimmed baseball cap. Mid-way through the session, I noticed pancake make-up around his right eye and a large purple bruise emerging underneath. When I asked him about it, he pulled his hands in tighter around his face and denied anything was different. Finally, I said, "Richard, I see a bruise under the make-up. I also see that you don't want me to see. But, I am wondering if you hurt yourself."

He looked at me then and said, "Okay, I might as well tell you the truth. I smacked myself after I lost my stomach meds and had to get a refill. I guess the cat's out of the bag now."

I thought about his earlier plea for someone to "really know me" and it seemed that he had desperately wanted me to see beneath the make-up, to see how much pain he was in. Richard told me that when he gets angry with himself – which is whenever he loses or breaks something – he hits himself in the face and swears at himself. I wondered out loud if he was taking up where his father left off. "Can others lose and break things without deserving such harsh punishment?" I asked. He said, "Yes." When I asked him why he did not allow himself room for human error, he said, "A series of small fuck-ups leads to one fucked-up person."

I was so struck by the extent to which Richard continued to "see himself" through his father's disdainful gaze – a gaze he had so internalized that he worked to eradicate his own face by covering it or damaging it with his own hands. Winnicott (1971) writes that "Psychotherapy . . . is a long-term giving the patient back what the patient brings. It is a complex derivative of the face that reflects what is there to be seen" (p. 117). Mirroring back, according to Winnicott, is a way to give the patient the space to find his or her own self, and . . . to be able to exist and to feel real. Feeling real is more than exist-ing; it is finding a way to exist as oneself, and to relate to objects as oneself, and to have a self into which to retreat for relaxation.

(p. 117)

I had been seeing Richard, but I had not been showing him *that* I was seeing or *what* I was seeing.

And that day he wanted to make absolutely certain that I would see. Suddenly, in an abrupt, but clearly habitual movement, his clenched fists (first his right, then his left) delivered strong blows to either side of his face. I heard the dull and sickening thud of knuckles on cheekbones before I even registered visually what he was doing. "There, you can see how I actually do it," he said.

I felt sick to my stomach and I felt tears welling up from somewhere deep below my throat. But he had become suddenly analytical: "Do you know others who hurt themselves?" he asked. Somehow, I talked rationally with him for a minute about people who are feeling so much internal/emotional pain that one way they try to manage it is to externalize it by hitting themselves. He said, "Yes, I guess that makes sense." We sat in silence. I wanted very much to reason him out of self-destruction, to argue and to analyze us to a safer place – but then I pictured us retreating back to our corners, gearing up for the next round of blows, and the consequences of falling into this same pattern seemed so much more dire, so much more literal.

Benjamin (1990) looks at the "creative, even desperate, acts the analyst may take in the interaction to restore intersubjective space" including "speaking – 'acting' – in such a way that we manage to bring our sub-jectivity back into place forcefully yet carefully enough to create externality" (p. 205). We had managed to do this before through "acting" (role-playing); this time, I drew from a deep felt response that was mine. I shared with him that seeing him hit himself gave me a pain deep in my stomach. "Right here," I pointed. I told him that it made me feel so much sadness to see him hurting so deeply that he feels he deserves such punishment.

He looked at me and I could see that same hint of a smile behind his eyes. Then he stated just as ration-ally that his life felt like a "living hell" and he wondered sometimes if he should even exist. When I asked him if he thought he was suicidal, he said no. He said that he was still holding out "some hope" that he would feel better some day and, besides, he said, "I am apparently in above-average physical health, no chronic diseases, so that is something to be grateful for."

That session occurred sometime in the middle of the year and was probably the session in which we most directly encountered one another. We would periodically connect and then he would retreat again into his repetitive phrases and I into my anxious searching for a method.

Toward the end of the year as I started counting down our final ten sessions, he informed me that he would not be at our next session because he had scheduled a doctor's appointment during our time. I told him that I would keep our hour open and that he could come late and then I stood, perhaps a little open-mouthed, as he walked out the door. This would be the first time that Richard would not show up at 2:00 on the dot. (Sometimes, in looking at the check-in screen on EPIC, I would notice that he would arrive up to forty minutes early for our appointments. Was this his reaction to my leaving? Maybe, I was secretly hoping, he was acting out. At least then I could say that he was having a reaction to me.)

The day became significant not just because of his uncharacteristic schedule change. At 2:00 the next week I walked out in the lobby to find Richard waiting, still, for the nurse to get him prepped for his doctor's visit. He was frustrated, irritated, explaining that this was the only time he could get an appoint-ment with his doctor and it was conflicting with our session and that was "pissing [him] off." So I sat in the waiting room with him while he waited. It was "our" scheduled time; it seemed like the right place to be. I watched him shield his face from the others in the lobby and I moved closer to him in what felt like a protective gesture. I wanted to believe that I could and should somehow insulate him from the world around him – particularly this one of discipline and surveillance.

Even as I worked to shrink Richard's and my world, the clinic's historic uniqueness had been draw-ing outside attention all year, especially with then-President George W. Bush's new Medicare plan in the drafting phases. The clinic had become a site of surveillance, co-opted in the service of various competing political agendas on a state and national scale. On that particular day as I sat with Richard in what felt like the already-too-big lobby, a US Congressman and his entourage walked into the clinic, wholly unannounced. Richard had been looking at me but now he locked his hands firmly around his face and began to rock a little. I sat and watched him, telling him that I wanted to sit with him until the nurse called him and that I would wait in my office for him after his appointment. I looked up to see the politician watching us.

Richard came back to my office with about twenty minutes left in our session. (Just as I closed the door, the Congressman's entourage entered the mental health section of the clinic, on an impromptu tour. I could hear one of the administrators speaking loudly of the role of the mental health department. Knowing what I knew of this administrator and his investment in strategic changes, I was resentful, distracted, and suspicious.) Richard blocked my view of his face and rocked. He had not done this in my office in a long time. But, was that true? It seemed like he had been looking me straight in the face for months – I was sure of it. He answered my questions abruptly, perfunctorily, resentfully mostly with, "I don't knows."

(Meanwhile, I found myself trying to eavesdrop on the Congressman. Would he take note of the cramped conditions? Of the diversity of clients walking through here? What kind of effect could he have on the state's community mental health resources? On individuals like Richard?) Richard. I was back again. And we had seven weeks left. What were we going to do? How could we make something of our goodbye?

I heard him saying, "Nothing has helped me. I just want you to understand me." As I heard his statement break through the din of my questions and the fog of distraction that the politician's presence brought, I felt a wave of sadness, followed quickly by a very familiar feeling of impotence when I realized that our time was running out.

XI

He rode over Connecticut
In a glass coach.
Once, a fear pierced him,
In that he mistook
The shadow of his equipage
For blackbirds.

Richard started putting his hands down – yes, I remember now – around the time that we started role-playing and discovering his theatrical talents. I learned things about him that I never imagined I would know – things like what he looks like when he is on the verge of smiling, like how good he is at imitating voices, like how quickly he can shift in and out of character. I learned a lot about his past, particularly his relationship with his father. I learned that he punches himself in the face (although I don't think he did it again after the episode in my office). But did I understand him? If I understood him, maybe I would have known how to say goodbye. If I understood him, maybe I would have known how he needed to say goodbye. Or maybe understanding him meant really getting that he "doesn't make social connections" – as he told me again and again. I even imagined role-playing a goodbye with him. But then I wondered, would I just have been doing it for me – to role-play what it would have been like to have been seen by my patient as someone with whom he might possibly have connected?

If I really had understood him, wouldn't I have remembered – the moment that the Congressman walked into the clinic – the recurring dreams he had been telling me since September? In the dream he is walking through the first house he lived in as a young boy. He is both a boy and a man and he is moving from room to room in the house trying to make sure that everything is just exactly as it used to be – that every piece of furniture, every detail is exactly in place. He feels comforted when he finds the familiarity but also anxiety that he will discover something out of place. He eventually moves to the basement, which is a 1950s style rec room. Now he is firmly a child, standing two feet shorter than all the adults who crowd the room. The adults are politicians – important people. He cannot be seen or heard above the pronouncements. He suddenly feels lost, alone.

When the Congressman walked into the clinic that day, I was trying to help Richard narrow his field of vision – to "protect him," I felt. So determined was I that I, like him, began to block out the world around us. I had wanted to create a world for him in my office, one space in which he could be safely seen and insulated from all that frightened him in the world. Instead, I had at various times, gotten lost in the tiny claustrophobic world of a shared fear and anxiety that he would not be "cured." Rather than being separate-but-connected beings, we had at times collapsed into his very limited field of vision where everything must be the same. How could I ever actually have protected him or presumed that this was what he needed?

There are always politicians in the basement, politicians who infiltrate the walls of familiarity, politicians who speak in promises: of solutions, of money, and achieving goals that lay far outside the realm of Richard's extremely tenuous and fractured self. Politicians who, in their very posture, promise something beyond. Until I worked in this clinic, at this particular moment in the clinic's history, I wanted to believe in the possibility, and the efficacy, of creating a kind of insulated safe space between patient and therapist – which was really a collapsing of space. The clinic reminded me, in very real ways (frustrating and enervating ways, celebratory and energizing ways), of the vital importance of opening up *the space between* my patients and to allow in the tension of difference and to live out sincerely the promise of mutual recognition or, in Gadamer's terms, a shared real experience.

XII

The river is moving.
The blackbird must be flying.

Clay and I finally took our first walk outside of the clinic together in April. And somehow, but not surprisingly, a number of the clinic staff knew about it by the time Clay walked into the lobby that Thursday morning. My new supervisor touched my elbow in the hallway as I walked past the Mental Health Lead's office to meet him. She said, "I hear you and Clay are walking today. Treat this session as a systematic desensitization exercise." I nodded, wondering if she was telling me this now (and in this relatively 'public' space) for the benefit of the Mental Health Lead and the increasingly standardized treatment plan policy or if she was registering my own anxiety about Clay and me broadening our field, and, perhaps feeling some of her own anxiety.

"You're going for a walk with a client?" The Mental Health Lead stepped out of her office.

"He's agoraphobic," my supervisor responded.

I left them talking with each other as I went to find Clay.

I could feel Linda at the front desk, and other patients in the lobby watch us leave.

As we began the steep walk down to the first set of elevators that would carry us down to (but, alas, not, as we had fantasized months before, along) the waterfront, the voices of my supervisor and the Mental Health Lead resonated in my head. I tried to anchor our movement in "technique" by periodically and diligently asking Clay (as we got into the elevator, got out of the elevator, crossed train tracks, and stopped traffic at the crosswalk), "How is this feeling?" – uncertain about what I was supposed to do with his responses.

Once we got to the waterfront, Clay pointed ahead of us to a tall metal structure sticking up out of the water amidst piers and creosote pilings. I had always wondered about this structure; it had been erected around the same time the waterfront suddenly sprouted new luxury condominiums and hotels in the late nineties. During that same period in the city's history, I had been working on my dissertation for my doctorate in American literature and had spent considerable time walking along this stretch of waterfront, ostensibly taking a break from my work, but studying and lamenting the various construction projects that seemed to be anesthetizing the waterfront, I never knew quite what to make of this obelisk-like structure Clay was pointing to now.

Clay, standing beside me, spoke the same words I had muttered sarcastically many times during that period of writing and walking: "Objet d'art." We turned and smiled at each other – and I felt a kind of mutual recognition between us.

At that moment, I lost track of "technique" and looked around at the expanded context in which we were moving together – a context in which my history and his history could somehow intersect in their difference. (I remembered that Clay would have been homeless, suicidal, drinking and struggling to survive down here on the streets during the years I was using this space in my struggle against doctoral student writer's block).

Rather than continuing to ask him questions that seemed congruent with his diagnosis as "phobic" and my attendant clinical justification for being out on the waterfront with him on this misty spring day, I began asking him, "What are you seeing?"

As we walked Clay drew a rich history of the waterfront in which he had occupied an ever-shifting place over the past twenty years. He pointed to the thirty-foot sailboats he used to sail before he had had psychotic breaks. We sat to rest on the very park bench where he used to sleep at night when he became homeless and suicidal. He told me that he was feeling safe, "protected" by me, and yet, rather than feeling like a maternal protective force, I had this interesting sense of walking with a benevolent elder who was guiding *me* through his city, which was also my city but was becoming a different city altogether through our shared experience.

When we returned to my office that day, I reminded him that we had only a few weeks left before my departure and he said, "I was thinking that I would like to continue therapy. I have also realized that I would like to see someone who will continue to feel motherly to me – that's something I think I've never really had until now."

As our field had broadened – psychologically, emotionally, and, indeed, geographically – it had also become imbued with a shared intersubjective sense of safety. He no longer felt like "the clinic's" to me and he was speaking in terms of *his* choices and *his* desires. Orange, Atwood, and Stolorow (1997) write that,

> The intersubjective field of the analysis, made possible by the emotional availability of both analyst and patient, becomes a developmental second chance for the patient. New more flexible organizing principles can emerge, now accessible to reflection, so that the patient's experiential repertoire becomes enlarged, enriched, and more complex.
>
> (p. 8)

The emotional availability we shared seemed to unfold through, in Jessica Benjamin's (1990) terms, "a reopening of intersubjective space" to a "third" (p. 205). She describes this "third" as intrinsic to establishing an intersubjective space, which restores "recognition" and "creative tension" after the collapsing that occurs when one person's subjectivity seems to be at stake. Instead, we had each found a space in which to play and to reopen our intersubjective space: "it is as if we were sight-reading an unknown score. We make it up as we go, yet it feels as though we are oriented to something outside. It feels discovered as well as invented" (Benjamin, p. 206).

When it felt as if there were no room in the clinic in which to explore new possibilities for authentic being, Clay and I had moved outside.

XIII

It was evening all afternoon.
It was snowing
And it was going to snow.
The blackbird sat
In the cedar limbs.

There are as many ways of leaving a clinic as looking at it. Leaving is, in fact, simply another way of looking – not an ending, but a speculation.

"When I first saw you," Matthew, one of the Friday group members told me during our third-to-last session, "I thought you were some snooty professor lady who got bored of her university job. I could not imagine what you were doing here and what you thought of us. It seemed like this was a really big step down for you. I bet you won't ever even come back downtown once you leave here." As he spoke, I found myself getting hooked into the stereotype he had drawn (and thus his rejection) because it seemed to hold out the promise now of a revisioning (a recognition): "I used to think this way about you, now I know better." However, somehow, in those few statements, he deftly moved from the caricature that he had initially drawn of me (as a "snooty" outsider) to a reiteration of the caricature (you may have stepped inside and stayed for a little while but now you will go back to being an outsider). And so when he relegated me to the outside, I was caught off-guard, a little lost in my own urge to self-defend, until I told him that I had been afraid at first that I would never actually be invited inside. In the end of group that day, Matthew reminded me that he was going to give me a sketch on my last day – as sketch that, as it turned out, he was making of me. I wondered that day what I would look like.

After that group, Kate, my co-leader, and I talked. We talked about Matthew and his many and varied distancing mechanisms. Over a period of less than ten years, he lost every one of his family members. He does not want to have to experience loss, we speculate. Then Kate told me that she is feeling a particular kind of loss and regret in thinking about my departure. "We have spent so much time dealing with all the upheavals in the clinic this year that I feel like we have not spent as much time as we could have in clinical consultation – in really exploring all the ways we could have worked together as group co-leaders. We have really used the clinic as a distraction, I think. That's kind of a shame. I wish we could have been having different kinds of conversations throughout the year." I left that conversation feeling something akin to what I felt with Matthew – as if something, some ground that I had been exploring, learning to navigate, over the period of the last nine months, had just been pulled out from under me.

In the second-to-last Friday group session, Patty reached under the table and pulled out a hand-made afghan ("African") and handed it across the table to me, saying my name for the first time all year. "I didn't wrap it." I had no words. I stood up and moved over to her side of the table to hug her; she let me give her a half hug but she was already turning and then she was out the door. "This is my last day of group," she said to Kate as she walked into the hallway and out the staff door of the clinic.

I met with Richard K. that same afternoon. "Is this our last session?" he asked, face a little red as he walked in the door.

"No, we have one more next week."

"I have some really bad news. This will make you really sad. I had a follow-up appointment with the psychiatrist and she told me that I am clinically depressed. That means *chronically* depressed. She wants me to take anti-depressant medication."

The sentence "This will make you really sad" echoed through my head even as I asked him questions about his follow-up appointment with her and fought off the urge to argue with him about the difference between "chronically" and "clinically." He told me that they had a thirty-minute appointment scheduled, she asked him how depressed he felt on a scale of zero to ten, he said six or seven, she diagnosed him, prescribed for him, then sent him away. "After *twenty* minutes," he added.

I suddenly wondered if the problem with a *chronic* diagnosis is that people stop listening. After I shared this with him, he looked straight into my eyes, and told me things he has never told me before about the ways in which his parents abused him, and the ways he responded. "They would start whispering to each other whenever I walked into the room, so I started doing things like taking my dinner plate out to the picnic table and eating there, even in the middle of winter."

I was so struck by this image that I laughed in disbelief. Then I said, "I'm not laughing at you, I am laughing because you had such a brilliant response to their horrifying behavior."

He said to me, simply, directly, "I know you are not laughing at me."

That night I dreamed that I was getting on a small plane to take a "regional flight." Richard was standing next to me and he put his arm around my shoulders. "Why won't you lean on me?" he asked, a little demanding. I said, "Because it was never like that. I must have given you the wrong idea." I turned back as I boarded the plane, and I saw that he looked sad, betrayed by a broken promise.

The process of saying goodbye, akin to the process of writing this story, reminds me that both psychotherapy and writing are tactics. What a tactic "wins it cannot keep," de Certeau says (p. 37). When I remember this, I no longer think in terms of breaking my promises or losing my place. The process of psychotherapy is about creating something much more enduring and flexible than promises or places, it is about opening up spaces. It is my hope that this story, rather than closing the book on my internship year, also opens up spaces for further tactical operations within disciplined places or at least spaces for real shared experiences among clinicians and especially between clinicians and patients, even as these places work to inscribe neat definitive conclusions or, in the clinic's parlance, "graduations" and "terminations."

When I reminded Anna, the Clinic Manager, of my imminent departure date, she wrinkled her forehead, said, "Aww. . . . That went by quickly! . . . Oh, wait, does EPIC know you're leaving?" She turned to her computer and I walked away as she worked to terminate my appointment book.

References

Atwood, G., Brandchaft, B., & Stolorow, R. (1987). *Psychoanalytic treatment: An intersubjective approach*. Hillsdale, NJ: The Analytic Press.

Atwood, G. & Stolorow, R. (1984). *Structures of subjectivity: Explorations in psychoanalytic phenomenology*. Hillsdale, NJ: The Analytic Press.

Benjamin, J. (1990). Recognition and destruction: An outline of intersubjectivity. In L. Aron & S. Mitchell (Eds.), *Relational psychoanalysis: The emergence of a tradition* (pp. 181–209). Hillsdale, NJ: Analytic Press, Inc.

Caruth, C. (1995). Recapturing the past: Introduction. In *Trauma: Explorations in memory* (pp. 151–157). Baltimore: Johns Hopkins University Press.

de Certeau, M. (1988). *The practice of everyday life*. Berkeley: University of California Press.

Foucault, M. (1995). *Discipline and punish: The birth of the prison*. New York: Vintage Books.

Gadamer, H. G. (1998). *Truth and method* (2nd rev. ed) (J. Weinsheimer & D. Marshall Trans.). New York: Continuum. (Original work published 1960).

Heidegger, M. (1962). *Being and time*. (Macquarrie & Robinson, Trans.). New York: Harper and Row.

May, R. (1983). *The discovery of being: Writings in existential psychology*. New York: W.W. Norton and Co.

Orange, D., Atwood, G., Stolorow, R. (1997). Intersubjectivity theory and the clinical exchange. In *Working intersubjectively: Contextualism in psychoanalytic practice* (pp. 3–18). Hillsdale, NJ: The Analytic Press.

Stern, D. (1997). The analyst's unformulated experience of the patient. In *Unformulated experience: From dissociation to imagination in psychoanalysis* (pp. 185–201). Hillsdale, NJ: The Analytic Press.

Stevens, W. (1990). Thirteen ways of looking at a blackbird. In H. Stevens (Ed.). *The palm at the end of the mind: Selected poems*. New York: Vintage Books.

Winnicott, D. W. (1971). *Playing and reality*. London: Tavistock Publications.

29

EUDAIMONIC WELL-BEING AND EDUCATION

Denis Francesconi

Introduction

Nowadays, the concept of well-being and its synonyms – quality of life, happiness, health, flourishing, thriving, fulfilling and many others that are listed in the last chapter of this book – can be easily found in popular magazines as well as scientific journals. The increment of this area over the last two decades has led to the creation of what has been called the *science of happiness* (Kahneman *et al.* 1999; Diener 2000; Seppala 2016).

Modern studies on well-being and happiness cover a wide spectrum of scientific investigation, from the biological level (Berridge and Kringelbach 2011; Lewis *et al.* 2014), to the personal level (psychology, Seligman 2013), to the macro level (policy studies and big data, (OECD 2015). The neuroscientific aspect focuses mainly on the pleasure and reward neuronal circuits and how to reinforce, limit or suppress them (Kringelbach and Berridge 2010; Berridge and Kringelbach 2015). The psychological level mostly focuses on the subjective well-being (SWB), its inherited and/or malleable aspects, and its concrete applications (Diener 1984; Diener and Suh 2000). The policy level makes use of big data sets to discover how different factors such as schooling, health or income interact in shaping collective well-being (Costanza *et al.* 2014).

Each of these areas are already vast and well-structured. Educational reflection on happiness and well-being in modern society and science has also been brought forward (White 2007; Suissa 2008) but it does not seem to have reached the same magnitude and critical mass of other disciplines. In order to contribute to the debate within educational science and to suggest a possible approach, this paper relies on the distinction between hedonic and eudaimonic well-being as proposed in the seminal work by Ryan and Decy (2001) and presents the strong historical connection of the latter with education.

In their paper, Decy and Ryan identify a new trend in psychology, called positive psychology, and show how this marks a fundamental switch from a standard psychological approach, usually driven by rehabilitative/re-educational efforts, to more educational ones. In other words, from a position aimed at reconstituting the positive psychophysical states – or at least socially acceptable ones – from negative states, to a position of promoting positive psychophysical states from socially normal or even already positive ones. They affirm that modern psychology should concentrate on the promotion of flourishing and human potential realization (Ryan and Deci 2001, p. 141). A concrete example of this approach is the creation of the *Character Strengths and Virtues: A Handbook and Classification* (Peterson and Seligman 2004). This manual is intended to be a professional tool to support the work of positive psychologists alongside or even beyond the standard psychopathological manuals. It is the positive counterpart to the more traditional Diagnostic and Statistical Manual of Mental Disorders (DSM), which focuses on what can go or has already gone wrong.

This strategic move, from rehabilitation to flourishing as a new field of study and application of psychology – in this case called positive psychology – seems to make sense and to be innovative within psychology itself. In education, however, it makes less sense and is less relevant because, by definition, etymology and history, education and flourishing are synonyms. The terms are tautological. If positive psychology has recently discovered the positive side of the spectrum of human development, this is certainly not new to educational theory. This is probably why, even though a lot of attention has recently been focused on new and sometimes trendy ideas, concepts and words such as well-being, happiness and flourishing, they have received little attention in educational science: they say little to nothing new to educational scientists and professionals since they already belong to educational theory and practice. That does not mean that educational researchers should skip and avoid this contemporary debate. On the contrary, they must be able to tackle it and to build an interdisciplinary dialogue. This only means that in educational research the contemporary debate should be placed within the historical framework to help separate concrete new advances from what is simply terminological renovation. For instance, the birth of what has been called *positive education* (Kristjánsson 2012), following the positive psychology movement, leaves many questions unanswered about epistemological grounding and the methodological and practical novelty of such a new label.

In the next section, I look at the strong connection between eudaimonic well-being (*Eudaimonia*) and education (*Paideia*), suggesting that eudaimonic well-being education must be intended as *care for the self* (*cura sui*) in both ancient and contemporary traditions (Foucault *et al.* 1988; Foucault 2006). I will stress that well-being and flourishing are not necessarily the same – for instance, hedonic well-being does not need to refer to flourishing – and that eudaimonic well-being is intrinsically related to the concepts of self-realization and flourishing, thus being intrinsically educational.

Hedonic vs. eudaimonic well-being

What kind of well-being are we talking about when we talk about well-being? A widely accepted position marks a clear differentiation between hedonic and eudaimonic well-being.

From the etymological point of view, hedonism (*hēdonē*) is generally translated as pleasure, with acceptable extensions to delight and self-indulgence. Theoretically, hedonism can be defined as the culture of pleasure, a way to live, a school of thought, a cultural tradition that supports maximizing pleasure and reducing suffering. This tradition has had important representatives and many followers throughout Western history. Hedonism can be further divided in two sub theories: psychophysical pleasure ("liking") and desire ("wanting"). In the first one, well-being is mostly understood as a short-term, immediate, instinctive, physical and sensorial pleasure to be reached via psychophysical effort. The second one has a motivational component assigned to rewarding stimuli, it is the will, the intention to do something in order to achieve psychophysical pleasure. "Liking", unlike "wanting", is a pleasure immediately gained from consumption or sensorial contact with a stimulus, while the "wanting" of incentive salience is a motivational magnet and can also be merely imaginary. It is the quality of a stimulus that makes it a desirable and attractive goal, transforming it from a mere sensory experience into something that commands attention, induces approach and causes it to be sought out (Berridge and Robinson 1998).

A cigarette for a smoker is a typical example of a hedonic pleasure experience, with the following characteristics: time-space limited, moto-sensorial dimension, often recursive (especially in addictions). Addiction to pleasure is a classic: based first on "I like", then on "I want", finally on "I need", the will of something turns into the need, even if the person may still perceive it as a will, thus agency is deactivated and passivity takes place. At this point the person is dethroned by the needed object. The will to repeat the pleasurable experience causes specific actions, however in the medium-term wanting and liking diverge: wanting persists, liking disappears. In the longer term wanting also disappears and only the need – the *I have to* – remains (Berridge and Robinson 1998).

Even if hedonic pleasure is often at the base of any addiction, not all hedonism ends up becoming an addiction. In certain cases, hedonism can also be elevated to the intellectual level of a kind of self-education – like in Epicurus – and transformed from mindless psychophysical slavery into a philosophy and a way of life; in other cases, it can become a form of aestheticism or bohemian lifestyle. We can cite Marquis de Sade, Oscar Wilde and Gabriele D'Annunzio among the representatives of this kind of hedonism. In this case, happiness as immediate pleasure still plays a crucial role, but is framed within a larger sophisticated intellectual perspective. A famous phrase of Wilde well explains the awareness of intentionally self-induced dependence to pleasure: "I can resist everything except temptation."

The main issue that educational theory must face with hedonic well-being is not pleasure itself or the search for pleasure (all of this can definitely be object of teachings) but the intentional loss of intentionality, command and capacity of self-government typically involved in hedonism as pure pleasure. The intentional loss of intentionality, being among the highest levels of self-development, is not easy to teach and reproduce, so it should be carefully brought into educational discourse and practice. The issue of hedonism-eudaimonia and its difference in connection with self-control and education is well exemplified by Socrates and Callicles in the Gorgias (491–492) (Plato Gorgias):

CALLICLES: *What do you mean by his 'ruling over himself'?*
SOCRATES: *A simple thing enough; just what is commonly said, that a man should be temperate and master of himself, and ruler of his own pleasures and passions.*
CALLICLES: *What innocence! YOU mean those fools – the temperate?*
SOCRATES: *Certainly: anyone may know that to be my meaning.*
CALLICLES: *Quite so, Socrates; and they are really fools, for how can a man be happy who is the servant of anything? On the contrary, I plainly assert, that he who would truly live ought to allow his desires to wax to the uttermost, and not to chastise them; but when they have grown to their greatest he should have courage and intelligence to minister to them and to satisfy all his longings. And this I affirm to be natural justice and nobility. (. . .) Nay, Socrates, for you profess to be a votary of the truth, and the truth is this: that luxury and intemperance and licence, if they be provided with means, are virtue and happiness – all the rest is a mere bauble, agreements contrary to nature, foolish talk of men, nothing worth.*
SOCRATES: *There is a noble freedom, Callicles, in your way of approaching the argument; for what you say is what the rest of the world think, but do not like to say. And I must beg of you to persevere, that the true rule of human life may become manifest. Tell me, then: you say, do you not, that in the rightly-developed man the passions ought not to be controlled, but that we should let them grow to the utmost and somehow or other satisfy them, and that this is virtue?*
CALLICLES: *Yes; I do.*
SOCRATES: *Then those who want nothing are not truly said to be happy?*
CALLICLES: *No indeed, for then stones and dead men would be the happiest of all.*

Letting pleasure and desire rule behaviour is opposed to the eudaimonic approach to well-being. Etymologically, eudaimonia means good spirit (*èu*=good, *dàimōn*=spirit), the good god, which nowadays can be translated as good potential, talent, character or mind. Behaving in a eudaimonic way means behaving for self-realization, for the actualization of one's own potential. It can also be translated as flourishing or thriving. Eudaimonia must be intended as a meaningful, existential, programmatic will or intention to guide present and future action accordingly to self-realization. In this case, very much differently from hedonic well-being, agency, self-control and consciousness not only play the important role of planning behaviour but they are also the target of behaviour itself. This is exactly the opposite of what happens with hedonic pleasure, where there is no temporal horizon except the one for the immediate satisfaction of emergent desire or need. Eudaimonia can be intended as happiness by being *meaningfully engaged into the lived-world*, involved in a significant experience, having existential ends and practical daily goals, looking prospectively at life and not only in a utilitarian and instinctual way. This is the Aristotelian definition of happiness as eudaimonia (Aristotle's *Nicomachean Ethics*) and it is close to what Ryan and Decy call 'life satisfaction' (Ryan and Deci 2001).

Eudaimonic well-being and education

What would an education on happiness be? Aristotle says that

> For this reason also the question is asked, whether happiness is to be acquired by learning or by habituation or some other sort of training, or comes in virtue of some divine providence or again by chance. Now, if there is any gift of the gods to men, it is reasonable that happiness should be god-given, and most surely god-given of all human things, inasmuch as it is the best. But this question would perhaps be more appropriate to another inquiry; happiness seems, however, even if it is not god-sent but comes as a result of virtue and some process of learning or training, to be among the most godlike things; for that which is the prize and end of virtue seems to be the best thing in the world, and something godlike and blessed.
>
> (*Nicomachean Ethics*, 1, 9)

Thus, for Aristotle, happiness is the ultimate 'godlike and blessed' purpose of human existence. From his perspective, as well as in Roman and Christian traditions, happiness can only be acquired through the exercise of virtue, a learning to be well, happiness being the 'prize and end' of virtuous behaviour.

In another passage in his *Nicomachean Ethics*, Aristotle describes happiness and virtue as such:

> the function of man is to live a certain kind of life, and this activity implies a rational principle, and the function of a good man is the good and noble performance of these, and if any action is well performed it is performed in accordance with the appropriate excellence: if this is the case, then happiness turns out to be an activity of the soul in accordance with virtue.
>
> (*Nicomachean Ethics*, 1, 7)

The Aristotelian definition of eudaimonia clarifies how eudaimonic well-being is educational per se. Eudaimonia, indeed, implies an embodied pragmatics of life, a tendency towards self-development, an 'activity of the soul in accordance with virtue'. I want to focus here on the idea that happiness is an activity, an exercise and a practice, while simultaneously being the result one derives from practice, and from conducting a good life. The autotelic and heterotelic natures of happiness coincide in eudaimonia.

Thus, we must look at the problem of how this kind of happiness can be brought into schools (White 2007; Suissa 2008). Here I stress three characteristics that eudaimonic well-being education should have: it must be based on and derived from the concept of care of the self (*cura sui*), have a long temporal dimension (it is projectural), and be based on reflective ethics.

First, I claim that eudaimonic well-being can only be derived by working on oneself as a craftsman (*techne tou biou*, the craft of living) and by taking care of the self (*epimeleia heautou, cura sui*). In this sense, in order to be happy, it is necessary to discover and follow our inclination, potential, talent and to intentionally work on those as if we were the masters of ourselves (Foucault *et al.* 1988; Foucault 2006). This position, however, must not be intended in the form of solipsism. As suggested by Nussbaum and Sen (1993), the possibility to follow one's own talent does not depend exclusively on the subject itself, but also on the socio-ecological niche around the subject that describes the set of chances available to the subject's set of capacities. This entanglement defines the possibilities to reach any result and even any further chance to extend and augment these possibilities. The capability approach, in this sense, is the most concrete and serious attempt to describe happiness as a function of the entanglement of the subject-system capacities. The role of schools in improving students' – and even teachers' – awareness about subject-system entanglement here is crucial and must be further promoted.

While classical and liberal education (Paideia) has always taken seriously into consideration the concept of eudaimonia (Jaeger 1986), the same cannot be said about modern education and school systems where eudaimonic well-being is definitely not at the top of the agenda. Recently, we have witnessed attempts to study students' well-being as part of the well-known Programme for International Student Assessment (PISA) (OECD 2017). While important indications can be derived from such big data sets, it appears to be clear that any effort to uncover human potential through educational diagnosis-evaluation-assessment and then to foster it through mass educational interventions might be reductionist and might miss a crucial point. Eudaimonic happiness occurs while living life, consists in the *exercise of life*, not through successful school performance. It is an existential issue, not a cognitive one. It has to do with the person, not with the brain (not only with the brain). If we agree on the fact that we get to know our talents only by experiencing them in real life, that we craft our life only by living it through our embodied embedded mind, then surely we also need to agree on the urgency of the creation and implementation of different educational approaches, methods and practices (Francesconi and Tarozzi 2012).

Second, eudaimonia is related to a temporally extended perspective. For Aristotle, happiness is a final end or goal that encompasses the totality of one's life. It is not something that can be gained or lost in a few hours or minutes, like a pleasurable sensation. It transcends the immanence of momentaneous situations. Happiness as eudaimonia has a longer temporal dimension than hedonism and is in this way projectual (*pro jectus*, to throw forward), while hedonism has a sort of here-and-now dimension. Hence, eudaimonic well-being is a goal and not a temporary state, it implies a teleology, a tension towards an end. As Aristotle suggests "for as it is not one swallow or one fine day that makes a spring, so it is not one day or a short time that makes a man blessed and happy" (*Nicomachean Ethics* 1, 7).

Third, the idea of good, appropriate, ethical behaviour is contained within the very etymological root of the word eudaimonia: the particle *èu*, indeed, means good. This particle transforms happiness into virtue and also helps to mark the difference from the hedonistic version of happiness. The effort of self-realization cannot solely be understood as a pragmatic tension towards life's goals. The reflective dimension must be also included as a form of constant monitoring of subject-system entanglement and trajectory. Re-flectere means to bend again over the lived experience in order to extract intuitions, meaning and indications for future actions. The ethical, meaningful dimension is not simply within the action itself but emerges from the reconsideration and subsequent planning of actions.

The educational system should be adapted to where it can embrace and promote eudaimonic well-being and its characteristics. When doing that, we need to consider the use of appropriate practices and interventions: for instance, body-mind and contemplative practices (Francesconi 2009), reflective techniques (Schön 1987) or other methods, which do not often appear in school curricula. Teacher education programs, as well, should be redesigned in order to teach teachers basic concepts about happiness and clarify the difference, for instance, between hedonism and eudaimonia. Such teacher education programs should also promote the role of teachers as educators instead of information providers or facilitators, and should transmit competencies for the promotion of their own psychophysical well-being. Moreover, we should also consider changes in school design and instructional design to favour the concept of schools as dynamical ecological niches where *learning to be well* prevails over or at least equalizes with *learning to do* or *learning to know*.

Conclusion

In this chapter, I have remarked on the necessity of an educational approach to contemporary well-being theories, reminding that any educational theory, if really educational, is already charged *de facto* with a well-structured perspective on the topic of happiness. Based on historical philosophical affinity between

Eudaimonia (happiness) and Paideia (education), I have proposed a reflection on eudaimonic well-being compared to hedonistic well-being, suggesting that the first one possesses more historical connections with education-paideia. With this being said, it is important that educational applications of hedonic well-being should also be further investigated.

I suggest that a deeper discussion on the issue of eudaimonic well-being and contemporary education is needed to avoid both colonization from other disciplines – 'neurofication' or 'psychologization' – and reductionism, due to a mere hedonistic or performance-based conception of happiness.

Happiness as eudaimonia is the exercise of virtue, is virtue in practice, is the crafting of the self, and this kind of exercise is a form of learning to live – in this case learning to live *well* – which deserves more attention and should be better supported in contemporary education systems.

References

Berridge, K.C. and Kringelbach, M.L., 2011. Building a neuroscience of pleasure and well-being. *Psychology of Well-Being*, 1 (1), 1–3.

Berridge, K.C. and Kringelbach, M.L., 2015. Pleasure systems in the brain. *Neuron*, 86 (3), 646–664.

Berridge, K.C. and Robinson, T.E., 1998. What is the role of dopamine in reward: Hedonic impact, reward learning, or incentive salience? *Brain Research Reviews* [online], 28 (3), 309–369. Available from: www.sciencedirect.com/science/article/pii/S0165017398000198.

Costanza, R., Kubiszewski, I., Giovannini, E., Lovins, H., McGlade, J., Pickett, K.E., Ragnarsdóttir, K., Roberts, D., De Vogli, R., and Wilkinson, R., 2014. Development: Time to leave GDP behind. *Nature News*, 505 (7483), 283.

Diener, E., 1984. Subjective well-being. *Psychological Bulletin*, 95 (3), 542–575.

Diener, E., 2000. Subjective well-being: The science of happiness and a proposal for a national index. *The American Psychologist*, 55 (1), 34–43.

Diener, E. and Suh, E.M., 2000. *Culture and subjective well-being*. Cambridge, MA: MIT Press.

Foucault, M., 2006. *The hermeneutics of the subject: Lectures at the Collège de France, 1981–1982*. New York, NY: Picador.

Foucault, M., Martin L.H., Gutman, H., and Hutton, P.H., 1988. *Technologies of the self: A seminar with Michel Foucault / edited by Luther H. Martin, Huck Gutman, Patrick H. Hutton*. London: Tavistock.

Francesconi, D., 2009. Embodied mind between education and cognitive sciences. *The International Journal of Interdisciplinary Social Sciences: Annual Review*, 4 (10), 19–28.

Francesconi, D. and Tarozzi, M., 2012. Embodied education. *Studia Phaenomenologica*, 12, 263–288.

Jaeger, W., 1986. *Paideia: The ideals of Greek culture / by Werner Jaegar; translated from the second German edition by Gilbert Highet. Vol. 1, Archaic Greece, the mind of Athens*. 2nd ed. New York, NY, Oxford: Oxford University Press.

Kahneman, D., Diener, E., and Schwartz, N., 1999. *Well-being: The foundations of hedonic psychology*. New York: Russell Sage Foundation.

Kringelbach, M.L., and Berridge, K.C., 2010. The functional neuroanatomy of pleasure and happiness. *Discovery Medicine*, 9 (49), 579–587.

Kristjánsson, K., 2012. Positive psychology and positive education: Old wine in new bottles? *Educational Psychologist*, 47 (2), 86–105.

Lewis, G.J., Kanai, R., Rees, G., Bates, T.C., 2014. Neural correlates of the 'good life': Eudaimonic well-being is associated with insular cortex volume. *Social Cognitive and Affective Neuroscience* [online], 9 (5), 615–618. Available from: http://scan.oxfordjournals.org/content/9/5/615.short.

Nussbaum, M. and Sen, A., 1993. *The quality of life*. Oxford: Oxford University Press.

OECD, 2015. *How's life? 2015*. Paris: OECD Publishing.

OECD, 2017. *PISA 2015 results (Volume III)*. Paris: OECD Publishing.

Peterson, C. and Seligman, M.E.P., 2004. *Character strengths and virtues: A handbook and classification / Christopher Peterson & Martin E.P. Seligman*. Washington, DC: American Psychological Association; Oxford: Oxford University Press.

Ryan, R.M. and Deci, E.L., 2001. On happiness and human potentials: a review of research on hedonic and eudaimonic well-being. *Annual Review of Psychology*, 52, 141–166.

Schön, D.A., 1987. *Educating the reflective practitioner*. San Francisco, CA: Jossey-Bass.

Seligman, M.E.P., 2013, ©2011. *Flourish: A visionary new understanding of happiness and well-being*. New York, Toronto: Free Press.

Seppala, E., 2016. *The happiness track: How to apply the science of happiness to accelerate your success*. New York, NY: Harper-One, an imprint of HarperCollinsPublishers.

Suissa, J., 2008. Lessons from a new science? On teaching happiness in schools. *Journal of Philosophy of Education*, 42 (3–4), 575–590.

White, J., 2007. Wellbeing and education: Issues of culture and authority. *Journal of Philosophy of Education*, 41 (1), 17–28.

Acknowledgments

The author was supported by Fondazione Cassa di Risparmio di Trento e Rovereto.

30

EIGHTEEN KINDS OF WELL-BEING ALTHOUGH THERE MAY BE MANY MORE

A conceptual framework illustrated with practical direction for caring

Kathleen T. Galvin and Les Todres

Our bodies know what well-being is. We recognise well-being in many different forms and nuances when it is present, and recognise its absence in suffering. When asked the question 'how are you?', if we take a moment, as human beings, we can sense very concretely our state of well-being or otherwise, even if we are not able to find the best words to say all of it. This experiential sense of well-being can be articulated in many different ways, as indicated by many chapters in this volume. The task of a previous chapter (Todres & Galvin, Chapter 8) introduced a theory of well-being as 'Dwelling-mobility', and attempted to capture the range of well-being experiences within a coherent existential whole. We asked the question: what is it about the essence of well-being that makes all kinds of well-being possible? Guided by Mugerauer (2008) and drawing on Heidegger's later work on homecoming (for example, Heidegger, 1959/1966, 1969/1973, 1971/1993, 1971, 1977) we articulated the deepest experience of well-being as a unity of dwelling and mobility. In this earlier philosophically focused chapter we indicated how our well-being theory was inspired by a particular interpretation of Heidegger (Mugerauer, 2008), an interpretation that considers the trajectory of Heidegger's work as a whole including both the continuities and discontinuities of his earlier and later works. This interpretation was central to our more applied concerns about the phenomenon of well-being. Here we also followed Heidegger in the *Zollikon Seminars* (Heidegger et al., 2000) in which an ontological level of analysis is seen to have important potentially practical ontic insights for our everyday lives. It is in this spirit that we have attempted to translate these ideas into its consequences for understanding human well-being and the practical implications this may have for caring science.

Mobility or a sense of movement describes all the ways that one can have access to the feeling of possibility. Metaphorically we can describe it as a sense of adventure, a sense of moving into wider horizons, 'a new dawn'. The essence of mobility

> lies in all the ways in which we are called into the existential possibilities of moving forward with time, space, others, mood and our bodies. We could say that it is a kind of Eros or energy that can give a feeling of flow, a sense of aliveness and vibrant movement.
>
> (Todres & Galvin, Chapter 8, p. 84, this volume)

By dwelling, we mean a sense of 'at homeness' with what has been given. There is a sense of rootedness, of settling into what is there, a 'letting be' and a certain peaceful attunement. The essence of dwelling lies in all the ways that we existentially 'come home' to what we have been given in time, space, others, mood and our bodies. The feeling of this 'coming home' is one of acceptance, 'rootedness' and peace. In our previous chapter we elaborated these two dimensions of dwelling and mobility as separate kinds of well-being in their own right, but also considered how the deepest possibility of well-being was best expressed as a paradoxical unity of dwelling and mobility, what we called 'dwelling-mobility'.

In dwelling-mobility, there is both 'the adventure' of being called into existential possibilities as well as 'the being at home with' what has been given. It carries with it a sense of rootedness and flow, peace and possibility. In dwelling-mobility there is an integration of peace and possibility or stillness and movement.

A typology of well-being

We have indicated previously that the unity of dwelling-mobility has within it a sense of both mobility and dwelling. Thus experiences of possibility and peace, flow and rootedness are not necessarily separate experiences even though they may be articulated as logically discrete. The nature of embodied experience is that it is able to hold multiple qualities at the same time. This unity of dwelling-mobility indicates well-being in its deepest fullness, but does not have to be experienced in this fullest sense to be of benefit to people: there can be different kinds and levels of well-being that can be derived from this unity, depending on emphasis and focus. It is in this spirit that we have derived eighteen variations of well-being experience. In the following Figure 30.1 we present what we call 'the dwelling-mobility lattice':

Figure 30.1 'Dwelling-mobility' lattice

	MOBILITY	*DWELLING*	*MOBILITY-DWELLING*
SPATIALITY	Adventurous horizons	At homeness	Abiding expanse
TEMPORALITY	Future orientation	Present-centeredness	Renewal
INTER-SUBJECTIVITY	Mysterious interpersonal attraction	Kinship and belonging	Mutual complementarity
MOOD	Excitement or desire	Peacefulness	Mirror-like multidimensional fullness
IDENTITY	I can	I am	Layered continuity
EMBODIMENT	Vitality	Comfort	Grounded Vibrancy

An explanation of this framework

On the left-hand side of Figure 30.1 we name a number of experiential domains within which well-being can be emphasised (spatiality, temporality, etc.). These experiential domains are centrally informed by the phenomenological-philosophical tradition in which Husserl, Heidegger, Merleau-Ponty and others have delineated fundamental lifeworld constituents that are implicated in human experience (Husserl, 1970; Merleau-Ponty, 1962; Heidegger, 1962; Boss, 1979). So for example, one can think of well-being in terms of the way it can be experienced spatially, temporally, interpersonally, bodily, in mood, and in terms of the experience of personal identity. Although each of these domains of experience are implicated in one another, one can still usefully refer to these qualities as emphases (Ashworth, 2003), and this can help us to delineate different well-being possibilities. Along the horizontal rows, the two emphases of well-being (dwelling and mobility) are delineated, together with a third possibility when intertwined or unified (dwelling-mobility). Indeed, ontologically, this intertwined phenomenon is primary and the separate emphases of dwelling and mobility are variations that exist in 'stepped down' ways ('figure-ground' emphases within a unity). So, considering each of the qualities of well-being as both separate and intertwined (dwelling, mobility, the unity of dwelling-mobility), one can see these qualities more clearly as a 'structure' with different emphases or variations in everyday life. For example, one can think of a well-being possibility where mobility is emphasised, a well-being possibility where dwelling is emphasised and a well-being possibility where they are integrated. By considering the relative interaction of these two dimensions (experiential domains and well-being possibilities) one can derive a number of kinds and levels of well-being that are afforded to human existence. In this framework we have derived eighteen terms that each describe a particular quality of well-being such as 'present-centeredness' when dwelling and temporality interact, or 'I can' when identity and mobility interact. Although these variations are all implicated in one another, their distinct experiential emphases in terms of figure and ground can be usefully delineated and named. For example, one may experience a kind of well-being in which spatial dwelling is in the foreground; here, one may feel particularly tuned into the physical environment's quality that engenders a sense of 'at homeness' as a foreground experience. This emphasis is 'never alone' or apart from other possible well-being variations. So the mood of dwelling (that has a quality of 'peacefulness') may also be there, but in the background, and not explicitly focused upon. Nevertheless, we will now show that it is helpful to articulate each of the variations of well-being as discrete emphases. We call this framework a 'lattice' because the various kinds of well-being are dynamically intertwined and layered. The term 'lattice' attempts to indicate this woven nature and to express the dynamic possibilities of their figure/ground relationships within their larger unity. We now describe each variation of well-being experience. We believe that these discrete emphases are both experientially meaningful, as well as having value when one comes to think about practical directions. Further, in order to make comparisons between the eighteen variations of well-being, we address similar topics within each variation. Although this may appear formulaic and perhaps repetitive to read, we do this for the sake of rigour and to be able to show how the various elements are similar or different across variations, so in each case we consider how that dimension is essentially defined, give an example of how it may be lived, and provide a possible health care application.

Spatial mobility: adventurous horizons

There is a well-being experience that emphasises 'adventurous horizons'. When adventurous horizons are bright, a person is tuned into the spatial possibilities of their environment that offer movement (either metaphorically or literally) in ways that are valued or wanted. So for example, adventurous horizons in a literal sense may occur 'on the road' where one feels invited to explore new places and things; there is a 'sense of adventure' provided by the spatial possibilities of the situation. A sense of 'adventurous horizons' in a metaphorical way may occur through, for example, reading a novel in which descriptions of place open up a feeling of adventure as imagined movement; however there may be many more ways to experience a sense of horizons opening.

In relation to the implications of this 'well-being emphasis' for care, one could ask the question: what adventurous horizons in this person's physical environment can be offered and supported as either a literal reality or as a focus for possible experiential engagement? One example of offering adventurous horizons as a possible experiential focus that is not literal may occur in the case of a person who is physically disabled. Here, some time may be spent in which carers find out about the kind of imaginative journeys that could be meaningful to a person, and engage in help that could open up such a possibility either through access to paintings, or films and so on. Alternatively, literal possibilities may include outings that achieve something of the essence of this felt sense in a way that is possible. Another example might simply be the sense of adventurous horizon in which a person experiences the feeling of spatial mobility by looking out at the stars or a sunset. Well-being as a sense of 'adventurous horizons' is thus anything that offers a place of promise.

Spatial dwelling: at homeness

There is a well-being experience that emphasises 'at homeness' or a sense of 'being at home'. When there is a sense of 'being at home' a person may be tuned into the spatial possibilities of their environment that offer settling or stillness (either metaphorically or literally) in ways that are valued or wanted. So for example, a sense of at homeness in a literal sense may occur 'on my favourite easy chair in front of the fire'. Here, literally, one is in physical surroundings that are familiar and comfortable; there is a sense of at homeness provided by the spatial possibilities of the situation. A sense of at homeness in a metaphorical sense may occur through, for example, having familiar objects and personal things close to hand, that connect a person to their familiar sense of place and belonging; this returns one spatially to a sense of at homeness as an experience of welcome 'dwelling'. In relation to the implications of this 'well-being emphasis' for care, one could ask the question: what sense of 'at homeness' in this person's physical environment can be offered and supported as either a literal reality or as a focus for possible experiential engagement? One example of offering welcome 'at homeness' as a possible experiential focus that is not literal might be where a person is being treated in a clinical environment. Here, there is a danger that the person may feel dislocated or alien, and some effort may be spent bringing in objects and things into the environment that provide a sense of familiarity and belonging. This could range from plants and other natural items to personally significant objects that connect the person with their familiar sense of place. Well-being as a sense of at-homeness is anything that offers a place of settling or peace.

Spatial dwelling-mobility: abiding expanse

There is a well-being experience that can hold both spatial mobility and spatial dwelling together; an experience that can straddle both adventurous horizons and at-homeness. We call this experience 'abiding expanse'. In 'abiding expanse', a person is tuned into the spatial possibilities of their environment that offers at the same time 'settled at homeness' as well as 'adventurous horizons', either metaphorically or literally in ways that are valued or wanted. In this unity, there is an experience of abiding expanse; being deeply connected to a familiar place that offers itself as a stepping out point for possible literal or metaphorical adventures or journeys. So, for example, one person may have a sense of abiding expanse, in both literal and metaphorical ways, at a window where she feels both safe and settled inside, as well as invited out by the path disappearing into the distance. In relation to the implications of this well-being emphasis for care, one could ask the question: what possibilities of 'abiding expanse' can be offered in this person's physical environment and supported as either a literal reality or as a focus for possible experiential engagement?

One example of facilitating 'abiding expanse' as a possible experiential focus is where a person is physically disabled. Here, instead of just facilitating imaginative journeys in different ways or bringing familiar objects into the environment, the carer pays attention to designing the physical environment in such a way as to facilitate a creative tension between home and adventure. One might offer the possibility of spatial experiences in which there is a transition between the familiar and unfamiliar in a way that is both nourishing and interesting. For example, a carer and the physically disabled person may expend some effort arranging a 'liminal' space near a window where the person can feel both at home with familiar things to hand, as well as the possibility of following the flights of birds as they venture to warmer climes. Well-being as a sense of abiding expanse is any place that stretches between home and adventure.

Temporal mobility: future orientation

There is a well-being experience that emphasises a future orientation or future possibilities. When there is a sense of future orientation, a person may be tuned into the temporal possibilities of moving forwards into a future (either as a sense or literally) in ways that are valued or wanted. So, for instance, a sense of future orientation in a literal way may occur when one is able to identify and progress one's valued projects. Here, a person may be energised by life possibilities that call from the future and which motivate them in a way that constitutes a sense of purpose. This sense of meaningful purpose constitutes this kind of well-being because it can provide a quality of flow and continuity to the ongoing progression of one's life in time. Without this possibility one may feel 'stuck', as if frozen in time without meaningful invitations 'into the future'. A well-being future orientation may occur for example, as one looks forward to a celebration that is due to happen with others. Here, there is a well-being dimension in the anticipation of what is to be; a very human kind of joy. Well-being as future orientation does not need to be as special as this in order to act as a resource. One can imagine possibilities for achieving change in small ways that are welcome, anything that can provide a sense of new things happening and that constitute 'a breath of fresh air'. In relation to the implications for care, one can ask the question: what future orientation could be welcomed by this person, no matter how small? One example of a literal entry point into the possibility of facilitating future orientation could be where a carer considers, together with a person, those small changes that might 'unstick' a sense of deadening routine or situation. Well-being as a sense of temporal mobility is anything that offers an invitation into a welcoming future.

Temporal dwelling: present centredness

There is a well-being experience that emphases 'present centredness'. When a person is absorbed in the present moment, they are tuned into a kind of temporal focus that offers 'at oneness', an intimacy, a sense of belonging or a deep connection with what is happening in the moment in ways that are valued or wanted. So for example, a sense of present centredness often occurs in marginal literal situations where one's attention 'is grabbed', such as in sports and other absorbing challenges. Here, people are 'in the zone'. An example in an everyday sense of temporal dwelling may be when one is enchanted by beautiful music or the taste of good food. In these and other situations, which may be very personal, one is 'brought home' to the very simple event of 'just being', and there is a completeness and satisfaction in this moment of temporal dwelling. In relation to the implications of this well-being emphasis for care, one can ask the question: what welcome present-centred experience can be facilitated and supported as a possible focus for experiential engagement? One example of offering a present focus to experience could be very simple such as the mere directing of a person's attention to something that is already there as a source of comfort, such as the gentle sound of rain on the roof or the rise and fall of breathing. Another example is where a sense of temporal dwelling is offered by helping the person to engage in activities of possible dwelling such as through painting, or through spending time in the garden. Well-being as a sense of present centredness is anything that offers absorption as a moment of welcome 'being here'.

Temporal dwelling-mobility: renewal

There is a well-being experience that can hold a sense of temporal mobility and temporal dwelling together; an experience that unifies future orientation and present centredness at the same time. We call this experience 'renewal'. In 'renewal', a person is tuned into a temporal range that carries with it both the novelty of being called into the 'newness' of the future, as well the settledness of being absorbed in the present moment. There is simultaneously a welcome invitation from the future as well as a 'being here', present with whatever is happening. This is a 'rooted flow', a sense of the present that strongly grounds the movement towards the future. The word 'renewal' indicates something of the freshness, aliveness and uniqueness of the present moment which has never before quite happened like this, as well as a sense of possibility and potential movement that leans towards a future that opens up. Here, one is both intimately 'at one with the present moment', as well as energised by life's future possibilities; it is a dwelling that leans forward. So for example, a person may experience a feeling of being connected to their life's desires and their future possibilities through an activity, such as climbing towards the top of a mountain, as well as experiencing the 'nowness' of this 'complete moment' as it is unfolding. In relation to the implications of this well-being emphasis for care, one could ask the question: what possibilities for renewal can be offered in this person's situation? Here, one avenue of exploration concerns how meaningful ritual has characteristics that can mark the importance of the present moment, as well as signal the potential to move into a new phase or possibility as 'renewal'. So for example, in a situation of a person undergoing the kind of surgery that will involve the loss of a body part, a carer could facilitate something like 'a ritual' or some space and time by which the person is encouraged to honour that part of the body and its role in the past, and then move on to include some acknowledgement of what the new phase of life may open up. Well-being as a sense of renewal is any welcome 'joining' between the depth of the present and the openness of the future.

Intersubjective mobility: mysterious interpersonal attraction

There is a well-being experience that emphasises 'mysterious interpersonal attraction'. When such attraction is present, a person is tuned into the interpersonal possibilities that offer movement (either metaphorically or literally) in ways that are valued or wanted. There is an 'eros' in which a person's 'otherness' is an attraction beyond any simple knowing. Indeed, the essence of this attractiveness is precisely in the mystery of otherness. This well-being possibility in the interpersonal realm constitutes an energised openness towards the other which can be called 'desire'. Such desire or attraction, when experienced as well-being, constitutes a kind of radiance and a 'leaning towards'. So for instance, a sense of mysterious interpersonal attraction may occur where one cannot quite name why it is that you wish to find out more about another person. The essence of this mysterious interpersonal attraction is not, however, in finding out or knowing that person, but in the sheer energy of the 'beyondness' of someone or something partially hidden in the unknown; this interpersonal unknown is always in a sense 'wild' (in the sense of undiscovered or exotic), an aliveness that energises an interest to reach towards the other, something that the spontaneous innocence of a baby's grasp understands. This gravitation towards the other is not only 'eros' but can also be 'agape': a respectful caring interest in the other's difference and uniqueness. In relation to the implications for care, one can ask the question: what mysterious interpersonal attraction can be welcomed by this person as a source of interest in the world? One example of a literal entry point into the possibility of facilitating 'the spark' of the call from the mystery of otherness is where a carer surprises an animal lover who is withdrawing because of illness by bringing a new cat onto the scene. Well-being as a sense of mysterious interpersonal attraction is anything that offers an invitation into the mystery of being.

Intersubjective dwelling: kinship and belonging

There is an interpersonal well-being experience that emphasises a sense of kinship and belonging. Here a person feels at home with another or others. This sense of familiar interpersonal connection constitutes relaxed situations of meeting in ways that can make us feel that we belong there. In such a metaphorical or literal situation of 'kinship' there is a sense of 'we' rather than 'I' and 'you'; an effortless being together with one another, a sense of familiar security and togetherness.

So for example, a sense of interpersonal kinship and belonging may occur literally where one has built up a long history with someone that one has come to love and know. However this sense of kinship and belonging can also occur in a more metaphorical way as when we meet a 'kindred spirit' with whom we feel immediately compatible on various levels such as personality, heritage, interest and so on. In these situations of intersubjective dwelling there may be a kind of reconnecting with where we had left off previously, a long time ago, almost as if we share a kind of eternal presence with the other person. This may constitute the sense that not much time has passed once we are together again: there is an eternal return to dwelling in this interpersonal present. In relation to the implications of this well-being emphasis for care, one can ask the question: what forms of kinship and belonging can be facilitated and supported as a possible focus for experiential engagement? One example of a literal entry point into the possibility of facilitating a sense of kinship and belonging is where a carer, sensitive to the cultural background of a person, helps to connect that person with others from their shared background and to possible events, objects, music and traditions from their heritage. Within this context, heritage can be healing in that it provides cultural homecomings and shelter. Alternatively a carer could facilitate a sense of kinship and belonging in a more metaphorical sense by engaging in shared stories in which the person re-members and 'joins with' ancestry and shared histories that give a sense of continuity, familiarity and belonging. Alternatively, some people may need interpersonal kinship experiences that move beyond the cultural level to include interests and affinities that are very specific and not necessarily related to cultural heritage. So for example 'clubs' and social networks have become much more important as the history of community life becomes more fragmented. Well-being as a sense of kinship and belonging occurs in any of the ways that one can find an 'at homeness' with others.

Intersubjective dwelling-mobility: mutual complementarity

There is an experience that can hold a sense of both intersubjective mobility and intersubjective dwelling together; an experience in which there is both the qualities of mysterious interpersonal attraction as well as kinship and belonging. We call this experience 'mutual complementarity'. In 'mutual complementarity' a person is tuned into the possibility of being with another or others in such a way that there is 'homelike-oneness' with the other, as well as an energetic separation or attractive mystery, 'calling' from the other. Here, there is a paradoxical quality of both familiarity and strangeness in which we are reciprocal but complementary to one another. The 'mutuality' is one of kinship and belonging, the complementarity is one of 'a giving' in which one is 'more' when together than when apart. So for example two or more people may have a sense of mutual complementarity when there is a partnership constituted by a shared equality, together with the ongoing learning that may come from each other's difference. This is a creative tension of 'sameness' and difference'. The difference is given by a 'not knowing' in which the other appears as a mysterious depth that can be surprising and which brings something new to the relationship. At the same time a certain 'sameness' or familiar 'sharedness' is given by a familiarity based on a shared recognition of places where 'we meet' and that we have 'in common'. In this creative tension there is both the intimacy of feeling at home with the other, as well as a sense of the novelty that each brings to the other in a mutual and complementary way. Mutual complementarity as an intersubjective well-being experience is thus a journey of companionship that is both 'at home' and 'in adventure'. In relation to the implications of this well-being emphasis for care, one can ask the question: what forms of mutual complementarity can be facilitated and supported as a possible focus for experiential engagement? One example of a literal entry point into this possibility is where a carer encourages a couple who feel at home together but who are 'in a rut', to discover either things they do not yet know about each other or to pursue something new together. Alternatively a carer could facilitate a sense of mutual complementarity in a more metaphorical sense by helping a person engage with their cultural history in new ways that give new directions for that person's life, such as, an engagement with the cuisine of their culture that they had not previously known about. This opens up both an intersubjective reconnecting as well as a sense of new direction; something old and something new. Well-being as a sense of mutual complementarity can occur in any way that one finds the 'attractive unknown' in the ones that are close, and with whom we feel we belong.

Mood mobility: excitement or desire

There is a well-being experience that emphasises the mood of excitement or desire. Here, well-being as a mood or felt attunement is emphasised, but specifically, as a mood which has the quality of movement and buoyancy. In everyday terms this mood may be characterised as one of excitement or welcome desire. So for example, there may be a sense of excitement when one is about to leave for a much-longed-for holiday or special event. A sense of such excitement or desire in a metaphorical sense may occur when there is a feeling of possibility; a feeling that the world is inviting one into horizons that connect with the desires of one's heart. This energised feeling constitutes the mood of motivation, a kind of 'life force' or vitality that sustains the feeling that life is worth living. In relation to the implications of this 'well-being emphasis' for care, one can ask the question: what sense of excitement or desire in this person's situation can be offered? One example of offering an invitation to the mood of welcome excitement or desire may be in a situation where older people are living in a residential care setting. Here, such older people may be provided with opportunities to celebrate important events or seasons. In this example one is helping to focus attention on the possibility of a sense of celebration that brings with it a mood that has, in various ways, been available to us all as part of the heritage of being human. Well-being as a mooded sense of excitement is thus anything that motivates a felt connection to a person's meaningful life desires.

Mood dwelling: peacefulness

There is a well-being experience that emphasises the mood of peacefulness. Here, well-being as a mood or felt attunement is emphasised, but specifically as a mood that has the qualities of stillness, settledness or reconciliation. In everyday terms this mood may be characterised as one of peace and welcome 'pause'. So for example, there may be a sense of peacefulness when one has fulfilled a task or responsibility that required some effort and commitment. We would like to note that the process of settling or 'coming to accept' things may be challenging, and that the direction of acceptance may be a journey that includes sadness, patience and concern. A person can come to the mood of dwelling in multiple ways, but in the end, the mood of dwelling is one of peacefulness in spite of everything. A felt sense of peace may also be experienced in less literal situations through an attunement of mind, or through a more general comportment towards the world. Here, a person is able to accept 'what has been given' for what it is, and to experience the concomitant feeling of peacefulness that arises with such 'letting-be-ness'. Peace as a felt sense is thus the mood of dwelling or 'at homeness'. In relation to the implications of this well-being emphasis for care, one can ask the question: what sense of peace or settledness is possible for this person? One literal example of offering an invitation to the mood of peace may be where a carer suggests, for example, that a person keeps 'a book of abundances' in which they note daily something that they can appreciate or accept 'just as it is'. A less literal example may be where a carer introduces practices that help focus a person's attention on the possibility of accepting things as they are, where it may be possible to do so. One can perhaps begin to encourage someone to do this by first noticing and appreciating simple changes in life such as the rhythms of day and night, and of the seasons, and the mood that this may bring. One could then move onto more complex mindful practices for life in which the possibility of peacefulness and 'letting be-ness' is progressively achieved as a general mood or comportment towards life's changes. Well-being as a mooded sense of peacefulness occurs whenever there is a felt acceptance of things, circumstances and changes.

Mood dwelling-mobility: mirror-like multidimensional fullness

There is a well-being experience characterised by a highly complex mood that participates in both the energetic quality of enthusiasm and interest, as well as the settled quality of being at home with oneself and the world. We call this paradoxical mood 'mirror-like multidimensional fullness'. We have called this mood 'mirror like' because it contains a settled openness that is large enough to reflect whatever is happening in a 'letting be' kind of way. At the same time we have called this mood 'multidimensional fullness' because it is a fullness of mood which can be many things such as sadness, love and happiness. It can be many things because this mirror-like mood does not need to separate itself from whatever is happening right now. In not separating itself, the mood is one of 'union with', but a 'union with' the fluidity that is alive and unfolding, rather than a union with a finished circumstance. The paradoxical quality of the mood of 'mirror-like multidimensional fullness' is, metaphorically speaking, like that of being at both the centre and the periphery of a cyclone at the same time. There is a mood of both stillness and of being 'on the move' simultaneously. The mood is one of fullness in the sense that one feels complete and that nothing is missing; it is far from a sense of deficient emptiness. So for example, a person may experience a mood of mirror-like multidimensional fullness when they are 'drinking in' the novelty of new sights and sounds, and feeling complete 'there' in this moment. The paradoxical quality of this complex mood thus includes fullness and completeness, novelty and surprise, appreciation and serenity and so on. The Japanese Haiku tradition evokes something of this mood in stanzas such as:

> *how touching*
> *to exist after the storm*
> *chrysanthemum.*

(Basho, 1692–94/2008)

In relation to the implications of this complex well-being mood for care, one could ask the question: what possibilities are there for such a complex mood that is one of 'giving oneself emotionally' to this moment, in both an enthusiastic and reconciled way? Sometimes this mood may occur spontaneously in a patient with a chronic illness after having 'gone through a lot'. Suddenly she feels something more than just acceptance and peace about her condition. She feels, without there being a reason, enthusiastic about sipping a simple cup of tea early in the morning. She is not enthusiastic in the sense of looking forward to anything, but in the sense that there is nothing more important to be or do, but just to fully 'give herself' to appreciating what is available now, even though there may be pain and uncertainty. This mood cannot be directly facilitated, and often comes in surprising and unexpected ways; it is the mood where hard earned 'songs of experience' meet the child-like presence of 'songs of innocence'. It is not so much that professionals and carers can help make this happen, but that they can prevent this possibility from happening by not recognising or understanding the value of this mood, and therefore in such situations could mistakenly bring the person back prematurely to projections about the future, or back to a narrative definition of themselves. So, well-being as a sense of multidimensional fullness is characterised by the enthusiastic mood of 'giving oneself' to an experience without narrative implication, and because of, rather than in spite of, the limits of this timeless moment.

Identity mobility: 'I can'

There is a well-being experience that emphasises a sense of one's personal identity as 'I can'. When such an emphasis of personal identity is experienced, the person will experience themselves as being 'on the move' (either metaphorically or literally) in ways that are valued or wanted. Relating to their sense of personal identity, there is a sense of 'being able to', a degree of confident personal competence in which one feels able to move into the kind of future and its expanding horizons that are consistent with a knowledge of one's personal possibilities and self-belief. This sense of 'I can' can range from being very simple and literal to very complex and metaphorical. So, for example, this self-sense of 'being on the move' can be as simple as a toddler developing the self-belief that they can consistently walk to the corner. At a more complex and metaphorical level, this sense of 'I can' may occur when one has been able to develop a tacit sense of optimism that dreams can be realistically achieved on the basis of one's hard work and personal capacities.

At its most existential level, there may be a very general sense that there is always 'a more' to one's identity, and a feeling that one's personal capacities lie in possible potentials that have not yet been named or realised. There is thus a very close relationship between 'I can' identity mobility and a sense of personal agency. This well-being possibility in the realm of identity constitutes an energised openness about the possibilities of the self. In relation to the implications of this well-being emphasis for care, one could ask the question: what possibilities for self-efficacy are there in this person's life that are meaningful to the person and that can be offered and supported as either a literal reality or as a focus for possible experiential engagement? One example of facilitating a greater sense of self-efficacy may be with a person who has lost their confidence in being able to engage in past activities because of an illness. Here they can be encouraged to set small relevant goals, and over time, experience a gradual build up of 'I can' successes. This 'I can' mobility–identity then becomes somewhat restored, and can constitute a source of well-being. An example that is less literal is where a more general sense of self potential is facilitated. Here, a psychotherapy patient who had been overly identified with personal historical experiences of failure may rediscover aspects of themselves, or previously unknown aspects of themselves that had been obscured by their self definition of failure. This is usually done psychotherapeutically in a non-linear way where, instead of focusing on the problem, one helps the person to explore things about themselves and their potential that they may have forgotten. There are many ways in which this can be facilitated, for example, through art, writing and through pursuing dormant passions. Well-being as a sense of 'I can' is thus any experience where one's personal identity is felt to be capable of 'being able to' and of being able to achieve what one values.

Identity dwelling: 'I am'

There is a well-being experience that is in touch with one's sense of personal identity as 'I am' in its most general sense. When such an emphasis of personal identity is in focus, a person may experience themselves as someone who is simply supported by histories and contexts that are continuous with one's sense of self, and which does not need to be excessively questioned or 'at stake'. This is not an 'I am' as if it was an objectified definition of oneself; rather it is an 'I am' that, at its depth, feels connected to a sense of being which is given to us in its most foundational sense. When one is tuned into this sense of identity, there is a sense of 'being there' before all the specific layers of self definition that have been built up are brought into play. So, this sense of 'I am' is not 'I am this or that'; it really is just the feeling of 'being' very generally, or present, as 'someone who belongs here right now', and who is able to take 'nourishment' and some security from this sense of ontological identity. At its depth one can call it an 'ontological security': that one's identity (in a very general way) is supported by 'merely being' rather than 'having to be' something or someone. The well-being focus of the 'identity dwelling' emphasis of 'I am' is experienced as a familiar continuity, a sense of effortless connectedness, a certain peacefulness or lack of dilemma of who and what I am: a kind of being at home with one's self. In relation to the implications of this well-being emphasis for care, one can ask the question: what effortless or peaceful sense of 'I am' is possible for this person? One literal example of facilitating a greater sense of 'I am' that has an 'identity dwelling' quality, may be where one helps a disabled person connect with identity resources to which they feel continuous with, and belong to, beyond the particularity of 'I am disabled'. In this example a practitioner may facilitate the possibility of an experiential engagement in which the person recognises their continuity with cultural, geographical or historical connections with which they may identify such as a place, or a sense of belonging with 'my people'. A more existential example of deep 'identity dwelling' may be where a person who has been recently diagnosed with a terminal illness spontaneously realises, within the midst of their anguish, an inexplicable feeling that 'I am still here, and much more than my illness', and that 'my sense of being here' is vast and indefinable. At this existential level, such experiences cannot be predicted or determined, and seem to involve a kind of 'breakthrough' to a sense of self as 'simply being'. Such an ontological sense of the foundation of personal identity is a well-being resource in which a certain timeless dimension of one's depths relieves the narratives of our lives. Well-being as a sense of 'I am' is thus an experience where our sense of personal identity is felt to be connected to resources and contexts far beyond oneself, but which nevertheless, are continuous with what is most deeply one's own.

Identity dwelling-mobility: layered continuity

There is a well-being experience that can hold a sense of identity mobility and identity dwelling at the same time; an experience that unifies 'I can' with 'I am'. We call this experience 'layered continuity'. In 'layered continuity' a person may experience their own identity, not in any particular thing-like way, but as a sense of continuity with different layers of 'I can', as well as a continuity with the general sense of simply being here before all the specific layers of self definition are brought to the fore. In this rare and paradoxical experience, both one's specific sense of identity, as well as one's strong sense of 'just being' in a foundational sense, are both in the foreground. Here, one's sense of identity is inclusive of a sense of all the historical details and connections that make up the 'I can', as well as the sense of ontological security of 'I am'. This sense of inclusion of both these identity resources is experienced as a layered continuity in which one is empowered by both the multiple resources of one's uniqueness as well as that level of identity that opens out to one's most anonymous and transpersonal ground. This layered continuity is thus continuous with both personal and transpersonal layers of self. Jung indicated this ambiguous experience of both the unity and multiplicity to one's identity when he said:

> I am all these things at once and cannot hold up the sum . . . and it seems to me that I have been carried along. I exist on the foundation of something I do not know. In spite of all uncertainties I feel a solidity underlying existence and a continuity in my mode of being.
>
> (Jung, 1961/1995, p. 392)

The well-being experience in layered continuity lies in its inclusive qualities of 'I am all this and more'. So for example, a person may have a feeling of the 'layered continuity' of who they are in unguarded moments when the need to assert or protect any sense of self definition is in abeyance; self definition is not at stake and a sense of oneself as 'layers' that spontaneously shine through without the need to 'be achieved' is supportively experienced.

In relation to the implications of this well-being emphasis for care, one could ask the question: what possibilities are there for experiencing such a complex identity within this person's life situation? Again, such experiences cannot be predicted or determined, and seem to involve a kind of 'breakthrough' to an ambiguous sense of self as 'layered continuity'. An example of experiencing layered continuity may be in a person who has been through much effortful and self-conscious treatment regimes. After a long period in which she was struggling with her sense of self as 'a patient' trying to take 'full responsibility' for her recovery, she spontaneously realised that there was not much more that she could do. Something deep within her relaxed; a letting go of the 'responsible one' and a 'letting in' of the deep need to simply be cared for. Suddenly in this moment, a sense of her layered continuity was restored; she felt unconcerned about any definition of herself that she had been upholding, and felt the well-being experience of 'I already am and I already can, even though I do not know who that is in specific terms – I am many layers'. Well-being as a sense of layered continuity is any experience where one's personal identity is felt to be both already achieved in its essence, as well as felt as a sense of self that is 'able to' in a general sense.

Embodied mobility: vitality

There is a well-being experience that emphasises a sense of bodily 'vitality'. When there is such a sense of vitality a person may be tuned into an embodied energy that carries with it a quality of movement in ways that are valued or wanted. So for example a sense of embodied mobility may occur in a literal way, actualising the power of one's own body to move in various ways and towards different desired outcomes. This is a literal 'bodying forth'. Therefore, one important source of the kind of well-being that is given to bodily existence is an active power to move in, and with, one's world and others. At a more existential level, a sense of vitality can refer to energised bodily feeling that can occur without literal physical movement, such as in imagination, eroticism or any other generalised desire where one feels the energy of this motivation as a palpable bodily experience; it is an incarnate sense of vitality. This sense of vitality constitutes a kind of well-being because it essentially provides life-forward and life-positive qualities of 'being an actor' or 'agent' in the world; of extending one's power freely, a 'life force' in the world through bodily sensation and capacity. Without this possibility one may feel depleted and lacking in bodily energy and functional capacity. In relation to the implications of this well-being emphasis for care, contexts one could ask the question: what possibilities for bodily vitality can be offered and supported to this person as either a literal reality or as a focus for possible experiential engagement? A literal example of the possibility of restoring a sense of vitality may be where a physiotherapist works with a person to maximise a dysfunctional limb so that literal movement is enhanced. An example of facilitating a sense of vitality in a more metaphorical or existential way may occur in the case of a person who is experiencing an embodied listlessness and lethargy. Here, a carer may understand that this bodily listlessness and lethargy is not disconnected from the person's felt sense of 'how' or 'where' their life is going, where they feel blocked, and where there may be possibilities for moving forward.

With such an understanding, the carer may help the person to first see a link between their bodily sense of lethargy and the blocked life projects that are announced. Second, the carer may help the person to then focus their energies on meaningful possibilities that are relevant to them. If this is successful, the sense of existential movement achieved will concurrently constitute the more bodily felt level of 'movement' that we are calling vitality. Well-being as a sense of vitality thus occurs as the bodily sense of refreshed possibilities in literal and metaphorical ways.

Embodied dwelling: comfort

There is a well-being experience that is in touch with one's sense of 'comfort' as a bodily experience. When such a sense of bodily comfort is felt, a person may literally experience their body as warm, full, relaxed, still, satiated, rooted. Here one feels a welcome simple sense of 'being at home' in one's body, simply feeling the support or nourishment of the reliable rhythms of one's natural bodily functions, as in the gentle rise and fall of the breath or the relaxation of the body at rest. In bodily comfort there is a certain unforced sense of familiarity and intimacy with the internal natural and organic rhythms announced by the body. There are also silent and unseen rhythms that we take for granted but which support the palpable sense of comfort. Such natural comfort is, in a sense unthought or pre-reflective. The comfortable body is simply there in its reliable givenness. Here, one is unpreoccupied with the body. The body does not announce itself as a bodily 'dilemma'; it 'just is' and is in 'letting be' mode. We know comfort through a kind of trust rather than through a purposeful search. At its depths such bodily comfort is connected to natural rhythms beyond oneself such as the rhythms of day and night, warmth and coolness, and other fleshly contexts that are familiar to a body that feels comfortable in its context. We can also think of the comfort of bodily dwelling in a more metaphorical way as in Mary Oliver's (2004) expression 'your *soft animal body*', a body 'curled up' or 'folded in' with sources of nourishment and support, sustaining a bodily sense of well-being. Metaphorically we could say that the body knows that it comes from primordial darkness, intimate with rhythms within rhythms, lapping on this fleshly shore. Bodily comfort as well-being is something the body deeply knows as a tacit, self-evident foundation to healthy being. Comfort constitutes a kind of well-being because it essentially provides an embodied dwelling in which there are qualities of 'non purposeful natural presence' as a foundation for being there. Such comfort is a bodily 'gravitas' that makes possible an embodied openness to the world. Without comfort as a well-being possibility, one may feel a sense of *dis*-ease, a preoccupation with the palpable bodily sense that 'something is wrong'. In relation to the implications of this well-being emphasis for care, one can ask the question: what possibilities for bodily comfort are available to this person at either a literal or existential level? A literal example of the possibility of restoring a sense of comfort will be familiar to many readers. Here for example, a carer may aim to bring comfort to a paralysed person through being sensitive to the need for a change of position, and to facilitate a welcome refreshment through bathing, clean linen, a warm drink, and with attention to minimising noise and bright light. A more existential example of promoting a sense of comfort may occur in the case of an immigrant who is experiencing bodily restlessness and insomnia. Here, a professional may understand this restlessness and insomnia in a way that is not disconnected from the person's felt sense of 'trying to find a way back home', where home in a literal sense is no longer available. With such an understanding, the professional may help the person to find bodily reminders of feeling at home, perhaps through familiar foods or other possible ways that connect the person to the bodily feeling of comfort of what home is like for them. If this is successful to some degree, the sense of existential settling that is achieved may also constitute the more bodily level of comfort that provides enough security to perhaps 'settle' and sleep. Well-being as a sense of comfort thus occurs as the bodily sense of 'feeling at home' and settling in literal and metaphorical ways.

Embodied dwelling-mobility: grounded vibrancy

There is a well-being experience that can hold a sense of embodied mobility and embodied dwelling at the same time, an experience that unifies vitality with comfort. We call this experience 'grounded vibrancy'. In grounded vibrancy a person's bodily existence is felt as an intertwining of gentle energised flow, unified with a bodily sense of feeling deeply at home and settled. In this complex experience, there may be a bodily sense of both 'being' and 'becoming' at the same time; a sense of fullness that solidly anchors the body and with it, a 'humming' vibrancy that is attracted to unfinished horizons. This paradoxical quality of grounded vibrancy contains both a sense of the freshness of renewal and great possibility, as well as a sense of the deep continuity that belongs to feeling 'at one with' oneself and the world. This bodily well-being experience can be expressed more poetically as a 'well-spring, a bubbling brook at its source, out of the ground'. The bodily feeling where being and becoming 'are humming' can constitute a welcome and effortless bodily tension or oscillation between the body's 'quest' (the attraction to unfinished horizons) and satiation (the comfort of bodily fulfilment). The body's 'quest' is given by a certain kind of vitality that is the essence of the feeling of 'being attracted'. At the same time a bodily sense of comfort is experienced at a deeper level in the background. This background bodily sense of completeness and tranquility holds and empowers a bodily vibrancy that is 'ticking over' with potential, and a readiness to live forward. In relation to the implications of this well-being emphasis for care, one could ask the question: what possibilities are there that would allow a person to experience grounded vibrancy? Because of the complexity of this experience, its circumstance cannot be determined or predicted: situations that facilitate either comfort or vitality can make way for it. But there is something 'extra' to the comfort or vitality. So, for example, we were told a story by one of our friends about a man with dementia. He is outside with his carer on a hot day, and sees an ice-cream van. He does not know what to call it, but points, and his carer buys him one. He tastes and his eyes light up. He looks for words but can't find them, so exclaims: "This is a good one!!" Here, there is a deep bodily satisfaction and recognition as well as an enthusiasm that links the body's 'satiation' to the vibrant world of a 'hot-summer's-day-full-of-ice-cream-potential'. Well-being as a sense of grounded vibrancy is any bodily experience where variations of rest and comfort are intertwined with variations of alertness and vitality.

Conclusion

Although we have given examples of specific possible ways that each of the well-being emphases can be facilitated within a caring context, such experiential possibilities should not be understood in a deterministic way as if certain conditions will inevitably lead to certain well-being experiences. Within the human realm, experiential well-being possibilities can happen unpredictably in spontaneous and unexpected ways. The conditions for well-being, such as economic, political, social, health-related and institutional, may provide either a support or an obstruction to well-being, but these conditions are not always sufficient or necessary for the experience of well-being to occur. This existential view of well-being is thus consistent with a resource-oriented approach in which the possibilities for well-being experiences can be revealed or focused upon from the perspective of its widest literal and deepest existential contexts. By considering the multidimensional facets of well-being as articulated in this framework, we may widen and complexify the range of possible resources that are available for the alleviation of suffering. Here, suffering is much more complex than illness, and well-being is much more complex than health. In our view it is this multidimensional complexity that defines the deepest scope of contributions to caring professions within a caring science domain.

We would also like to say something about the deepest possibility of well-being as a developmental calling beyond the context of caring science, (the focus of this present chapter). There is obviously a relationship between 'existence' and 'caring', but well-being as an existential call far exceeds the vocation of caring science. Beyond the scope of this chapter, the existential theory of dwelling-mobility also has implications for a broader quest towards well-being as an existential task. For example, a further development of the theory could focus on an articulation of the deepest possibilities of well-being as 'an existential pull' in people's lives. Future elaboration of the theory would then focus on the developmental processes by which human attention can be widened in such a way as to sustain multiple intertwined dimensions of well-being as an increasingly available conscious resource at the foundation of experiential life. Although we have indicated eighteen kinds of intertwined variations of well-being that may provide a direction for caring, it is possible to imagine the unfolding of many more variations and nuances in a range of situations and contexts.

Having acknowledged the existential developmental task that is given by the call of well-being, we would like to finally come back to the importance of our theory of well-being for the project of caring science. In the midst of suffering, a felt experience of well-being is particularly important to people as an inner resource when they are facing health-related challenges. Carers can then become much more attuned to the importance and value of this felt experience for the person. The wider 'vocabulary' for well-being experiences that are offered here may contribute to an emerging cultural discourse that wishes to put well-being as a value more centrally at the forefront of public life.

References

Ashworth, P.D. (2003) An approach to phenomenological psychology: The contingencies of the lifeworld. *Journal of Phenomenological Psychology*, 34, 145–156.

Basho. (1692–1694/2008) *The Complete Haiku Translated with an Introduction Biography and Notes by Jane Reichhold*. London: Kodhansha International.

Boss, M. (1979) *Existential Foundations of Medicine and Psychology*. Trans. S. Conway and A. Cleaves. New York: Jason Aronson.

Heidegger, M. (1959/1966) *Discourse on Thinking*. Trans. John M. Anderson and E. Hans Freund. New York: Harper & Row [*Gelassenheit*, 1959].

Heidegger, M. (1962) *Being and Time*. Trans. J. Maquarrie and E. Robinson. Oxford: Basil Blackwell.

Heidegger, M. (1969/1973) *Art and Space*. Trans. Charles H. Seibert. Man and World, vol 6, no. 1 pp. 3–5 [*Kunstund Raum*, 1969].

Heidegger, M. (1971/1993) 'Building, Dwelling, Thinking' Reprinted in *Basic Writings: Martin Heidegger*. Edited by David Farell Krell. London: Routledge, pp. 343–364.

Heidegger, M. (1971) *Poetry, Language, Thought*. Trans. A. Hofstadter. New York: Harper and Row.

Heidegger, M. (1977) *The Question Concerning Technology and Other Essays*. New York: Harper and Row.

Heidegger, M., Boss, M., Mayr, F.K., & Askay, R.R. (2000) *Zollikon Seminars: Protocols-Conversations-Letters (SPEP Studies in Historical Philosophy)*. Evanston: Northwestern University Press.

Husserl, E. (1970) *The Crisis of European Sciences and Transcendental Phenomenology: An Introduction to Phenomenological Philosophy*. Evanston: North Western University Press.

Jung, C.G. (1961/1995) *Memories, Dreams, Reflections*. Edited by A. Jaffe. London: Fontana Press.
Merleau-Ponty, M. (1962) *Phenomenology of Perception*. Trans. C. Smith. London: Routledge & Kegan Paul.
Mugerauer, R. (2008) *Heidegger and Homecoming: The Leitmotif in the Later Writings*. Toronto: University of Toronto Press.
Oliver, Mary. (2004) *Wild Geese: Selected Poems*. Bloodaxe World Poets Series 2. Northumberland, UK: Bloodaxe Books.

Acknowledgement

We would like to thank Karin Dahlberg for helpful conversations and comments. An earlier version of this chapter was published in Galvin, K.T. & Todres, L. *Caring and Well-Being: A Lifeworld Approach*. Routledge.

INDEX

Note: Italicized page numbers indicate a figure on the corresponding page

abiding expanse 327
Aboriginal Australia 25
action-theoretic theory 168–169
actual living 92–94
additive theories of well-being 79
aesthetics of well-being: aesthetic thinking 246–247;
    competence development 243–244; creative people
    248–249; introduction to 10–13; reason and wisdom
    244–245
aesthetic thinking 246–247
agencies of well-being 194–200
amyotrophic lateral sclerosis (ALS) 125–126
androcentric theory 73
angels and well-being 40–43
animals and well-being 202
anthropology of well-being 27–28
anthroposophic medicine 142–146
anti-establishment neighborhoods 36
archaeological fieldwork 117–119
architectural dimensions of well-being 6
Arden, Paul 275
Århus University Hospital in Denmark 60
Aristotle (Greek philosopher) 8, 21, 68, 77, 194, 243, 320
arousal measurements 208
arts-based approaches to well-being 12
Asclepian Sanctuary 114
Atkinson, Sarah 250
atomism 148
Authentic Happiness Theory (Sumner) 77

Bacon, Francis 93
bad mind (malicious intent) 24
Baldwin, James 36
Barry, Jane 105–106
Bauman, Zygmunt 197

Bayley, John 18
Beamish Museum 116
Beck, Ulrick 199
Beckmann, Max 40
behaviorist model of treatment 305
Being and Time (Heidegger) 85, 86–87, 296
being-at-home concept 55
being-in-the-world concept 55–56
Bentham, Jeremy 76
Berlin: City of Stones (Lute) 35
Berlin: Symphony of a City (film) 35, 43
Better Places to Live (Jowell) 112
big Pharma 199
bio-cultural character of neighborhoods 45
bio-statistical theory of health and disease 168–170
Blue Riders *(Blau Ritter)* 40
bodily comfort 335–336
body as it is lived *(Leib)* 174
body-mind relationship 275
body's 'quest' 334–335
Boorse, Christopher 167–170
Braidotti, Rosi 127
Brentano, Franz 26
Brun Norbye, Anne-Katrine 24–25
Buddhism 8, 194
Bunkše, Edmunds 114
Bury, Michael 136–137
Buytendijk, F.J.J. 137

Calhoun, Chelshire 70
Callicles 319
capabilitarians 91–92; *see also* universalism and
    capabilities
care argument 171
care ethics 71–72

Carel, Havi 138
caring and well-being 4–5, 178
Carlson, Allen 18, 20
Carroll, Noel 20
Cartesian dualism 61
case vignettes 156–157
Casey, Edward 6
cems rituals 25
Centre for Evidence-based Medicine 233
Chambers, Emma 253
character of well-being 26–27
*Character Strengths and Virtues: A Handbook and
    Classification* (Peterson, Seligman) 317
childhood and capabilities 98
child mortality 183
child well-being 185
Christian spirituality 156
Christopher Day Parades 39
Cider with Rosie (Lee) 134
circadian rhythms 43
Claxton, Guy 271
clinical decision-making 235
clinical internships: behaviorist model of treatment
    305; co-creating new intersubjective space 298–302;
    emotional availability 313–314; endings *vs.* speculation
    315–316; ethos of the clinic 307–308; everydayness
    297–298; facility requirements 306; introduction to
    292–293; lack of structure 293–295; meaning-making
    302–304; operational considerations 306–307; patient
    flow/appointment scheduling 306–307; provider/
    patient ratios 306; real experience *vs.* expectations
    309–312; shared real experience 312–313; transition
    from teaching 295–297
co-constitutive dimensions 34–35
co-creating new intersubjective space 298–302
cognition and aesthetic thinking 246
Coleman, Leo 25
Collaborating Centre 236
collaborative drawings: art workshops 252–254;
    conversations through drawing 260; examples of
    260–264, *261, 262, 263*; *face2face* project 252, 255,
    258; identity 257–260, *259*; looking 255–257, *256*;
    mirroring 254–255; summary of 264–266, *265, 266*;
    well-being and 250–252
comfort as embodied dwelling 335–336
community well-being 19
complex values 232
compositional theories of well-being 79
conaissance, defined 61
Concerning the Spiritual in Art (Kandinsky) 40
confined present 137
conflicting values 232
conventional medication 142
conversations through drawing 260
corporeal being 5
cosmo-centric well-being 3
Council of Europe 112

creative people 248–249
Csikzentmihalyi, Mihali 196
cultural relativism 95–97
cultural story to well-being 23
Culture White Paper (2016) 113
Cyborg Manifesto 6, 125, 126–129

Daimler Benz Offices 46
D'Annunzio, Gabriele 319
Daudet, Alphonse 139
de Beauvoir, Simone 68, 72
de Certeau, Michel 296–297, 303
decision-making 234, 235
dede rank 25
Defence Archaeology Group 118
Deleuze, Gilles 127
descriptive theories of well-being 78
designed gardens 113–114
desire-fulfillment theories of well-being 1, 78
Diagnostic and Statistical Manual of Mental Disorders
    (DSM) 317
Diaries of Jane Somers (Lessing) 103
Dillon, Robin 73
disabilities and ambiguities: Cyborg Manifesto 125,
    126–129; introduction 124–125; lived voice 125–126
disability movement 227
Disaster Relief Act (Japan) 53
disciplinary perspective of well-being 5–10
disease, defined 168
disease-oriented notion of quality of life 7
diversity, defined 231
downpression (oppression) 24
dualism 4, 58, 61, 136, 148–149, 195
Duet for Pain film 252
Durkheim, Emile 27, 196
dwelling-mobility well-being: embodied dwelling-
    mobility 336; existential dwelling 87–88; existential
    mobility 86–87; homelessness 86; identity dwelling-
    mobility 334; introduction to 5, 84–85; kinds and
    levels of 89–90; ontological possibility of well-being
    85; summary of 88–89; unity of dwelling-mobility 173
dwelling well-being: embodied dwelling 335–336;
    existential dwelling 87–88; intersubjective dwelling
    329–330; mood dwelling 331–332; spatial dwelling
    327; temporal dwelling 328–329; *see also* homes/
    residences and wellbeing
dys-appearance 136

Early Intervention Foundation 183
Earth and sense of well-being 44–47
eco-centric well-being 3
ecological health and well-being: ecology and 142;
    empirical study 142–148; green and white caring
    147–148; health and caring 141–142; introduction
    to 141; lived experience 143; meaning of the
    environment 147; peacefulness and letting be
    144–146; summary of 152–153

economic well-being 2
education *see* eudaimonic model for well-being education
efendi rank 25
ego and Self relationship 160
Elmet Archaeological Services Ltd 118
embodied connectivity in visual/tactile arts: body-mind relationship 275; discussion about 275; embodied responses 273–274; group context 276; HeART of Stroke 272–274, 276; identity and impact 276; improvisation and philosophical enquiry 275; introduction to 269–271, *271*; role of materials 274–275; sensory knowledge 271–272
embodied dwelling 335–336
embodied dwelling-mobility 336
embodied mobility 334–335
embodied routes to well-being: animals and 202; emerging ideas 207–208; emotional changes 208; emotions and 206; equine assisted interventions 202–204, 205–206, 208–209; introduction to 201; learning to be well 204–205; summary of 209–210; well-being overview 201–202
emotional availability 313–314
emotional well-being 2, 20, 28, 206, 217
empirical theories of well-being 78
Encountering Pain Conference (2016) 264
Enemy of the People (Ibsen) 194
Enlightenment 244
environmental dimensions of well-being 6, 19
Epicurus (Greek philosopher) 194
epistemic authority 79, 81
equine assisted interventions (EAI) 202–204, 205–206, 208–209
equine assisted psychotherapy (EAP) 203
equine facilitated learning interventions (EFL) 203
ethics *see* values-based practice
ethnic inequalities 185–186
ethnographic versions of well-being 28
eudaimonia (perfect life) 165, 319
eudaimonic model for well-being education: hedonic *vs.* eudaimonic well-being 318–320; introduction to 13, 317–318; overview of 320–321; summary of 321–322
eudaimonism 1
European Union 187
eurythmy therapy movements 147
everydayness 297–298
evidence-based practice 233–234
existential dwelling 87–88
existential mobility 86–87
existential theory of well-being 5, 28, 86
existential vulnerability 144
Expressionism 40

face2face project 252, 255, 258
fairy-tale case example 158–159
family and sense of home 52
Federal Refugee Act (1999) 39

Feldman, Fred 76
female genital mutilation 96
feminine virtues 72
feminist perspective of well-being: care ethics 71–72; as communal pursuit 70–71; introduction to 4, 68; oppression and 68–69; relational conception of the self 69–70; self-respect and 72; self-understanding and 73
Finnegan, Alan 118
Fitbit technology 118
Foucault, Michel 243, 296, 303
Fox, Edward Long 113
Framework Convention on the Value of Cultural Heritage for Society (Faro Convention) 112
freedom and aesthetic thinking 247
Freeman, Lauren 70
frequent attenders, defined 59
Fukuda, Tokuzo 51, 53–55
Fukushima Daiichi nuclear power plants *see* disabilities and ambiguities; Great East Japan Earthquake

Gadamer, Hans-Georg 292–293, 297, 309
Galen (Roman philosopher/physician) 169
GalGael project 117
Gallwey, W. Timothy 135
Galvin, Kathleen T. 114–115, 131
Gapminder 183, *184*
'Gegnet' notion 5, 84–85, 88–89
general health questionnaire (GHQ) 217
geographical story to well-being 23
Gesler, Wil 114
Ginzberg, Ruth 68–69, 70
Global Financial Crisis (2008–2010) 187
globalization 248
Godel, Kurt 196
gods and well-being 40–43
good health and well-being 133–139
good life notion: dimensions of 164–165; happiness 165–166; home/residence 23–24; introduction to 8; sense of well-being 26
Grant, Mary 276
Gray, John 24
Great East Japan Earthquake (2011): home and welfare 52–53; human reconstruction 53–55; introduction to 6, 51, 124–125; others as mortal beings 55–56; summary of 56–57; *see also* disabilities and ambiguities
Great Hanshin earthquake (1995) 53
Great Kanto earthquake (1923) 54
Greek ethics 243
green caring 147–148
green skyscrapers 46
Grønseth, Anne Sigfrid 27
Grosse Hamburger Strasse Memorial 39
grounded vibrancy 334–335
Guiding Principles 236–237, *237*

haikus 279–290
Hämer, Hardt-Waltherr 36

happiness as life-satisfaction 77

happiness gene 196

happiness notion 165–166, 317; *see also* eudaimonic model for well-being education

Happy Museum Project (HMP) 116

Haraway, Donna 6, 124–128

harmony and aesthetic thinking 247

Harris, Mark 24

Hartig, Terry 114

Haslanger, Sally 68

Haybron, Daniel 225

health: behaviors 187–188; bio-statistical theory of health and disease 168–170; defined 168, 170; general health questionnaire 217; good health and well-being 133–139; within illness 138; maternal mental health 9; mental health 235–237, *237*; quality of life and 167–170; subjective health 169–170; *see also* ecological health and well-being; perinatal well-being; psychosomatic health

HeART of Stroke 272–274, 276

Heat Wave (Klinenberg) 107

heavens and sense of well-being 43–44

Heavens over Berlin, The (film) 40–41

hedonic *vs.* eudaimonic well-being 318–320

hedonism 1, 77

Heidegger and Homecoming (Mugerauer) 85

Heideggerian (Martin) analysis of well-being: being-in-the-world concept 55–56; everydayness. 296–297; homecoming notion 84; introduction to 3, 34–35, 324; notion of 'Gegnet' 5, 84–85, 88–89; things ready-to-hand 19; *see also* Dwelling-Mobility well-being

Heisenberg, Werner 196

Herder, Johann Gottfried von 19

heritage and well-being: archaeological fieldwork 117–119; Human Henge project 113, 119; introduction to 112–113; museum collections 116–117; pilgrimage roads and designed gardens 113–114; summary 119–120; therapeutic landscapes 114–117

Heritage in Hospitals project 116

Heritage Lottery Fund 112, 118

Hermeneutics of Medicine and the Phenomenology of Health, The (Svenaeus) 85

High, Mette 24

high-profile monuments 39

Hill, Caroline Ellis 272

historical story to well-being 23

Hoagland, Sarah 71–72

Hobbes, Thomas 76

holistic thinking 245

Holocaust Memorial 39

homelessness 86, 117

homes/residences and wellbeing: being-at-home concept 55; family and sense of home 52; homecoming notion 84; introduction to 17–21, 51; meaning of home 52–53; spatial dwelling 327; *see also* dwelling well-being

homeworld 104–105

Human Development Index 195

Human Development Report 195

human experience of well-being 2–5

Human Henge project 113, 119

human-immersion-in-world 103, 105–108

human reconstruction 53–55

human story to well-being 23

human universality 32–33

Husserl, Edmund 60–61, 104

hybrid view of social policy 225–227

IBA (*International Bauausstellung*, International Building/Construction Exposition) 36

Ibsen, Henrik 194

identity: collaborative drawings 257–260, *259*; dwelling-mobility 334; embodied connectivity in visual/tactile arts 276; as 'I am' 333–334; as 'I can' 332–333; introduction to 19; place-based identity 55

immersion-in-place 108–109

immortals and sense of well-being 40–43

improvisation and philosophical enquiry 275

income inequality 188–190, *189*

individual diversity 32–33

individual notion 2

individuation notion 155–156, 160–161

inequalities in well-being: child mortality 183; child well-being 185; between countries 183–184, *184*; within countries 185–186, *186*; ethnic inequalities 185–186; future directions 190–191; health behaviors 187–188; income inequality 188–190, *189*; introduction to 9, 182–183; material deprivation 187; policy-oriented research 190–191; rainbow diagram *186*, 188; reverse causality 187; summary of 191; theories of 186–190

infallible epistemic authority 80

Inner Game of Tennis, The (Gallwey) 135

intersubjective dwelling 329–330

intersubjective mobility 329

intersubjectivity in the clinical situation 296, 298–302

In the Land of Pain (Daudet) 139

Irigaray, Luce 254–255

Iwasaki, Kaori 125

Jackson, Michael 25

James, Henry 17, 18

James, William 18, 194

Japanese Red Cross Society 54

Japan Federation of Bar Associations (JFBA) 53

Jewish Museum 39

Jowell, Tessa 112

Jubilee Sailing Trust 271

Jungian notion of well-being 7

Jungian thinking about well-being: case vignette 156–157; fairy-tale case example 158–159; individuation notion 155–156, 160–161; introduction to 154–155; phenomenology of individuation

160–161; psychology of consciousness *vs.* unconscious 155; summary of 161

Kaiser Wilhelm Memorial Church 40
Kandinsky, Wassily 40–41
Kant, Immanuel 244, 245, 247
Klinenberg, Eric 103–104, 107–108
Kobe University 130
Kopf, Gereon 225
Korsgaard, Christine 226
Kuranko of Sierra Leone 25
Kyrost cheese 24

Lamb House at Rye in England 17
layered continuity 334
learning to be well 9
Lee, Laurie 134, 139
Lessing, Doris 106–107
life course and capabilities 97–99
Life-Threads Model 272
life values 18
lifeworld approach 174
lifeworld analysis 7–8, 104–105, 174; *see also* phenomenological perspective of well-being
lightdarkness cycle 43
linguistic commensuration 26
Livability Holton Lee 115
lived body notion 3–4, 60–63
lived experience 143
lived obliviousness 103, 108–109
lived voice 125–126
looking and collaborative drawings 255–257, *256*
Lute, Jason 35

Malpas, Jeff 6, 105
Marchand, Trevor 25
Marcus, Clare Cooper 114
Marquis de Sade 319
Marx, Werner 39
Maslow, Abraham 196
masonic communication 25–26
Master, The (Toibin) 17
material deprivation 187
maternal mental health *see* perinatal well-being
McCausland, Onya 264
meaning-making in clinical internships 302–304
Medicaid 292
Medical Outcomes Survey Short-Form 36 (SF-36) 216
Medicare 292, 311–312
mental health 235–237, *237*
Mental Health Act (2007) 236
mental well-being 2
Merleau-Ponty, Maurice: cyborg embodiment 128–129; ecology and well-being 141–142; introduction to 19, 58; ontological understanding of human existence 149–152; phenomenology and lived body 60–63
Mid Niigata prefecture Earthquake (2004) 53

Mies, Maria 55
Mietskasernen (large tenement blocks) 35, 36
Mill, John Stuart 32, 77, 194
Miller, Jean Baker 73
mind-body-world phenomenon 4, 62–63
minority communities 117
mirroring and collaborative drawings 254–255
mirror-like multidimensional fullness 331–332
mobility well-being: defined 324; embodied mobility 334–335; existential mobility 86–87; intersubjective mobility 329; mood mobility 331; social mobility 9; spatial mobility 326–327; temporal mobility 328; *see also* dwelling-mobility well-being
Modern Ameliorist Program (MAP) 194, 195, 200
Modern Man in Search of a Soul (Ryff) 155
Modified Visual Analogue Scale (MVAS) 117
mood dwelling 331–332
mood mobility 331
mortals 35–39, 55–56
motility 135, 175
Murdoch, Iris 18, 21
musculo-skeletal pain 255–257
museum collections 116–117
Museum Wellbeing Measures Toolkit 116
mutual complementarity 330

Naess, Arne 142
Nancy, Jean-Luc 290
narrative theories of well-being 78
National Office of Vital Statistics 194
National Portrait Gallery (NPG) 11, 252–254
National Trust's Brockhampton Estate 118
natural attitude 104
naturalism 127
neo-positivism 244, 248
neurofication 322
NHS Forest initiative 115–116
NHS Rotherham Commissioning Group 118
Nicomachean Ethics (Aristotle) 68, 320
Nietzsche, Friedrich 32
Niger child mortality rates 186
Noddings, Nel 55–56, 71–72
non-reflexive theories of well-being 78
normal function, defined 168
normative theories of well-being 78
Nussbaum, Martha 5, 77, 91–92, 94–99, 197

object-awareness 20
Objective List theories 77
objective theory of well-being 79–81
Oedipal layer 157
Oliver, Mary 335
Omand, Helen 253
ontological possibility of well-being 85
ontological understanding of human existence 149–152
Operation Nightingale 118
oppression and feminist well-being 68–69

Orr, Gregory 290
others as mortal beings 55–56
Ovington, Catherine 276

Pain: Speaking the Threshold project 252
PAIN CARDS tool 11
Pain under the Microscope (Padfield, Omand) 265–266
Palmer, Parker 276
Parelli Natural Horsemanship program 205
Parfit, Derek 10, 76–77, 222–225
Parkinson's disease: embodied presence of 174–176;
    introduction to 7–8, 173–174; life world analysis 174;
    relational presence of 176–178; self-understanding
    178–180; summary 180
paternalistic well-being 80
peacefulness 144–146, 331
peace of soul 32
perceptions of pain 257–258
perfectionistic well-being 80
perinatal well-being: assessment of 216; conceptualising
    of 214–215; defined 216; discussion about 218–219;
    emotional well-being measures 217; general health
    questionnaire 217; introduction to 9, 214; Quality of
    Life and 216–217; summary of 219; Well-being in
    Pregnancy (WiP) Questionnaire 217–218
personal competences 244
phenomenological perspective of well-being:
    human-immersion-in-world 103, 105–108;
    immersion-in-place 108–109; introduction to 6,
    28, 103–104; lifeworld analysis 7–8, 104–105;
    lived body and 60–63; lived obliviousness 103,
    108–109
Phenomenology of Perception (Merleau-Ponty) 61
philosophical taxonomies of well-being: better
    distinctions 77; compositional *vs.* additive theories 79;
    empirical *vs.* normative theories 78; introduction to
    21, 76; Parfit's taxonomy 10, 76–77; reflexive *vs.* non-
    reflexive theories 78; subjective *vs.* objective 79–81;
    summary of 81, 275
philosophical thinking 246
phronesis, defined 244
physical well-being 2
pilgrimage roads 113–114
place-based identity 55
Plato (Greek philosopher) 243
pluralism 77, 96
poetry and/as wellness: examples of 279–290;
    introduction to 11–12, 279; summary of 290
political authority 79, 81
population-based approach to well-being 8–9
Positive and Negative Effects Schedule (PANAS) 117
positive psychology: horsemanship and 209; introduction
    to 13; Modern Ameliorist Program 196; perinatal
    period and 215, 218; psychological well-being and
    154; standard psychological approach *vs.* 317–318;
    well-being and 201
positive education 318

positivism 148, 244, 248
posttraumatic stress disorder (PTSD) 59
'practical wisdom' (life knowledge) 245
preference-satisfaction levels 92
present-centeredness 326, 328
professional perspective of well-being 5–10
Programme for International Student Assessment (PISA)
    320
psychological (eudaimonic) well-being 154
psychologization 322
psychology of consciousness *vs.* unconscious 155
Psychology of the Sickbed, The (van den Berg) 7, 133
psychosomatic health: anomaly of 58–60; introduction
    to 58; multi-dimensional phenomenon of 63–64;
    phenomenology and the lived body 60–63
psychotherapy, defined 310
Purpose Principle 237
Pym, Barbara 18

Quality of Life (QoL): care and rehabilitation 170–171;
    care argument 171; dimensions of Good Life
    164–165; health and quality of life 170; health-related
    quality of life 167–170; introduction to 163–164,
    202; perinatal well-being 216–217; questions about
    166–167; subjective health 169–170

rainbow diagram for health and well-being *186*, 188
rationality and self-interest 223–224
Rawls, John 9, 70, 76, 222, 223
real experience *vs.* expectations 309–312
reason and aesthetics of well-being 244–245
Reasons and Persons (Parfit) 10, 76, 222
reattribution theory 60
Rebuttal on Health, A (Boorse) 168
reconstruction schemes 52
recovery programs 52
reductionism 148, 224–225
reference class 168
reflective lifeworld research (RLR) 143
reflexive theories of well-being 78
relational conception of the self 69–70
renewal and well-being 328–329
Research Center for Urban Safety and Security 130
Research Clinic for Functional Disorders and
    Psychosomatics 60
resettlement policy 52
resource-based approach to well-being 93
Respect Principle 237
revealing/hiding in collaborative drawings 255–257,
    256
reverse causality 187
revisionary theories of well-being 78
rhythmical movement of existence 149–150
Richard Rogers Partnership 46
Rogers, Carl 196
Rose, Emma 114
Rosti, Giovanni 264

Ruttmann, Walter 35
Ryff, Carol 154–155, 160

saihan amdral (wonderful life) 24
samrddhi, defined 24
Santiago de Compostela 113
Saville, Jenny 251
Sayer, Andrew 96–97
Scarry, Elaine 20
Scharoun, Hans 38–39
school philosophy 245
Science-Driven Principle 235
science of happiness 317
Second Sex, The (de Beauvoir) 68
self-interest: hybrid view of social policy 225–227;
    introduction to 222–223; rationality and 223–224;
    reductionism problems 224–225; summary of
    227–228
self-respect and well-being 72
self-understanding and well-being 73
Seligman, Martin 196
Sen, Amartya 92–94
Sennett, Richard 36
sense of well-being: anthropology of well-being 27–28;
    case study 29–32; character of well-being 26–27;
    Earth and 44–47; heavens and 43–44; immortals and
    40–43; individual diversity *vs.* human universality
    32–33; introduction to 23; mortals and 35–39; social
    anthropology 23–26; summary of 47–48
sensing-sensible 134
sensorimotor activity 134–135
sensory knowledge 271–272
service-user bias 227
Shankland, David 25
shared notion of well-being 2, 3
shared real experience 312–313
Short Warwick Edinburgh Mental Wellbeing Scale 119
showing/masking in collaborative drawings 255–257,
    256
Sidgwick, Henry 9, 222, 223
situated knowledge 127
Skin Conductivity Responses (SCR) 206, 208
slavery 96
sleep-wake rhythms 43
Smith, Adam 9, 222, 223
social anthropology 23–26
social competence 203
social contextualization of well-being 28
social housing units 45
social mobility 9
social-natural systems 3
Social Security 292
social story to well-being 23
social-structural habituations 28
social well-being 2
socioeconomic inequalities 187–188
Socrates 319

soft animal body 335
sole epistemic authority 80, 81
somatic fixation 58
somatic marker hypothesis (SMH) 206
Some Tame Gazelle (Pym) 18
sophia, defined 244
spatial dwelling 327
spatial mobility 326–327
spatial-temporal multiplication 38
spiritual well-being 2
splendor of the simple 41
Stanley, Pauline 276
Steiner, Rudolf 142
Steven, Wallace 292–293
Stevenson, Robert Louis 139
støler (mountain summer dairy-farms) 24
Stonehenge 113
story and well-being 12
STreSS model (Specialized Treatment for Severe Bodily
    Distress Syndromes) 60
Structure of Behavior, The (Merleau-Ponty) 61
subjective health 169–170
subjective theory of well-being 79–81
subjectivist notion of quality of life 165
subject-object dialogue 130
subsistence concept 55
substantiation of well-being 32–33
survival-based account of well-being 70
Swedish Health and Medical Services Act (1997)
    163

tabes dorsalis 139
tactile arts *see* embodied connectivity in visual/tactile
    arts
Tamil refugees in northern Norway 27–28
technique follows understanding 294
techno-scientific studies for feminism 127, 129
temporal dwelling 328–329
temporal mobility 328
TERM program (The Extended Reattribution and
    Management Model) 60
terra incognita 137
therapeutic eurhythmy 142
therapeutic landscapes 114–117
Therapeutic Landscapes (Williams) 115
Tiberius, Valerie 225
Tiergarten, Berlin 44–45
Todres, Les 114–115, 131
Toibin, Colm 17
Tokyo Electric Power Company (TEPCO)
    125, 130
Tonks, Henry 253
Topology of Terror monument 39
Townsend, Patricia 251
Transcendental Meditation 8, 194
transparent account of well-being 80
*Trouble With **Being Human**, The* (Bauman) 197

Tsuchiya, Masashi 125–126
typology of well-being 325

UK Department of Health 236
Ulrich, Robert 114, 115
understanding follows technique 294
UNICEF 185
United Nations Development Programme 195
unity in diversity 246
unity of dwelling-mobility 173
universalism and capabilities: approach to actual living
   92–94; capabilities approach to actual living 92–94;
   cultural contexts 95–97; introduction to 91–92; life
   course and 97–99; Nussbaum, Martha, and 94–99;
   summary of 99
University College London Hospital (UCLH) 11, 252
urban dynamics 39, 43
urban ecology 44, 45–46
urban nature parks 45
urban renewal 36–37
utilitarianism 80, 93, 248

values, defined 230–232, *232*
values-based practice: introduction to 230; in mental
   health 235–237, *237*; overview of *233*, 233–234, *234*;
   summary of 238–239; in surgery 234–235; values,
   defined 230–232, *232*
van den Berg, J.H. 7, 133–134, 136–137
van Ormand Quine, Willem 196
Viney, William 276
Visible and the Invisible, The (Merleau-Ponty) 150
visual analogue scales (VAS) 217
visual arts *see* collaborative drawings; embodied
   connectivity in visual/tactile arts
vitality as embodied mobility 334–335
Volksgarten (people's gardens) 44
Volkspark (people's park) 44

Ward, Phil 29–32
Wardle, Huron 23
Water of Life fairy-tale 158–159
welfare in Japanese society 53
Well, H.G. 139

well-being: aesthetic nature of 10–13; agencies of
   194–200; collaborative drawings and 250–252;
   disciplinary and professional 5–10; embodied
   dwelling 335–336; embodied dwelling-mobility
   336; embodied mobility 334–335; explanation of
   325, 325–326; good health and 133–139; homes/
   residences and 17–21; human experience of 2–5;
   identity as 'I am' 333–334; identity as 'I can' 332–333;
   identity dwelling-mobility 334; intersubjective
   dwelling 329–330; intersubjective mobility
   329; introduction to 1–2, 324–325; mirror-like
   multidimensional fullness 331–332; mood dwelling
   331–332; mood mobility 331; overview of 201–202;
   peacefulness 331; present centredness 328; renewal
   328–329; spatial dwelling 327; spatial mobility
   326–327; summary of 336–337; temporal dwelling
   328–329; temporal mobility 328; typology of 325; *see
   also* sense of well-being
Well-being in Pregnancy (WiP) Questionnaire
   217–218
Well-Being Measures Toolkit 117
well-being-of-person-or-group-in-place 103
Well-being of World 34
Well-being Outcomes Framework 116
Wender, Wim 40–41
Western metaphysical tradition 85
white caring 147–148
Wilde, Oscar 319
Wilkinson, Richard 188
Williams, Alan 167
wisdom and aesthetics of well-being 244–245
Wittgenstein, Ludwig 196
wonder of all wonders 60
Woolf, Virginia 133, 134–135, 136, 139
World Health Organization (WHO) 214, 250
World Heritage Site of Stonehenge 112
'world-wisdom' *(Weltweisheit)* 245

Yoga 8, 194

Zakrzewska, Joanna 250
Zaner, Richard 135
Zollikon Seminars (Heidegger) 85